Gary McCleane
Howard Smith
Editors

Clinical Management
of the Elderly Patient
in Pain

Pre-publication
REVIEW . . .

"This is a very comprehensive book which describes the clinical management of the elderly patient. It describes drug treatment options with differing application routes, oral, transdermal, and spinal. Besides the pharmacological approach to treating chronic pain, some chapters describe the psychological background and psychological approaches into chronic pain. This book is recommended—it gives the reader an easy approach to the treatment of chronic pain in the elderly."

Jacques E. R. Devulder, MD, PhD
*Professor of Anaesthesiology
and Pain Treatment,
Ghent University Hospital,
Belgium*

Clinical Management of the Elderly Patient in Pain

THE HAWORTH MEDICAL PRESS®
Haworth Series in Clinical Pain and Symptom Palliation
Senior Editor Howard Smith

Clinical Management of the Elderly Patient in Pain
  edited by Gary McCleane and Howard Smith

Cholecystokinin and Its Antagonists in Pain Management
  by Gary McCleane

Titles of Related Interest

Pain and Palliative Care in the Developing World and Marginalized Populations: A Global Challenge edited by M.R. Rojogopal, David Mazza, and Arthur J. Lipman

Aging, Spirituality, and Palliative Care by Elizabeth MacKinlay

Chronic Pain: Biomedical and Spiritual Approaches by Harold G. Koenig

Concise Encyclopedia of Pain Psychology by Roger B. Fillingim

Autogenic Training: A Mind-Body Approach to the Treatment of Fibromyalgia and Chronic Pain Syndrome by Micah R. Sadigh

The Concise Encyclopedia of Fibromyalgia and Myofascial Pain by Roberto Patarca-Montero

Clinical Management
of the Elderly Patient
in Pain

Gary McCleane
Howard Smith
Editors

The Haworth Medical Press®
An Imprint of The Haworth Press, Inc.
New York • London • Oxford

For more information on this book or to order, visit
http://www.haworthpress.com/store/product.asp?sku=5356

or call 1-800-HAWORTH (800-429-6784) in the United States and Canada
or (607) 722-5857 outside the United States and Canada

or contact orders@HaworthPress.com

Published by

The Haworth Medical Press®, an imprint of The Haworth Press, Inc., 10 Alice Street, Binghamton, NY 13904-1580.

PUBLISHER'S NOTE
The development, preparation, and publication of this work has been undertaken with great care. However, the Publisher, employees, editors, and agents of The Haworth Press are not responsible for any errors contained herein or for consequences that may ensue from use of materials or information contained in this work. The Haworth Press is committed to the dissemination of ideas and information according to the highest standards of intellectual freedom and the free exchange of ideas. Statements made and opinions expressed in this publication do not necessarily reflect the views of the Publisher, Directors, management, or staff of The Haworth Press, Inc., or an endorsement by them.

This book has been published solely for educational purposes and is not intended to substitute for the medical advice of a treating physician. Medicine is an ever-changing science. As new research and clinical experience broaden our knowledge, changes in treatment may be required. While many potential treatment options are made herein, some or all of the options may not be applicable to a particular individual. Therefore, the author, editor and publisher do not accept responsibility in the event of negative consequences incurred as a result of the information presented in this book. We do not claim that this information is necessarily accurate by the rigid scientific and regulatory standards applied for medical treatment. No warranty, expressed or implied, is furnished with respect to the material contained in this book. The reader is urged to consult with his or her personal physician with respect to the treatment of any medical condition.

Cover design by Kerry E. Mack.

Library of Congress Cataloging-in-Publication Data

Clinical management of the elderly patient in pain / Gary McCleane, Howard Smith, editors.
        p. cm.
    Includes bibliographical references and index.
    ISBN-13: 978-0-7890-2619-4 (hard : alk. paper)
    ISBN-10: 0-7890-2619-8 (hard : alk. paper)
    ISBN-13: 978-0-7890-2620-0 (soft : alk. paper)
    ISBN-10: 0-7890-2620-1 (soft : alk. paper)
    1. Pain in old age—Treatment. 2. Geriatric pharmacology.
    [DNLM: 1. Pain—drug therapy—Aged. 2. Aging—physiology. WL 704 C6405 2005]
I. McCleane, Gary. II. Smith, Howard S., 1956-

RB127.C57 2005
616'.0472'0846—dc22

                                                                                    2005023077

CONTENTS

Chapter 19. Treatment of Common Conditions   263
Gary McCleane

ABOUT THE EDITORS

Gary McCleane, MD, is a practicing consultant in pain management in Northern Ireland. His interests include the use of cholecystokinin antagonists in pain management and the use of tricyclic antidepressants and topical analgesics. He has published a number of studies examining the analgesic effect of CCK antagonists, capsaicin, topical TCAs, and anti-epileptics, including gabapentin, lamotrigine, phenytoin, fosphenytoin, and the novel anti-epileptic SPM 927. He has published a number of review papers examining current options for the treatment of neuropathic pain and cholecystokinin antagonists in human pain management.

Howard Smith, MD, is Academic Director of Pain Management in the Department of Anesthesiology at Albany Medical College, Albany, New York. He has served on the faculty at the University of Pittsburgh School of Medicine and Harvard Medical School as Director of Pain Medicine; Presbyterian University Hospital, University of Pittsburgh Medical Center, Pittsburgh, Pennsylvania; and Director of Cancer Pain, Beth Israel Deaconess Medical Center, Boston, Massachusetts, respectively. Dr. Smith also served as the Director of Pain Management and Director of Pain Fellowship at the Albany Medical College/Albany Medical Center Hospital. He is editor of the *Journal of Neuropathic Pain & Symptom Palliation* and the *Journal of Cancer Pain & Symptom Palliation* and is an editorial board member of the *American Journal of Hospice & Palliative Care.* Dr. Smith is the author of the forthcoming books *Drugs for Pain* and *A Women's Guide to Ending Pain.*

Clinical Management of the Elderly Patient in Pain
© 2006 by The Haworth Press, Inc. All rights reserved.
doi:10.1300/5356_a

CONTRIBUTORS

Charles Argoff, MD, is Consultant Neurologist, Cohn Pain Management Center, North Shore University Hospital, New York, New York.

Edmund J. Burke, PhD, is Clinical Assistant Professor, Department of PM&R and Psychiatry, Albany Medical College, Northeast Psychological Associates, Albany, New York.

Pradeep Chopra, MD, is Assistant Professor, Boston University Medical Center, Boston, and Director, Pain Management Center of Rhode Island, Providence, Rhode Island.

Steven P. Cohen, MD, is Associate Professor of Anesthesiology, New York University Medical School, New York, New York.

David Craig, MD, is Senior Lecturer, Department of Geriatric Medicine, The Queen's University of Belfast, Belfast, Northern Ireland.

Jennifer A. Elliott, MD, is Assistant Professor, Department of Anesthesiology, University of Missouri, Kansas School of Medicine, Kansas City, Missouri.

Guerman Ermolenko, MD, is Faculty/Teaching Instructor, Albany Medical College, Department of Psychiatry, Albany, New York.

Thomas M. Larkin, MD, is Lieutenant Colonel and Chief, Anesthesia Service, Walter Reed Army Medical Center, Washington, DC.

Mary E. Lynch, MD, is Director of Research, Pain Management Unit, Queen Elizabeth II Health Sciences Centre, and Associate Professor, Department of Psychiatry, Dalhousie University, Halifax, Nova Scotia.

Dennis Martin, DPhil, BSc (Hons), is a Senior Lecturer at the School of Health Science and Social Care, Collegiate Crescent Campus, Sheffield, UK.

Clinical Management of the Elderly Patient in Pain
© 2006 by The Haworth Press, Inc. All rights reserved.
doi:10.1300/5356_b

Peter Passmore, MD, is Senior Lecturer, Department of Geriatric Medicine, Queen's University of Belfast, Belfast, Northern Ireland.

Jana Sawynok, PhD, is Professor of Pharmacology, Department of Pharmacology, Dalhousie University, Halifax, Nova Scotia.

Preface

This is not a book about opioids and nonsteroidals, although they are mentioned. Nor is it about analgesics used in younger patients being used in smaller doses in elderly patients. Rather, it is hoped that it contains practical options for treating pain in elderly patients when other simple remedies fail to help.

At times this will involve using conventional analgesics in scaled-down doses, but at others it will involve using substances not yet fully recognized as possessing analgesic properties because they fit the bill in terms of possible analgesic actions, side-effect profiles, and lack of drug-drug interactions and because practical experience suggests they may be useful in the scenario described.

Given that our knowledge of pain management, and more particularly our understanding of the anatomy, biochemistry, and pathology involved in the generation and maintenance of pain, has increased enormously in recent years, the available pharmacological options have increased in number and range. At times the options presented in this book may appear unusual, and yet only by thinking outside the box can we hope to push forward the horizons of treatment. For example, no one would contest the statement that the tricyclic antidepressants, when given by mouth, can have an analgesic effect in patients with neuropathic pain. But fewer realize that they may also have analgesic effects when applied topically, and yet this property should be unsurprising when one learns that they have actions on sodium channels and adenosine receptors, both of which are found peripherally as well as centrally. How much better would it be to apply a tricyclic antidepressant topically in an elderly patient with a small patch of neuropathic pain rather than systemically, with all the well-documented side effects of systemic tricyclics?

So we will consider treatment that may be considered conventional, but also that which may appear more contentious. Where treatments in the latter group are considered, references are provided to allow those interested to satisfy themselves of the quality of evidence which suggests and underpins that particular treatment. Hopefully it will also stimulate them to have

Clinical Management of the Elderly Patient in Pain
© 2006 by The Haworth Press, Inc. All rights reserved.
doi:10.1300/5356_c

an increased level of awareness of how that line of evidence increases and matures with time. The understanding of pain and its treatment is a dynamic process. What we accept now as being indisputable sometimes evolves and becomes more questionable and vice versa.

When we consider treatment for elderly patients, we may do so without defining "elderly." Maybe what we are really considering is both those of advanced years and others who are less chronologically advanced but suffer from those conditions, often of a degenerative nature, that so frequently appear with increased age. Our need with these patients is treatment that is both effective and easily tolerated. The danger of prescribing treatment with potential sedative side effects, for example, to an elderly patient living alone is obvious. But then, using less risky treatments may not always be without problems. A topical treatment may give complete pain relief, but what use is it to a patient with thoracic pain who has osteoarthritis and cannot reach around to the thoracic area to apply the treatment? Therefore it is necessary to have a range of options and try to fit them to the individual patient, being aware of the patient's general state of health, concomitant medication, and home circumstances, for example.

This concept of having a list of possible options is important for another reason. Regardless of which pain-creating condition we consider, along with the age and health of patient, among the possible pharmacological options, none is guaranteed to be an effective analgesic or to be devoid of side effects. Even with some of the more straightforward pain conditions, such as postoperative pain, the numbers needed to treat, that is, the number of patients who receive the treatment before one gets a 50 percent reduction of pain on average, is not the hoped-for value of one. In reality, with many of the analgesics we currently use, it is around three. In the elderly patient, regardless of the pain condition, a similar situation exists. Furthermore, the "numbers needed to harm" is not infinity, but often in single figures, so even an effective treatment may not be suitable because of the side effects associated with its use. The tendency to incessantly increase dose despite the lack of effect when other options exist seems pointless. Therefore, when individual chapters are consulted, they should not be read in isolation. They are intended to be one piece in the jigsaw puzzle: only by consideration of all the pieces does a clear picture emerge.

To define the best set of options, we must consider the patient as a whole. Medication whose use is complicated by sedation or cognitive impairment may pose greater problems for the patient than the pain in its untreated state. Furthermore, cognitive impairment may reduce patients' ability to adapt their style of life to avoid those things that exacerbate their pain. For example, if a patient has a patch of allodynia on his back following shingles, use of strong opioids may precipitate sleepiness which confines the patient to bed, where further pressure is put on the sensitive area by lying down. This may manifest itself as restlessness and confusion, further exacerbating the original problem.

Polypharmacy is not uncommon in these patients. Awareness of potential drug-drug interactions should influence our choice of alternatives. Unfortunately, this involves keeping up-to-date with current treatments for a broad range of conditions. With the bewildering and ever-increasing array of pharmacological agents currently available, it is hard to be familiar with all of their parent pharmacological classes and modes of action. However, before instituting any pain treatment, we must be careful that our intervention does not interact or interfere with other concomitant treatments.

This book is not intended to be a reference book containing the latest thoughts on the understanding of the pathophysiology of pain. Rather, it is hoped that it will act as an interface between the specialist pain practitioner and that much larger body of clinicians faced with all the problems of satisfactorily managing pain in elderly patients. Inevitably, pain management continues to advance after this book is published, but we hope that it has enough commonsense, practical, patient-oriented options to make it a useful resource to already busy clinicians. By giving an insight into some novel options, perhaps interest in keeping abreast of developments will be encouraged. But at the end of the day, if a single patient has improved pain treatment in the sense that the quality of life is improved, then it has been worthwhile.

Gary McCleane

Chapter 1

Pain and the Elderly Patient

Gary McCleane

There is little merit in considering the treatment of pain in elderly patients unless it differs from that used in younger patients. If the treatment does differ, then it begs the question of whether the nature and severity of pain differ from that seen in younger patients and whether there may be underlying differences in nociceptive processing that account for this difference. Instinctively, one would expect that as age advances the incidence of pain caused by the consequences of degenerative conditions would increase, although many would feel that such pain is handled in elderly patients with a greater degree of stoicism. In this chapter, I consider some of the evidence for the differing perception, processing, and responses to pain when comparing elderly to younger patients without dealing with individual conditions or specific treatments, both of which are addressed in later chapters.

AN AGING POPULATION

In the year 2000, there were more than 400 million people aged 65 and over in the world with a projected increase to almost 1.5 billion by the year 2050. This represents a fourfold increase compared to the 50 percent increase for the global population as a whole. By that time, it is expected that 25 percent these elderly people will be over the age of 80. Epidemiological studies would suggest that the incidence of acute pain is similar across all age groups. Chronic pain seems to increase in incidence up to the seventh decade. When these older patients experience pain, it may be of a different nature and type than that found in younger people.

If we accept that a greater proportion of the population will be of advanced years and that at least some of them will experience both acute and chronic pain, then what factors may influence our treatment of their problems? Clearly the pharmacokinetics of analgesic drugs will be different in elderly

Clinical Management of the Elderly Patient in Pain
© 2006 by The Haworth Press, Inc. All rights reserved.
doi:10.1300/5356_01

patients compared to those of younger age. The elderly are more likely to have associated medical conditions and therefore a greater number of them will be taking medications other than those used just for pain relief. This may lead to an increased risk of drug-drug interactions and side effects related to medication.

From a practical perspective, assessment of pain and patient communication can be more difficult with elderly patients. Those suffering from dementia may have more problems communicating the type, location, and severity of their pain, and the assessor may have to rely more on nonverbal communication. Even young patients with more mental agility have difficulty remembering which medications they currently take, those used in the past, and the response or side effects produced by previous therapeutic trials. This issue is even more problematical in the elderly.

Access to treatment may be difficult. Conventionally, pain management clinics have been hospital based, and the elderly may have significant difficulty accessing these establishments. Furthermore, the treatment offered in many pain management clinics requires a hospital environment. It could be argued that we should concentrate our thoughts on how to make treatment more accessible to patients but also on developing treatments that are less reliant on a hospital environment. The development of home health care services, while placing extra burden on health care professionals and resources, may be rewarded by a substantial improvement in the quality of care offered to elderly patients with pain.

NEURAL DIFFERENCES IN THE AGED

Animal studies suggest that aging deeply influences several morphological and functional features of the peripheral nervous system. There is a loss of myelinated and unmyelinated fibers in the elderly, with the decrease in myelin being at least partially attributable to a decrease in expression of the major myelin proteins. Axonal atrophy is also more commonly observed. Nerve conduction and endoneural blood flow are reduced as age advances, and as nerve regeneration is less commonly observed, there may be a reduction in peripheral nerve function. Even when regeneration of damaged neurons occurs, these regenerated fibers have a smaller number of terminal and collateral synapses.

Spinal cord immunochemical studies reveal an increase in mRNA content of the neuropeptide tyrosine and galanin mRNA in dorsal root ganglia (DRG) neurons of aged rats. These animals have decreased cellular content of calcitonin gene-related peptide (CGRP) and substance P (SP) compared to younger animals, while their levels of somatostatin are similar.

The labeling intensity for encoding high-affinity tyrosine receptors (TrkA, TrkB, and TrkC) are decreased in the DRG neurons of aged rats.

In addition, there is a progressive loss of serotonergic and noradrenergic neurons in the superficial lamina of the spinal dorsal horn, and since serotonin and norepinephrine have important roles in the descending inhibitory control pathways, such loss may upset the natural endogenous pain-suppressing mechanisms.

At supraspinal levels, there is reduced neurotransmitter content and expression, decreased metabolic turnover, and a loss of neurons and dendritic connections throughout the cerebral cortex, midbrain, and brainstem.

If we accept, therefore, that the animal evidence would suggest that nerve structure and function may differ in young and old animals, it is not unreasonable to expect that this is reflected in the incidence and type of pain observed in elderly humans.

EFFECT OF AGE IN ANIMAL PAIN MODELS

A number of studies have examined the effect of age on the response to noxious stimuli in animal models. How far the conclusions of these studies can be extrapolated into human practice is debatable, but at least they suggest that there is a difference between young and old.

It is known that SP levels in the spinal cord of very old rats are lower than the levels in young rats. After injury to a peripheral nerve, immunoreactivity to the SP receptor (NK1, neurokinin 1 receptor) increases in the spinal cord ipsilateral to the injury and the increases correlate to the development of thermal hyperalgesia. After peripheral nerve injury, aged rats developed hyperalgesia and tactile allodynia more slowly than young rats and the thermal hyperalgesia correlated with increases in the number of NK1 receptors, with these receptors developing more slowly.

If rats have an incision inflicted on one of their paws and have their mechanical sensitivity tested with von Frey filaments and thermal responses assessed with a radiant heat source, both young and old animals respond in a similar fashion to the thermal stimulus. However, younger animals appear to recover more quickly from the mechanical allodynia produced by the paw incision when compared to the older animals. This suggests that modulation of A-fiber-mediated sensitization differs in young and old rats.

When considering isolated neuronal function, studies on spinal cord nociceptive neurons show that spontaneous firing rates are higher and the response to thermal stimulation is greater in aged as compared to adult rats. Furthermore, the size of the receptive field area of wide-dynamic-range neurons is larger and that of low-threshold neurons smaller in aged as compared to adult rats (see Figure 1.1). The increased nociceptive neuronal activity in aged rats correlates with the finding that paw withdrawal latency is significantly shorter in aged as compared to adult rats following heat stimulation of the paw. This, along with the loss of serotinergic and noradrenergic fibers in the spinal dorsal horn of aged rats, may contribute to the apparent diminution of descending inhibitory control of nociceptive processing in older animals.

EFFECT OF AGE ON HUMAN EXPERIMENTAL PAIN

It is hard to come to definite conclusions about the effect of age on human experimental pain because of the wide diversity of experimental techniques used. Furthermore, these experimental pain models often examine differing components of the endogenous pain-processing mechanisms. For example, some studies examine the effect of thermal stimuli while others examine hyperalgesia produced by capsaicin or visceral pain induced by esophageal balloon dilatation. Equating these particular induced pains with those observed in clinical practice is not always easy.

Perhaps the most clinically relevant issues are those of pain threshold and pain tolerance. Gibson (2003) reported that over 50 studies have examined

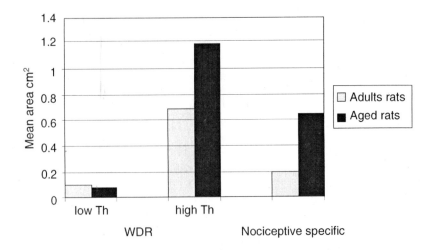

FIGURE 1.1. The mean sizes of receptive fields of nociceptive specific and wide-dynamic-range (WDR) neurons in aged and adult rats. *Source:* Iwata et al., 2002. Reprinted with permission from the American Physiological Society. *Note:* Th = threshhold.

age differences in sensitivity to experimentally induced pain and that the majority of these studies have focused on pain threshold. That is, 21 studies report an increase in pain threshold with advancing age, 3 a decrease, and 17 no change. When all results are examined meta-analytically, the effect size is 0.74 ($P < 0.0005$), indicating that there is definite evidence of an increase in pain threshold with advancing age.

When pain tolerance is considered, the ten studies examining the effect of age on pain tolerance show a definite age-related decrease in willingness to endure very strong pain. The decrease in pain tolerance is estimated at -0.45 ($P < 0.001$) across these studies.

In a study of the effect of age on the response to capsaicin-induced hyperalgesia, Zheng and colleagues (2000) reported that older adult rats take longer to report first pain (see Figure 1.2). Age had no effect on the magnitude of reported pain, flare size, or heat hyperalgesia. This heat hyperalgesia lessens rapidly in all age groups. However, punctuate hyperalgesia and mechanical pain thresholds remained at higher levels for considerably longer in elderly as opposed to younger adults.

Lasch and colleagues (1997) examined the effect of intraesophageal balloon dilation in healthy young and older adults. The volume of air inflated

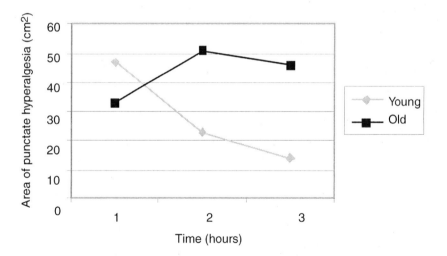

FIGURE 1.2. The time course of the area of punctuate hyperalgesia induced by capsaicin in young and old rats. *Source:* Reprinted from *Pain,* 85(1), Zheng et al., Age-related differences in the time course of capsaicin-induced hyperalgesia, pp. 51-58. © 2000, with permission from International Association for the Study of Pain®.

into the balloon before report of pain was measured. This volume was significantly higher in the older subjects. Indeed, many of the older subjects failed to report pain even after maximal balloon inflation, in marked contrast to the younger patients. It certainly seems that, using this experimental technique, pain threshold does increase with age. But this study also reminds us that pain is not always an entirely negative symptom. On many occasions, it provides a timely warning of impending problems. For example, if it requires a larger volume within a hollow viscus in an elderly patient before pain is experienced as compared to younger subjects, then the discomfort caused by an obstructive lesion in the bowel, for example, may take longer to become symptomatic in older patients, with all the consequences for the treatment and prognosis of the causative lesion. It is also clinically apparent that the incidence of silent myocardial ischemia increases with age. Whether this is due to increased pain threshold in the elderly, a pain-reducing effect of concomitant medication, or the effects of intercurrent illnesses is debatable, but probably all have some effect. Therefore, while our emphasis is on the management of pain in the elderly, we should not lose sight of the fact that thought must also be given to the absence of pain in these patients under circumstances where it normally would be present.

EFFECT OF AGE ON CLINICAL PAIN

I have already mentioned the increased incidence of silent myocardial ischemia in elderly patients as an example of how age may influence pain. Atypical presentation of an inflamed appendix where there may be an absence of localized right iliac fossa pain represents another example. So pain may be absent when one would normally expect it to be present; when pain does occur, it may be ill defined or poorly localized and may persist beyond a time that one would expect in younger individuals.

So differences in the neuroanatomy, physiology, and biochemistry of the nociceptive pathways may cause alterations in pain perception, while differences in the pharmacology of drugs in the elderly may alter expected responses to these drugs. Further compounding these problems is the perception of pain in elderly patients by their physicians. Yunus and colleagues (1988) compared elderly and young patients with fibromyalgia. They found that chronic headaches, anxiety, tension, mental stress, and poor sleep were all less common in elderly patients with this condition. But most important, in only 17 percent of the elderly patients in this study were the features of fibromyalgia recognized initially by their physicians prior to rheumatological referral. Many of these patients were exposed to inappropriate corticosteroid treatment in the mistaken belief that they had an inflammatory condition. We must remember that some elderly patients will present with a unique constellation of symptoms and signs and that only with adequate understanding of the relevance of their symptom complexes can a diagnosis be made and appropriate treatment given.

CONCLUSION

It is quite clear that the number of elderly patients will increase over the next decades and that the proportion of these individuals above the age of 80 will also increase. Animal and human study demonstrates a number of differences in the nociceptive processing mechanisms between young and older adults. Evidence suggests that as age advances, pain threshold also increases, but by the same token, pain tolerance decreases. Knowing that a higher proportion of elderly patients will have other health problems and be more likely to be taking a variety of medication, the treatment of pain in these individuals can be pose a number of difficulties. Allied to this are the problems for elderly patients in accessing treatment facilities. Significant challenges confront those who are tasked with treating pain in elderly patients.

BIBLIOGRAPHY

Barili P, De Carolis G, Zaccheo D, Amenta F. Sensitivity to ageing of the limbic dopaminergic system: A review. *Mech Ageing Dev* 1998; 106: 57-92.

Bergman E, Johnson H, Zhang X, Hokfelt T, Ulfhake B. Neuropeptides and neurotrophin receptor mRNAs in primary sensory neurons of aged rats. *J Comp Neurol* 1996; 11: 303-319.

Chakour MC, Gibson SJ, Bradbeer M, Helme RD. The effect of age on A delta and C fiber thermal pain perception. *Pain* 1996; 64: 143-152.

Corran TM, Farrell MJ, Helme RD, Gibson SJ. The classification of patients with chronic pain: Age as a contributing factor. *Clin J Pain* 1997; 13: 207-214.

Cruce WL, Lovell JA, Crisp T, Stuesse SL. Effect of aging on the substance P receptor, NK-1, in the spinal cord in rats with peripheral nerve injury. *Somatosens Mot Res* 2001; 18: 66-75.

Edwards RR, Fillingim RB. Age-associated differences in responses to noxious stimuli. *J Gerontol A Biol Sci Med Sci* 2001; 56: 180-185.

Edwards RR, Fillingim RB. Effects of age on temporal summations and habituation of thermal pain. Clinical relevance in healthy older and younger adults. *J Pain* 2001; 2: 307-317.

Gagliese L, Melzack R. Age differences in nociception and pain behavior in the rat. *Neurosci Biobehav Rev* 2000; 24: 843-854.

Gagliese L, Melzack R. Age differences in the response to the formalin test in rats. *Neurobiol Aging* 1999; 20: 699-707.

Gibson SJ. Age related differences in pain perception and report. *Clin Geriatr Med* 2001; 17: 433-456.

Gibson SJ. Pain and aging: the pain experience over the adult lifespan. In *Proceedings of the 10th World Congress on Pain* (pp. 767-790). Seattle: IASP Press, 2003.

Gibson SJ, Katz B, Corran TM, Farrell MJ, Helme RD. Pain in older persons. *Disabil Rehabil* 1994; 16: 127-139.

Gibson SJ, Voukelatos X, Ames D, Flicker L, Helme RD. An examination of pain perception and cerebral event-related potentials following carbon dioxide laser stimulation in patients with Alzheimer's disease and age-matched control volunteers. *Pain Res Manag* 2001; 6: 126-132.

Gloth FM. Geriatric pain: factors that limit pain relief and increase complications. *Geriatrics* 2000; 55: 51-54.

Harkins SW. Effects of age and interstimulus interval on the brainstem auditory evoked potential. *Int J Neurosci* 1981; 15: 107-118.

Harkins SW. Geriatric pain: pain perceptions in the old. *Clin Geriatr Med* 1996; 12: 435-459.

Harkins SW, Chapman CR. Detection and decision factors in pain perception in young and elderly. *Pain* 1976; 2: 253-264.

Harkins SW, Chapman CR. The perception of induced dental pain in young and elderly women. *J Gerontol* 1977; 32: 428-435.

Harkins SW, Davis MD, Bush FM, Kasberger J. Suppression of first pain and slow temporal summation of second pain related to age. *J Gerontol A Biol Sci Med Sci* 1996; 51: 260-265.

Harkins SW, Price DD, Martelli M. Effects of age on pain perception: Thermonociception. *J Gerontol* 1986; 41: 58-63.

Heft MW, Cooper BY, O'Brien KK, Hemp E, O'Brien R. Aging effects on the perception of noxious and non-noxious thermal stimuli applied to the face. *Aging* 1996; 8: 35-41.

Helme RD, Gibson SJ. The epidemiology of pain in elderly people. *Clin Geriatr Med* 2001; 17: 417-431.

Iwata K, Fukuoka T, Kondo E, Tsuboi Y, Tashiro A, Noguchi K, Masuda Y, Morimoto T, Kanda K. Plastic changes in nociceptive transmission of the rat spinal cord with advancing age. *J Neurophysiol* 2002; 10: 1086-1093.

Jourdan D, Boghossian S, Alloui A, Veyrat-Durebex C, Coudore MA, Eschallier A. Age related changes in nociception and effect of morphine in the Lou rat. *Eur J Pain* 2000; 4: 291-300.

Kenshalo DR. Somesthetic sensitivity in young and elderly humans. *J Gerontol* 1986; 41: 732-742.

Khalil Z, Ralevic V, Bassirat M, Dusting GJ, Helme RD. Effects of ageing on sensory nerve function in rat skin. *Brain Res* 1994; 641: 265-272.

Laporte AM, Doyen C, Nevo IT. Autoradiographic mapping of serotonin 5HT1A, 5HT1D, 5HT2A and 5HT3 receptors in the aged human spinal cord. *J Chem Neuroanat* 1996; 11: 67-75.

Lasch H, Castell DO, Castell JA. Evidence for diminished visceral pain with aging: Studies using graded intraesophageal balloon distension. *Am J Physiol* 1997; 272: G1-G3.

Lautenbacher S, Strian F. Similarities in age differences in heat pain perception and thermal sensitivity. *Funct Neurol* 1991; 6: 129-135.

Lucantoni C, Marinelli S, Refe A, Tomassini F, Gaetti R. Course of pain sensitivity in aging: pathogenetical aspects of silent cardiopathy. *Arch Gerontol Ger* 1997; 24: 281-286.

Lunenfeld B. The ageing male: demographics and challenges. *World J Urol* 2002; 20: 11-16.

Manfredi PL, Breuer B, Meier DE, Libow L. Pain assessment in elderly patients with severe dementia. *J Pain Symptom Manage* 2003; 25: 48-52.

Onodera K, Sakurada S, Furuta S, Yoneezawa A, Hayashi T, Honma I, Miyazaki S. Age-related differences in forced walking stress induced analgesia in mice. *Drugs Exp Clin Res* 2001; 27: 193-198.

Pakkenberg B, Gundersen HJ. Neocortical neuron number in humans: Effect of sex and age. *J Comp Neurol* 1997; 384: 312-320.

Ririe DG, Vernon TL, Tobin JR, Eisenach JC. Age-dependent responses to thermal hyperalgesia and mechanical allodynia in a rat model of acute postoperative pain. *Anesthesiology* 2003; 99: 443-448.

Tucker MA, Andrew MF, Ogle SJ, Davison JG. Age-associated change in pain threshold measured by transcutaneous neuronal electrical stimulation. *Age Ageing* 1989; 18: 241-246.

US Bureau of the Census. *International Data Base* 2002; Vol. 2002. Washington, DC: U.S. Department of Commerce, U.S. Bureau of the Census.

Verdu E, Ceballos D, Vilches JJ, Navarro X. Influence of aging on peripheral nerve function and regeneration. *J Peripher Nerv Syst* 2000; 5: 191-208.

Wong DF, Wagner HN, Dannals RF. Effects of age on dopamine and serotonin receptors measured by positron tomography in the living human brain. *Science* 1984; 226: 1393-1396.

Yunus MB, Holt GS, Masi AT, Aldag JC. Fibromyalgia syndrome among the elderly: comparison with younger patients. *J Am Geriatr Soc* 1988; 36: 987-995.

Zhang YQ, Mei J, Lu SG, Zhao ZQ. Age-related alterations in responses of nucleus basalis magnocellular neurons to peripheral nociceptive stimuli. *Brain Res* 2002; 948: 47-55.

Zheng Z, Gibson SJ, Khalil Z, Helme RD, McMeekin JM. Age-related differences in the time course of capsaicin induced hyperalgesia. *Pain* 2000; 85: 51-58.

Chapter 2

Acute and Chronic Pain in the Elderly

Pradeep Chopra
Howard Smith

Pain is defined by the International Association for the Study of Pain as an unpleasant sensory and emotional experience associated with actual or potential tissue damage, or described in terms of such damage. In the elderly, many complex issues may contribute to the emotional experience of pain, including a long history of various pain experiences, multiple chronic comorbid conditions, proximity to death, dependency issues, and family support issues.

Presbyalgos is defined as advanced age systematically influencing pain sensitivity and perception in the later years of life.

Over the last century, the life expectancy has increased from 48 to 76 years in the United States of America. An increasing number of people are living into the seventh, eighth, and ninth decades. Studies have shown a peak or plateau in the prevalence of pain by 65 years of age. There is then a decline in reported pain after 75 years, even though there is an age-related increase in diseases associated with pain (e.g., degenerative joint disease).

During this decade, the increase in the elderly population will be moderate. However, between 2010 and 2030 the baby boomer population will begin entering the over-65 generation. The expected population in this age group by 2030 will be between 19 and 21 percent of the total population.

Gerontologists have identified subgroups of the elderly population. The most frequently used grouping is by age:

1. *Young-old:* 65 to 75 years. This is a generally healthy and active group.
2. *Old-old:* 76 to 90 years. This subgroup is characterized by decreasing independence and increasing morbidity, with an increasing demand on health care services.
3. *Oldest-old:* 90 years and above. There is a high level of morbidity in this subgroup. They also present with difficult-to-manage pain.

Clinical Management of the Elderly Patient in Pain
© 2006 by The Haworth Press, Inc. All rights reserved.
doi:10.1300/5356_02

Studies have shown wide variations in the prevalence of pain in the elderly. One of the earliest studies, conducted by Crook, Rideout, and Browne, 1984, showed increased pain complaints with increasing age. It also showed that the prevalence of temporary pain was the same at all ages, with a decline in persistent pain over time on occasion in the same individuals. A review of major studies on the prevalence of chronic pain in the elderly by Helme and Gibson, 1997 suggested a peak or plateau in the prevalence of pain by age 65 and a decline in the old-old and oldest-old groups. The decline in pain in these groups is surprising considering the significant increases in diseases that cause increased pain, such as degenerative joint disease. The reasons for this wide variation for reporting of pain in the elderly may be due to methodological variations, number of subjects in each age group, and variation in response rates in the different subgroups of the elderly (especially the oldest-old; e.g., educational status, unreliability of the memory of pain, and early dementia).

One of the reasons for increased pain in the elderly, undoubtedly is the increased number of coexisting diseases. The incidence of postherpetic neuralgia, degenerative joint disease, spinal stenosis, osteoarthritis, osteoporosis, fractures, and stroke is significantly higher in this age group and continues to increase with advancing age.

In the old-old and oldest-old subgroups of the elderly, a decrease in pain reporting appears. This decline in pain reporting may be secondary to the elderly beginning to lose more and more of their independence. Elderly patients tend to be sequestered in institutions, as a result of which reporting of pain among the elderly in the community is lower. Some possible contributing factors for less reporting of pain in the elderly include loss of cognitive functions, a tendency to be stoic in dealing with pain, other significant life issues overshadowing pain complaints (e.g., loss of a partner or a loved one), preoccupation in dealing with their disability, and altered nociceptive pathways.

The effect of pain in patients with dementia is unclear. These patients have a loss of communication skills and cognitive function and eventually a failure of basic reflexes (e.g., gag reflex) in the later stages. Many of these functions are critical for pain expression. It is unclear if the reduced response to pain is due to decreased sensitivity to pain stimulus or if patients have an apathy to pain. They appear to have a loss of interest and decreased response to any noxious stimulus. The pain response in dementia may be a combination of different etiologies including loss of cognitive skills and indifference or anhedonia. As dementia becomes more advanced, caution should be used when relying on self-reporting of pain. Pain assessment in these patients should factor in direct observations such as facial expressions and input from significant others.

Age-related physiological changes may lead to decreased perception of nociceptive pain; however, this remains uncertain. There is a decreased density of myelinated and unmyelinated nerve fibers in the elderly. Nerve-conduction studies have shown prolonged latencies in the peripheral sensory nerves in healthy older persons.

Studies have reported that older patients report pain only after C-fiber activation. In comparison, younger adults use additional information from A-delta fibers when reporting pain. Furthermore, when the A-delta fiber input was blocked in young adults, age-related differences in pain threshold and subjective ratings of pain intensity disappeared. Therefore it is conceivable that analgesic strategies for the elderly should be directed toward modulation of the C-fiber input.

Cerebral event-related potential (CERP) is an electroencephalogram response study to any stimulus. There is a strong relationship between peak amplitude and subjective ratings of pain in response to increasing stimulation. It represents an integrated response to central nervous system (CNS) processing of afferent input. The CERP in response to noxious stimulus is altered with increasing age. This finding supports that there is slowing in the cognitive processing of noxious stimulus and decreased activation of cortical responses in the elderly.

ACUTE PAIN

Acute pain reporting in the elderly is strikingly different and consistent across all subgroups of the elderly population. Common acute processes in the elderly leading to acute pain include infection, inflammation (e.g., diverticulitis), ischemia (e.g., myocardial infarction), tissue insult, trauma, surgery, and osseous fractures. The elderly may report less pain associated with an acute pathology. Pain tends to be reported in an atypical manner, making the diagnosis of the condition difficult. Pathological conditions that produce pain in the young may instead present with mental status changes such as lethargy, confusion, restlessness, and anorexia in the elderly. Ambepitiya et al., 1993 reported that of the elderly who suffered acute myocardial infarction, 305 did not report any acute symptoms and another 30 percent had atypical symptoms. Atypical presentations have also been reported in acute intra-abdominal pathology.

Treatment of acute pain in the elderly carries with it the challenges of maximizing side effects. Continuous peripheral neural blockade (if feasible and appropriate) may provide optimal results in various situations. Traditional methods of acute pain management (especially in the perioperative period) such as intravenous patient-controlled analgesia (PCA) or epidural analgesics (with or without patient-controlled mode) are used in the elderly. It is often prudent to start with a lower dose (e.g., start low and go slow) when treating acute pain with these strategies in the elderly.

For example, intravenous PCA hydromorphone doses for adults typically range from 0.15 to 0.25 mg. However, in the elderly a starting dose of 0.1 mg is often utilized. When using epidural analgesia in adults, the concentrations may be fentanyl 4 mg/cm^3 or hydromorphone 20 mg/cm^3. In the elderly, a starting concentration for fentanyl would be 1 to 2 mg/cm^3 or hydromorphone 5 to 10 mg/cm^3.

The coping mechanisms adopted by the elderly with chronic pain are very different than mechanisms adapted by younger patients. The elderly tend to use passive coping strategies such as spiritual solace and mental distraction. Therefore it is conceivable that the elderly may respond well to behavioral and psychological strategies.

Cultural beliefs in coping with pain are very important in the elderly. Many of them believe that pain is part of growing old and accept it as a physiological change. Personal and cultural beliefs affect how the elderly accept pain. These beliefs may influence the way they self-report pain, seek treatment, and comply with treatment. Very often, mild aches and pains are attributed to the normal aging process and the elderly tend not to seek medical attention for them. The elderly as a group are reluctant to acknowledge the contribution of psychological factors in their pain experience. Physicians should initiate discussions with their elderly patients about any pain that they may be suffering and offer them therapeutic options. Exhibit 2.1 outlines some of the different types of barriers to pain management.

CHRONIC PAIN

Chronic pain perception may also be different in the elderly. Osteoarthritis in the elderly significantly limits their ability to function and to care for themselves. It is the leading cause of disability in people over the age of 65 years. In the United States alone, it affects over 20 million adults. The joints become swollen, painful, and stiff. When the hips and knees are affected, the ability to conduct activities of daily living is impaired. Because of restricted joint mobility, sufferers they lose muscle tone and strength. The pain limits their ability to walk, restricts their social interaction, and compromises their physical mobility, thus reducing their independence.

EXHIBIT 2.1. Barriers to effective pain management.

Elderly Patient

    Altered presentation (silent myocardial infarction)
    Multiple sources and types of pain
    Fewer autonomic signs of pain
    Pain normal with aging
    Fear of disease (heralding sign or progression)
    Fear of diagnostics/treatment
    Concern about drug addiction
    Do not want to be a bother
    Dementia
    Impaired communication
    Impaired perception

Health Care Provider

    Misconceptions
    Aging blunts/reduces pain perception
    Lack of education
    Cannot adequately assess (especially in impaired, for example if patient has dementia)
    Lack of training in using narcotic prescriptions
    Fear of narcotic drugs
    Concern about patient addiction/abuse
    Fear of regulatory constraints/laws

Health Care System

    Low priority for pain assessment and treatment
    Staff (overextended and untrained)
    Reimbursement issues
    Overbearing regulations

Source: Adapted from Jacox et al., 1994.

The Agency for Healthcare Research and Quality (AHRQ) has noted that the key to effectively managing osteoarthritis is to develop an effective physician-patient partnership. The partnership should:

1. *Promote proper use of medications.* Acetaminophen and nonsteroidal anti-inflammatory drugs (NSAIDs) including COX-2 inhibitors are often used for pain relief in osteoarthritis. These drugs may provide only a modest analgesic effect. In the elderly, NSAIDs have been

associated with increased morbidity. NSAIDs may lead to peptic ulcers, gastrointestinal bleeding, and affect joint cartilage metabolism.

2. *Encourage patients to change their behavior to improve symptoms or slow disease progression.* Encourage patients to understand their disease process and adjust their lifestyle accordingly. Regular exercise such as walking, aquatic therapy, and aerobics may help patients retain their mobility, prevent muscle loss, decrease depression, and help regain their confidence.

3. *Instruct patients on how to interpret and report symptoms accurately.*

4. *Help patients adjust to new social and economic circumstances and cope with emotional consequences.*

5. *Support patients' efforts to participate in treatment decisions and maintain normal activities.*

CANCER PAIN

Cancer pain in the elderly has always been challenging to manage. In addition to morbidity from the primary cancer, elderly patients may have comorbid conditions as well as multiple associated symptoms. Management of these symptoms results in polypharmacy, making patients more susceptible to adverse drug reactions because of age-related changes in absorption, metabolism, and excretion and increased drug-drug interactions.

Inadequate treatment of pain is a major issue. These patients may experience both nociceptive and neuropathic pain at multiple sites by several different mechanisms:

1. Pain from cancer: Invasion of the bone by a tumor accounts for 50 percent of the cases in patients with breast cancer, prostate cancer, and multiple myeloma. Pain due to nerve compression, soft tissue infiltration, or invasion of the gastrointestinal tract accounts for the other 50 percent of cases.

2. Pain from cancer treatment: Painful neuropathy associated with chemotherapy and radiation.

3. Pain unrelated to cancer or its treatment: Prevalence of pain due to other comorbid conditions such as osteoarthritis accounts for a significant number of elderly patients.

Exhibit 2.2 lists common cancer-related pain syndromes.

Management of cancer pain in the elderly must be based on a regular schedule or round-the-clock administration of analgesics rather than on an as-needed basis. This maintains a steady serum concentration. In addition

EXHIBIT 2.2. Common cancer-related pain syndromes.

1. Peripheral neuropathies
   - Nerve infiltration by tumor
   - Postsurgical
   - Radical neck dissection
   - Mastectomy
   - Thoracotomy
   - Nephrectomy
   - Limb amputation
   - Treatment related
   - Chemotherapy (e.g., taxol, cisplatin)
   - Radiotherapy
   - Acute and posttreatment
2. Bone metastases
3. Epidural metastases/spinal cord compression
4. Plexopathies
   - Cervical
   - Brachial
   - Lumbosacral
5. Abdominal pain
6. Mucositis

Source: Sutton, Demark-Wahnefried, and Clipp, 2003.

to maintenance analgesics, patients should also be given analgesics with rapid onset of action for breakthrough pain. The dose for the breakthrough analgesics is usually 15 to 20 percent of the baseline 24-hour dosing. It is vitally important to attempt to adopt the following principles when treating pain in the elderly:

1. Keep the analgesic regimen simple.
2. Minimize the number of analgesics.
3. Minimize the frequency of analgesic dosing (e.g., aim for once or twice per day dosing).

The World Health Organization has recommended a three-step ladder of analgesic therapy for cancer pain (Ventafridda et al., 1985) (see Figure 2.1). The first step consists of starting with nonopioid analgesics such as acetaminophen, aspirin, or nonsteroidal drugs for mild to moderate pain. If the

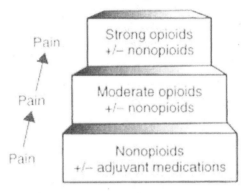

FIGURE 2.1. The World Health Organization ladder is tailored to the needs of patients with pain.

pain persists, then patients are to be maintained on nonopioid analgesics together with opioids for moderate pain such as hydrocodone, codeine, or combinations. Step 3 is considered when the patient continues to have unrelieved pain. In this step, strong opioids (e.g., morphine, fentanyl) for severe pain are started. Adjuvant medications are drugs that, although not labeled as analgesics, may exhibit analgesic potential. Examples of adjuvant medications include anticonvulsants and antidepressants. Adjuvant medications may be started with step one and can be modified or tailored throughout the treatment.

Pharmacological management of pain in the elderly must maintain a delicate balance between the risks of cognitive impairment and other side effects versus the clinical benefit. Consideration should be given to medications taken for other coexisting conditions and the possibility of drug interaction (see Table 2.1).

Acetaminophen is a relatively safe drug of first choice for treating mild to moderate pain in the elderly. The maximum dose of acetaminophen per day should not exceed 4000 mg. Acetaminophen in combination with other drugs such as hydrocodone helps potentiate the effects, thus allowing lower doses of both drugs and good pain control. All too often, patients take over-the-counter acetaminophen or in combination with cold medicines without realizing that they may be exceeding the maximum dose. Reduced doses must be used in patients with liver disease.

Other analgesic agents used in the elderly include anti-inflammatory agents (COX-2 inhibitors are associated with less gastrointestinal mucosal insult in the elderly), tramadol, and opioids.

TABLE 2.1. Adjuvant medications for chronic pain management.

Medication	Dosage	Indications/Comments
Nortriptyline (Pamelor)	10-25 mg p.o. at h.s.	Neuropathic pain
Desipramine (Norpramin)	Up to 50-150 mg/day in divided doses	Depression; side effects include anticholinergic effects, sedation, cardiac arrhythmias, orthostatic hypotension
Gabapentin (Neurontin)	900-3600 mg/day p.o. Start 100 mg/day then increase dose each day to 300 mg/day on the third day; then titrate to effect	Neuropathic pain (avoid abrupt withdrawal of all antiseizure medications)
Carbamazepine (Tegretol)	200 mg p.o. at h.s.; increase every 3 days as needed	Neuropathic pain; suspension available for rectal administration
Phenytoin (Dilantin)	1000 mg loading dose then 200-300 mg/day	Neuropathic pain
Dexamethasone (Decadron)	16-24 mg/day	Neuropathic pain
Prednisone	40-60 mg/day	Improves appetite, mood, and energy level; helps decrease edema associated with malignant tumors
Pamidronate (Aredia)	60-90 mg IV over 2 h each month	Effective for bone pain for several months
Calcitonin (Miacalcin)	One spray nasally each day	Effective for bone pain for weeks to a few months; take with calcium and vitamin D

Source: Abrahm, 2000.

Steps 2 and 3 of the WHO ladder are to either add an opioid or switch to a pure opioid for managing pain should the drugs in step 1 with or without adjuvants not work. The more commonly used drugs of this class are oxycodone, morphine, hydromorphone, and fentanyl. Opioids such as oxycodone and hydromorphone without significant active metabolites may exhibit advantages in the elderly, since renal function may be compromised

In conclusion, chronic pain is the single most common complaint in the elderly and has the greatest impact on quality of life. A comprehensive assessment must be done, followed by a multidisciplinary approach to treating the pain. A rational pharmacotherapeutic approach should be adopted, starting low and going slow at each dose level with frequent patient assessment and monitoring. The quality of life, prognosis, and frailty of the elderly population should be taken into consideration of the risk versus benefit of any therapy. Physical and behavioral medicine should be factored in when treating pain in the elderly.

BIBLIOGRAPHY

Abrahm JL. *A physician's guide to pain and symptom management in cancer patients.* Baltimore, MD: Johns Hopkins University Press; 2000.

AGS Panel on Chronic Pain in Older Persons. The management of chronic pain in older persons. *J Am Geriatr Soc* 1998; 46:635.

AHRQ. Managing osteoarthritis: Helping the elderly maintain function and mobility. *Research in action,* issue 4, AHRQ Publication No. 02-0023. Rockville, MD: Agency for Health Care Policy and Research, 2002.

Ambepitiya GB, Iyengar EN, and Roberts ME. Review: Silent myocardial ischaemia and perception of angina in elderly people. *Age and Aging* 1993; 22:302-307.

AMDA. *Chronic pain management in the long-term care setting.* Clinical practice guideline. Columbia, MD, 1999. Author.

Barberger-Gateau P, Chaslerie A, Dartigues J, et al. Health measures correlates in a French elderly community population: The PAQUID study. *J Gerontol* 1992; 472:S88.

Cherny NI, Foley KM. Current approaches to the management of cancer pain: a review. *Ann Acad Med Singapore* 1994; 23:139-159.

Cherny NI, Portenoy RK. Cancer pain management. *Cancer* 1993; 72:3393-3415.

Clark WC, Mehl L. Thermal pain: A sensory decision theory analysis of the effect of age and sex on d', various response criteria, and 50% pain threshold. *J Abnorm Psychol* 1971; 78:202.

Clinch D, Banjeree AK, Ostick G. Absence of abdominal pain in elderly patients with peptic ulcer. *Age Ageing* 1984; 13:120.

Crook J, Rideout E, and Browne G. The prevalence of pain complaints in a genderal population. *Pain* 1984; 18:299-314.

Farrell MJ, Gibson SJ, Helme RD. Chronic non-malignant pain in older people. In Ferrell B, Ferrell B (eds.): *Pain in the elderly.* Seattle, WA: IASP Press, 1996, p. 81.

Foley KM, Houde RW. Methadone in cancer pain management: Individualize dose and titrate to effect. *J Clin Oncol* 1998; 16:3213-3215.

Gagliese L, Melzack R. Chronic pain in elderly people. *Pain* 1997; 70:3.

Gibson SJ, Gorman MM, Helme RD. Assessment of pain in the elderly using event-related cerebral potentials. *In* Bond MR, Charlton JE, Woolf C (eds.): *Proceedings of the VIth World Congress on Pain.* Amsterdam: Elsevier Science Publishers, 1990, p. 523.

Gibson SJ, Helme RD. Age differences in pain perception and report: A review of physiological, psychological, laboratory and clinical studies. *Pain Rev* 1995; 2:111.

Griffin MR, Brandt KE, Liang MH, et al. Practical management of osteoarthritis. Integration of pharmacologic and nonpharmacologic measures. *Arch Fam Med* 1995; 4(12):1049-1055.

Harkins SW. Pain perceptions in the old. *Clin Geriatr Med* 1996; 12(part 3):435.

Harkins SW, Chapman CR. The perception of induced dental pain in young and elderly women. *J Gerontol* 1997; 32:428.

Harkins SW, Price DD, Bush FM, et al. Geriatric pain. In Wall PD, Melzack M (eds.): *Textbook of pain*, ed. 3. New York: Churchill Livingstone, 1994, p. 769.

Helme RD, Gibson SJ. Pain in older people. In Crombie IK, Croft PR, Linton SJ, et al (eds.): *Epidemiology of pain*. Seattle, WA: IASP Press, 2000, p. 103.

Helme RD, Gibson SJ. Pain in the elderly. In Jensen TS, Turner JA, Wiesenfeld-Hallin Z (eds.): *Proceedings of the 8th World Congress on Pain, progress in pain research and management*. Seattle, WA: IASP Press, 1997, p. 919.

Hochberg MC, Altman RD, Brandt KD, et al. Guidelines for the medical management of osteoarthritis. Part I. Osteoarthritis of the hip. *Arthritis Rheum* 1995; 38(11):1535-1540.

International Association for the Study of Pain. *Classification of chronic pai*. Seattle: DASP Press; 1994.

Jacox A, Carr DB, Payne R, et al. *Management of cancer pain*. Clinical Practice Guideline No. 9. AHCPR Publication No. 94-0592. Rockville, MD: Agency for Health Care Policy and Research, U.S. Department of Health and Human Services, Public Health Service, March 1994.

James FR, Large RG, Bushnell JA, et al. Epidemiology of pain in New Zealand. *Pain* 1991; 44:279.

Magni G, Schifano F, De Leo D. Pain as a symptom in elderly depressed patients. *Eur Arch Psychiatry Neurol Sci* 1985: 235:143.

McCracken LM. Learning to live with pain: Acceptance of pain predicts adjustment in persons with chronic pain. *Pain* 1998; 74:21.

Meyer BR, Reidenberg MM. Clinical pharmacology and ageing. In Evans JG, Williams TF (eds.): *Oxford textbook of geriatric medicine*. Oxford: Oxford University Press; 1992, pp. 107-116.

National Institute of Arthritis and Musculoskeletal and Skin Diseases. Handout on health: osteoarthritis. Web site: http://www.niams.nih.gov/hi/topics/arthritis/oahandout.htm.

Parmalee PA. Pain in cognitively impaired older persons. *Clin Geriatr Med* 1996; 12 (part 3):473.

Portenoy RK, Hagen NA. Breakthrough pain: Definition, prevalence and characteristics. *Pain* 1990; 41:273-281.

Ripmonti C, Groff L, Brunelli C, Polastri D, Stravrakis A, DeConno F. Switching from morphine to oral methadone in treating cancer pain: What is the equianalgesic dose ratio? *J Clin Oncol* 1998; 16:3216-3221.

Sengstaken EA, King SA. The problem of pain and its detection among geriatric nursing home residents. *J Am Geriatr Soc* 1993; 41 (part 5):541.

Smith H, Chen G. *Geriatric pain management issues. Progress in Anesthesiology:* Dannemiller Memorial Educational Foundation, San Antonio, Texas, December 2000.

Stein WM, Ferrell BA. Pain in the nursing home. *Clin Geriatr Med* 1996; 12 (part 3): 601.

Sutton LM, Demark-Wahnefried W, Clipp E. Management of terminal cancer in the elderly patients. *Lancet Oncol* 2003; 4(3):149-157.

Ventafridda V, Saita L, Ripamonti C, DeConno F. WHO guidelines for the use of analgesics in cancer pain. *Int J Tissue Realt* 1985; 7:93-96.

Wynne CF, Ling S, Remsburg R. Comparison of pain assessment instruments in cognitively intact and cognitively impaired nursing home residents. *Geriatr Nurs* 2000; 21:20-23.

Chapter 3

Pain Management and Pharmacological Differences in the Elderly Patient

Peter Passmore
David Craig

The fastest growing section of the UK population is individuals over 75 years. Consequently, physicians will treat larger numbers of elderly patients. The principles of drug therapy in this group are distinct and reflect age-related alterations in pharmacokinetics and pharmacodynamics set against a background of altered homeostasis. Moreover, these changes are often seen in the setting of polypharmacy and physiological compromise secondary to chronic disease. Knowledge of how such changes affect the older person can enhance treatment efficacy, improve awareness of potential drug-drug interactions, and help to minimize the incidence of adverse drug reactions.

EXTERNAL FACTORS

Physicians should attempt to minimize unnecessary drug use in older people. A clear relationship between number of prescribed medications and risk of adverse events has been established. Excessive and inappropriate prescribing may also increase the risk of drug-drug interactions. Indications must be clear and patients should receive regular review. Conversely, the underuse of appropriately prescribed treatment simply on the basis of age should also be avoided. Effective treatment is further aided by measures to improve compliance: communication, clear labeling, and use of once-daily treatments where possible.

Clinical Management of the Elderly Patient in Pain
© 2006 by The Haworth Press, Inc. All rights reserved.
doi:10.1300/5356_03

PHARMACOKINETIC ALTERATIONS

Drug Absorption

There is no quantitative difference in absorption in the older patient: slowed intestinal transit (which is a function of age and coexisting medications such as opioids or tricyclic antidepressants) improves absorption by providing a longer time for drug absorption. This is offset, however, by reductions in jejunal surface area and gastrointestinal blood flow. It is unclear whether carrier-mediated transport systems, such as occur with drugs such as gabapentin, are affected by aging. Data on the absorption of extended-release preparations in this population are similarly limited, and conclusions are based on clinical end-point data showing comparable efficacy with normal-release equivalents.

Transdermal routes of drug absorption appear equally efficient in older subjects compared to their younger counterparts. Dermal thinning may theoretically quicken penetration through the skin, although downstream effects relating to decreased skin perfusion and diminished cardiac output are equally relevant. Drug absorption via the transbuccal route may decrease if saliva output falls. Absorption via the transbronchial route is probably similar in older patients, although direct comparisons are rare.

The response to local anesthetics in the elderly is altered by several variables: decline in number of neurons, degradation of myelin sheaths, and concurrent slowing in signal conduction. Spinal anesthesia may be influenced by degenerative disease of the spine and intervertebral foramina. Epidural dose is generally lowered as hypotension and more intense motor blockade are common.

Intramuscular absorption (e.g., of opiates) is best avoided in the elderly as absorption is unpredictable due to less muscle and relatively more fat.

Drug Distribution

Physiological changes in older people affecting fat mass (increased), muscle mass (reduced), and body water (reduced) have important effects on drug distribution. Prescription of diuretics may additionally reduce blood volume. The relative change in body fat is greater in males. Fat acts as a depot for highly lipophilic drugs such as fentanyl and lidocaine, thus prolonging their duration of action. Water-soluble drugs (e.g., morphine sulphate) are less efficiently distributed and higher plasma concentrations are obtained with equivalent doses; opioid side effects resulting in respiratory depression and oversedation (with its attendant loss of protective reflexes and increased risk of falls) are not uncommon.

Free-drug availability is significantly augmented by decreases in serum albumin, particularly in those older patients with chronic disease and malnutrition. Such changes increase the potential for adverse effects associated with highly protein bound analgesics such as NSAIDs and antiepileptic agents with analgesic properties (e.g., valproate, phenytoin, carbamazepine). Levels of alpha1-acid glycoprotein, the serum carrier for basic drugs such as meperidine, appear unchanged in older people.

Drug Elimination

Older people are less effective at removing drugs from the bloodstream. The kidneys and liver become progressively less efficient at drug clearance and as already discussed, for lipophilic drugs, the volume of distribution increases in proportion to the relative accumulation of fat stores. Drug half-life, a ratio of the volume of distribution to clearance, is notably increased for several benzodiazepines and tricyclic antidepressants.

Lipid-soluble drugs such as lidocaine and narcotic analgesics are good examples of drugs that undergo significant first-pass metabolism during passage from the gastrointestinal tract to the liver. Peak plasma concentrations may rise as may the potential for dose-related side effects. This situation is further compounded when cardiac output is impaired through disease. Highly protein-bound drugs are less influenced by first-pass metabolism.

Although routine tests of liver function remain steady in old age, liver perfusion falls by approximately 40 percent and liver size by approximately 30 percent. These factors, rather than alterations in hepatic enzyme activity, appear most relevant. Notwithstanding, hepatic phase I reactions involving oxidation, hydrolysis, and reduction appear more strongly altered by age than phase II conjugation processes (acetylation, glucuronidation, sulfation, and glycine conjugation). In general, phase I reactions diminish irrespective of which microsomal cytochrome p450 enzyme is involved, although interindividual variation is again significant. Acetaminophen and diazepam, both processed through the CYP 3A4 and 3A5 enzymatic routes, are metabolized at equal rates irrespective of age. Carbamazepine, lidocaine, and fentanyl, in contrast, are subject to reduced metabolism by the same enzyme systems in older patients. Glucuronidation of morphine and glutathione conjugation of acetaminophen are examples of reduced and unchanged phase II reactions respectively. Age appears to have no effect on the frequencies of slow- and rapid-metabolizing genetic polymorphisms.

The most important pharmacokinetic effect of age is the reduction in renal clearance. As a general rule, renal blood flow falls by approximately 1 percent per year beyond the age of 50 years. Physicians should be encouraged to consider virtually all elderly patients as having renal impairment. Measurement of the glomerular filtration rate provides the only reliable index of renal function, as serum creatinine is closely related to muscle mass. Acute illness may further rapidly compromise renal clearance, especially if the patient is dehydrated (particularly with concomitant NSAID prescribing, and in such a situation the NSAID should be immediately discontinued). In the absence of dose modification, toxicity may occur when using, for example, lidocaine or morphine where renal elimination is impaired. Morphine-6-glucuronide, derived from the phase II conjugation of morphine and responsible for the majority of analgesic effects, produces prolonged effects and toxicity if allowed to accumulate. Gabapentin is excreted unchanged in the kidneys without appreciable metabolism in the liver, and its excretion is therefore decreased in elderly patients.

PHARMACODYNAMIC CHANGES

Whether the elderly demonstrate actual changes in intrinsic sensitivity at the receptor level is controversial both in terms of measurable alterations in receptor numbers and the efficiency of signal transduction following receptor binding. Increased brain sensitivity to narcotic analgesics at comparable drug concentrations has been reported in an electroencephalogram study in young and old subjects.

Altered drug sensitivity may also result from autonomic changes. Sensitivity to beta blockade and beta stimulation are both reduced. Beta-adrenergic receptor numbers fall, possibly due to downregulation by elevated serum norepinephrine levels, but less efficient postreceptor signaling is probably most relevant. Prescription of neuroleptics (typical and atypical) and some antiemetic drugs (e.g., prochlorperazine) may induce extra- pyramidal reactions due to reductions in central dopaminergic neuron counts, receptor numbers, and dopamine concentrations. Similarly, anticholinergic side effects emerge readily as muscarinic receptor numbers and acetylcholine levels fall with increasing age. Experiments in elderly rats suggest that the number of mu and kappa opioid receptor numbers fall while delta-opioid receptor numbers stay unchanged.

Decline in homeostatic counterregulatory mechanisms seen in older patients creates a less forgiving background once drugs enter the body. Older patients are thus less able to regain the original physiological steady state. The decline in homeostatic mechanisms is best exemplified by drug-induced orthostatic reactions set against a background of an already impaired autonomic reflex. Falls and syncope may result, leading to social isolation, fractures, and head injury. Implicated drugs (other than antihypertensives) include tricyclic antidepressants, neuroleptics, and opioids. Homeostatic changes increase the risk of gastric irritation and bleeding following exposure to NSAIDs. The risk of bleeding is four times higher in older versus younger individuals. Cyclooxygenase-2 (COX-2) inhibitors are less irritant to the gastric mucosa but appear equally capable of producing renal disturbance and fluid retention compared to nonselective NSAIDs.

CONCLUSION

Drug use in older people requires vigilance because of numerous alterations in pharmacokinetics and pharmacodynamics. Treating physicians are often reluctant to take risks, especially knowing the considerable variation in therapeutic and toxic outcomes among individuals. It is important not to deny older people adequate pharmacotherapy and relief of pain, and this can be mostly achieved by the judicious modification of dose appropriate to age and coexisting morbidities.

BIBLIOGRAPHY

Bressler R, Bahl JJ. Principles of drug therapy for the elderly patient. *Mayo Clin Proc.* 2003; 78:1564-1577.

Noble RE. Drug therapy in the elderly. *Metabolism.* 2003; 52:27-30.

Routledge PA, O'Mahony MS, Woodhouse KW. Adverse drug reactions in elderly patients. *Br J Clin Pharmacol.* 2004; 57:121-126.

Ruoff GE. Challenges of managing chronic pain in the elderly. *Semin Arthritis Rheum.* 2002; 32:43-50.

Turnheim K. When drug therapy gets old: Pharmacokinetics and pharmacodynamics in the elderly. *Exp Gerontol.* 2003; 38:843-853.

Vuyk J. Pharmacodynamics in the elderly. *Best Pract Res Clin Anaesthesiol.* 2003; 17:207-218.

Williams BR, Kim J. Cardiovascular drug therapy in the elderly: Theoretical and practical considerations. *Drugs Aging.* 2003; 20:445-463.

Chapter 4

Acetaminophen for the Elderly

Pradeep Chopra
Howard Smith

Acetaminophen is an analgesic and an antipyretic with a weak anti-inflammatory property. The chemical name is *N*-acetyl-*p*-aminophenol (APAP). The drug is known as paracetamol outside the United States. Acetaminophen is the active metabolite of phenacetin, which is a member of the aniline derivatives, also known as the coal tar analgesics. It is a white crystalline powder with a molecular weight of 151.16 and a pKa of 9.51 at 25°C (see Figure 4.1).

CLINICAL PHARMACOLOGY

Acetaminophen's mechanism of action is not well understood. Significant data suggest a central mechanism of action. Because of its high lipid solubility and its weak plasma protein binding, it can cross the blood-brain barrier easily. Various theories have been put forward to explain the mechanism of action of acetaminophen. Acetaminophen diminishes the thalamic evoked potentials elicited by nociceptive electrical stimulation. There may be some peripheral effect of acetaminophen by reducing prostacyclin synthesis.

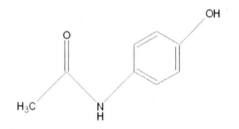

FIGURE 4.1. Acetaminophen molecule.

Clinical Management of the Elderly Patient in Pain
© 2006 by The Haworth Press, Inc. All rights reserved.
doi:10.1300/5356_04

At the spinal level, acetaminophen may have a direct action on a COX-2 variant or a COX-3 type of isoenzyme and inhibit prostaglandin E_2 release. It may act spinally to inhibit nitric oxide generation, which may impair the nociceptive potential of *N*-methyl-D-aspartate (NMDA) or NK-1 activation.

At the supraspinal level, it may inhibit the descending inhibitory pathways via indirect effects on serotonergic pathways. It may also affect the opioid systems, predominantly by modulating dynorphin release and mu receptor function.

ADVERSE EFFECTS

Acetaminophen is considered one of the safer analgesics. It should be used with caution in patients with preexisting hepatic damage and a history of chronic alcohol abuse (more than three alcoholic drinks per day). Acetaminophen is metabolized by the glutathione pathway. These patients have a potential for glutathione storage depletion. However, there is no absolute contraindication to use a short course of acetaminophen under medical supervision in patients with mild preexisting liver disease.

Some of the rare adverse effects of acetaminophen are agranulocytosis, anemia, dermatitis, allergic reactions, thrombocytopenia, hepatitis, sterile pyuria, and renal failure (with prolonged use of high doses in patients with preexisting renal impairment). Mild bronchospasm has been reported in less than 5 percent of patients with aspirin-sensitive asthma.

Acetaminophen has very few drug interactions. Caution is advised when used with the following drugs:

- Zidovudine—this drug is used in patients with HIV infection. As reported by Richman et al. (1987), concurrent administration of acetaminophen and zidovudine may lead to increased incidence of bone marrow suppression.
- Hepatotoxic and hepatic enzyme inducer drugs—there is an increased risk of hepatotoxicity with prolonged use of high doses of acetaminophen in patients taking these drugs.
- Coumadin—Acetaminophen used in doses greater than 2 g per day chronically may increase the anticoagulant effect. Prothrombin time is not affected by short-term use of acetaminophen.
- Salicylates and aspirin—Controversy surrounds the issue of increased risk of analgesic nephropathy when acetaminophen is taken chronically in a high dose in a preparation with combined analgesics. Some would consider a high dose of acetaminophen as 1.35 g per day or a

total ingestion of 1 kg per year for three years (when using a combined analgesic preparation).

• Difunisal—when taken concurrently with acetaminophen, the plasma concentration of acetaminophen is increased by 50 percent.

Although acute nephrotoxicity has been reported after massive overdose of acetaminophen, very little clinical evidence suggests that habitual appropriate use of acetaminophen causes nephropathy. The National Kidney Foundation's (2005) position has been to recommend the use of acetaminophen in patients with renal failure and it is also the nonnarcotic of choice for patients with preexisting kidney disease.

LABORATORY VALUES AFFECTED

Patients taking acetaminophen may have the following laboratory values altered:

• Blood glucose levels: Acetaminophen may cause falsely lowered values when blood glucose is determined using the oxidase method, but not when the glucose-6-phosphate dehydrogenase method is used.
• Pancreatic function: Acetaminophen taken prior to the bentiromide test will invalidate the results. It should be discontinued three days prior to the test.
• 5-Hydroxyindoleacetic acid (5-HIAA) determination: Acetaminophen may cause false positive results if the reagent nitrosonaphthol is used.

OVERDOSAGE

Acetaminophen toxicity may result from a single dose of 150 to 250 mg/kg or greater than 7.5 to 10 g within eight hours.

A minor portion of acetaminophen metabolism is by the cytochrome P-450 dependent N-hydroxylation to form N-acetyl-p-benzoquinone imine (NAPQI). This metabolite, without adequate levels of reduced glutathione available, directly arylates and oxidizes cellular proteins, leading to inhibition of enzyme activities. High doses of acetaminophen overwhelm the glucuronidation and sulfation pathways and deplete the glutathione pool.

Management of acetaminophen toxicity consists of vigorous supportive therapy and gastric lavage. The drug of choice is N-acetylcysteine. It is a glutathione precursor that replenishes the glutathione store in the liver. The earliest manifestation of acetaminophen hepatotoxicity is malaise, nausea, vomiting, and diaphoresis. It takes 48 to 72 hours for hepatic toxicity to develop. Liver damage from acetaminophen toxicity results in centrilobular hepatic necrosis.

N-acetylcysteine is available for oral use in the United States, whereas it is available in the intravenous form in Europe. It is ideally given within 8 hours or less of ingestion but should be given if less than 36 hours have elapsed since ingestion of acetaminophen. Treatment should be started immediately without waiting for acetaminophen levels, if the history is suggestive of acetaminophen toxicity. When administered orally, it is diluted to a 5 percent solution by mixing in water and should be given within one hour of preparing it.

The loading dose of oral *N*-acetylcysteine is 140 mg/kg followed by 70 mg/kg every four hours for 17 doses. Treatment is stopped if plasma acetaminophen levels indicate that the risk of hepatotoxicity is low.

Adverse effects of *N*-acetylcysteine are nausea, vomiting, diarrhea, skin rash, urticaria, and anaphylactoid reaction. Further information on acetaminophen overdose can obtained from the Rocky Mountain Poison Center, Denver, CO (telephone number: 800-525-6115).

DOSAGE AND ADMINISTRATION

The oral dose of acetaminophen is 325 to 1000 mg. Doses can be given every four to six hours. The maximum dose should not exceed 4000 mg per day.

The rectal dose is 650 mg. Rectal administration is suboptimal because its absorption may be affected by stool present in the rectum.

The extended-release acetaminophen formulation Tylenol Arthritis Extended Relief Caplets contains 650 mg of acetaminophen in a unique, patented bilayer. The first layer dissolves quickly (roughly about 325 mg), whereas the second layer is time released to provide eight hours of relief.

Acetaminophen is used mainly as an analgesic and antipyretic. It is a good alternative for patients in whom aspirin is contraindicated. There is no dose alteration when taken by the elderly. The American College of Rheumatology (2000) in their updated guidelines has recommended acetaminophen as the first-line pharmacological therapy because of its cost, efficacy, and safety profile.

Acetaminophen in the elderly has proven to have broad tolerability, reasonable efficacy, and a low side effect profile. It has very few drug interactions, an important consideration in the elderly, who are usually on several medications. The use of acetaminophen in the elderly is considered safe and without significant side effects when used appropriately.

BIBLIOGRAPHY

American College of Rheumatology. Subcommittee on osteoarthritis guidelines. *Arthritis Rheumatism* 2000; 43:1905-1915.

American Geriatrics Society Panel on Chronic Pain in Older Persons. Clinical practice guidelines: The management of chronic pain in older persons. *J Am Geriatr Soc* 1998; 46:635-651.

Benson GD. Acetaminophen in chronic liver disease. *Clin Pharmacol Ther* 1983; 33:95-101.

Bjorkman R, Hallman KM, Hender T, et al. Acetaminophen blocks spinal hyperalgesia induced by NMDA and substance P. *Pain* 1994; 57:259-264.

Bradley JD, Brandt KD, Katz BR, et al. Comparison of an anti-inflammatory dose of ibuprofen, an analgesic dose of ibuprofen, and acetaminophen in the treatment of patients of osteoarthritis of the knee. *N Engl J Med* 1991; 325:87-91.

Creamer P. Osteoarthritis pain and its treatment. *Curr Opin Rheumatol* 2000; 12:450-455.

De Param BJ, Gancedo SQ, Cuevas M, et al. Paracetamol (acetaminophen) hypersensitivity. *Ann Allergy Asthma Immunol* 2000; 85:508-511.

Henrich WL, Agodoa LE, Barrett B, et al. Analgesics and the kidney: Summary and recommendations to the Scientific Advisory Board of the National Kidney Foundation from an ad hoc committee of the National Kidney Foundation. *Am J Kidney Dis* 1996; 27:162-165.

Hochberg MC, Altman RD, Brandt KD, et al. Guidelines for the medical management of osteoarthritis: Part I. Osteoarthritis of the hip. Part II. Osteoarthritis of the knee. *Arthritis Rheum* 1995; 38:1535-1546.

Kuffner EK, Dart RC. Acetaminophen used in patients who drink alcohol: Current study evidence. *Am J Managed Care* 2001; 7:5592-5596.

Mehlisch DR, Sollecito WA, Helfrick JF, et al. Multicenter clinical trial of ibuprofen and acetaminophen in the treatment of postoperative dental pain. *J Am Dent Assoc* 1990; 121: 257-263.

National Kidney Foundation. Available online <http://www.kidney.org>; 2005.

Richman DD, et al. The toxicity of azidothymidine (AZT) in the treatment of patients with AIDS and AIDS-related complex: A double-blind, placebo controlled trial. *N Engl J Med* 1987; 317:192-197.

Rocha GM, Michea LF, Peters EM, et al. Direct toxicity of nonsteroidal anti-inflammatory drugs for renal medullary cells. *Proc Natl Acad Sci USA* 2001; 98:5317-5322.

Schnitzer TJ. Update of ACR guidelines for osteoarthritis: Role of the coxibs. *J Pain Symptom Manage* 2002; 23:524-530.

Smilkstein MJ, Knapp GL, Kulig KW, Rumack BH. Efficacy of oral N-acetylcysteine in the treatment of acetaminophen overdose: Analysis of the national multicenter study (1976 to 1985). *N Engl J Med* 1988; 319:1557-1562.

Smith H. Acetaminophen (bedside). In Smith H (ed.): *Drugs for pain,* 1st ed. Philadelphia: Hanley & Belfus, 2003, pp. 33-38.

Smith H. Acetaminophen (Bench). In Smith H (ed.): *Drugs for pain,* 1st ed. Philadelphia: Hanley & Belfus, 2003, pp. 19-28.

Steffe EM, King,JH, Inciardi JF. The effect of acetaminophen on zidovudine metabolism in HIV-infected patients. *J Acquir Immune Defic Synr Hum Retrovirol* 1990; 3:691-694.

Chapter 5

Opioids

Gary McCleane

Historically, the derivatives of the opium poppy, *Papaver somniferum*, have been the mainstay of pain management in patients of all ages. Since the isolation of morphine from opium in 1801 by Serturner and the synthesis of codeine by Robiquet in the 1850s, the range of available opioids has increased to the extent that the clinician is confronted by a bewildering array of agents active at the opioid receptors. Not only have the number of different opioids increased but so have the available modes of administration: we now have oral and parenteral formulations, and formulations that allow administration transdermally, intrathecally, rectally, via the oral mucous membrane, and even by inhalation. My concentration in this chapter is on oral and parenteral use, with other modes of administration considered in later chapters.

Although the use of so-called weak opioids such as codeine is extensive, the same is not true of the strong members of this class. It is universally accepted that strong opioids are useful in the management of acute pain and that related to terminal illness. However, their use in management of chronic pain not related to a terminal condition provokes much controversy. Consequently, any view expressed on their use reflects a personal opinion. In this chapter, an outline of the use of opioids in the elderly is given, with a personal view given at the end.

The pharmacological effects of the opioid analgesics are derived from their complex interaction with three opioid receptor types (mu, delta, and kappa). These receptors are found in the periphery, at presynaptic and postsynaptic sites in the spinal cord dorsal horn, and in the brainstem, thalamus, and cortex, in what constitutes the ascending pain transmission system, as well as structures that comprise a descending inhibitory system that modulates pain at the level of the spinal cord. The cellular effects of opioids include a decrease in presynaptic transmitter release, hyperpolarization of postsynaptic elements, and disinhibition. The antagonistic and partial

Clinical Management of the Elderly Patient in Pain
© 2006 by The Haworth Press, Inc. All rights reserved.
doi:10.1300/5356_05

agonistic effect at the opioid receptors of individual opioids varies, and this at least partially explains differing analgesic efficacy and side-effect profiles of individual members of this class. Combined with differing receptor affinities are ranges of serum half-life, lipid solubility, and presence of active metabolites, among many other factors, which contribute to the individual identities of members of this class.

As with so many other therapeutic agents, it is now clear that the activity of opioids is not solely related to their activity at one identifiable receptor type. It appears that opioids have a range of effects, which includes a non-competitive antagonistic effect at the N-methyl-D-aspartate (NMDA) receptor and action on calcium channels on nociception-specific neurons.

DOES AGE INFLUENCE THE DOSE OF OPIOID REQUIRED TO ACHIEVE ANALGESIA?

Instinctively, one would expect that smaller doses of opioid would be required to produce analgesia with advanced age. This may be because of alterations in the pharmacokinetics seen in older patients and because of the increased use of other drugs in elderly patients. However, the animal and human evidence that addresses the issue of the effective dose of opioids in relationship to age is contradictory. Jourdan and colleagues (2002, p. 813) conclude that in a rat model, aging animals "show a marked decrease in the effect of morphine with age," while Smith and Gray (2001, p. 445) conclude that "aged male rats are more sensitive to the antinociceptive effects of mu opioid antagonists than young male rats." Similarly the human evidence is contradictory, with Vigano and colleagues (1998, p. 160) stating that elderly cancer pain sufferers "require a lower amount of opioid analgesics than younger adults," while Aubrun and colleagues (2003) find in patients undergoing surgical procedures that the dose of morphine titrated to achieve analgesia is the same in elderly patients as compared to younger patients undergoing the same procedures.

PAIN AND ITS RESPONSIVENESS TO OPIOIDS

It is universally accepted that strong opioids are efficacious in reducing acute pain such as that occurring after surgery. Weaker opioids are commonly used for pain of a more chronic nature, including neuropathic pain. In the case of postoperative pain, McQuay and colleagues (1996) have shown that paracetamol alone is significantly more efficacious than codeine alone, while paracetamol given alone is almost as good as the combination of paracetamol and codeine. Presumably, however, side effects produced by the addition of codeine are significantly greater than those incurred by the use of paracetamol alone.

When the use of strong opioids is considered, much controversy exists. Although in the past many doubted the efficacy of strong opioids in the treatment of chronic pain conditions, the balance of evidence now suggests that strong opioids, be they morphine, fentanyl, oxycontin, or whatever, can reduce the pain of multiple sclerosis, osteoarthritis, rheumatoid arthritis, and even neuropathic pain, for example. However, if these agents are to be used successfully, then there must be a willingness to titrate the dose of the drug used to gain maximum effect and an appreciation that there may be a need to further increase the dose to achieve the same degree of pain relief as time progresses (due to tolerance). Along with this may come an increase in side effects as the dose escalates.

So the balance of evidence is that strong opioids are efficacious in a wide range of pain conditions, although the issue still exists as to whether in individual cases they are the best choice, given that there are so many other proven options available. A few comparative studies have been carried out that show, for example, that opioids and tricyclic antidepressants are both effective in reducing the pain of postherpetic neuralgia and because they have differing modes of action, both can legitimately be used either alone or in combination.

TYPES OF OPIOD

Codeine

Codeine is a weak opioid analgesic, so-called because of its weak affinity for the mu opioid receptor. It has a half-life of around 2.5 to 3 hours. Despite the widespread use of codeine, either on its own or in combination with other agents, it is likely that unaltered codeine has little intrinsic analgesic effect. It relies on in vivo O-demethylation to morphine to become active as an analgesic. This process is mediated by a cytochrome P450 enzyme, CYP2D6. Approximately 5 to 10 percent of Caucasians lack CYP2D6 activity and are termed poor metabolizers, while the remainder are termed extensive metabolizers. Poor metabolizers can expect little analgesia from the use of codeine alone.

Experimentally, codeine has been shown to reduce a number of pain-related parameters. It can increase pressure pain tolerance, pain threshold, and pain summation threshold, suggesting that it may be useful in clinical pain management.

Clinical studies have investigated the effect of codeine on its own and in combination with acetaminophen and nonsteroidal anti-inflammatory drugs. They suggest that codeine does have an analgesic effect in a range of pain conditions. Given that these studies must have included poor metabolizers, it is likely that the extent of analgesia observed overall may have been greater in individuals who were extensive metabolizers. The major drawback to these studies is the fact that they have investigated the analgesic effect of codeine administered over a short period of time. There are obviously clinical scenarios where pain is expected to be of short duration, but in many cases in the elderly patient the likelihood is that the pain will be of long duration. These studies fail to give reassurance that the analgesia apparent after short-term use is maintained with long-term use.

Dihydrocodeine

Like codeine, dihydrocodeine undergoes metabolism mediated by the CYP2D6 enzyme system. In contrast, dihydrocodeine does exhibit analgesic properties and its action does not depend on the presence of active metabolites. Therefore the issue of poor and extensive metabolizers is of less relevance than in the case of codeine.

Dihydrocodeine is metabolized to dihydromorphine, dihydrocodeine-6-O, dihydromorphine-3-O, and dihydromorphine-6-O glucuronide and nordihydrocodeine.

All of these metabolites have the greatest affinity for the mu opioid receptor, with dihydromorphine and dihydromorphine-6-O glucuronide having affinities at least 70 times higher for the mu receptor compared to the other metabolites. They also have an affinity for the delta receptor and to a lesser extent the kappa receptor. Both dihydrocodeine and dihydromorphine exhibit linear pharmacokinetics in extensive metabolizers.

Tramadol

Tramadol hydrochloride is a centrally active opioid analgesic with activity at the mu opioid receptor. It also causes inhibition of norepinephrine and serotonin reuptake and can therefore augment the descending bulbospinal inhibitory pathways. Results from placebo-controlled studies show that tramadol can reduce the pain from diabetic neuropathy, polyneuropathy, postherpetic neuralgia, and osteoarthritis. Evidence from use in postoperative analgesia suggests that it is more effective than codeine alone or in combination with acetaminophen. There is a clinical impression that analgesic tolerance is less common, or less rapid in onset, when tramadol and codeine are compared. Tramadol is commonly used in combination with other analgesics and nonsteroidal anti-inflammatories and the impression is of enhanced analgesia when these combinations are used. That said, confusion is possible when compound preparations are used, and the risk of inadvertent overdose with particular components of the combination is possible.

The issue of coprescription of other mu opioid receptor-active agents and of drugs such as the tricyclic antidepressants with documented effects on serotonin and norepinephrine has not yet been fully addressed.

Tramadol is available as normal-release and extended-release oral preparations. The analgesia from extended-release preparations is as good as normal-release tramadol with the advantage of a reduction in overall dose and a consequent reduction in the frequency and severity of side effects.

Meperidine

Meperidine is a relatively weak mu opioid agonist with marked anticholinergic and local anesthetic properties. With a half life of around three hours, it is most appropriately used for the treatment of acute pain of expected short duration. Its principle metabolite is normeperidine which has epileptogenic properties, which again would suggest use in the short rather than the long term.

Propoxyphene

Propoxyphene is synthetic analgesic with a half-life of 6 to 12 hours. Only its *D*-stereoisomer, dextropropoxyphene, has analgesic effects. Its principle metabolite, norpropoxyphene, has a half-life of 30 to 60 hours and may have a cardiotoxic effect. Propoxyphene has mu opioid agonist effects as well as some action on the NMDA receptor.

Pentazocine

Pentazocine is a semisynthetic derivative of the benzomorphinanes with a delta and kappa opioid action. The effect on these receptors may contribute to its dysphoric side effects. In addition to its delta and kappa agonist effects, it also possesses mu antagonistic effects and is therefore classified as a mixed opioid agonist/antagonist.

Morphine

Morphine is metabolized chiefly through glucuronidation by uridine diphosphate glucuronosyl transferase enzymes in the liver. Despite its long history in medical practice, morphine still remains the gold standard in terms of strong opioids. The use of morphine in patients with postoperative pain and pain related to terminal illnesses is well accepted. Its use in those with chronic pain not related to terminal illness and in those with neuropathic pain is more controversial. Mounting evidence now suggests that morphine, when titrated to effect, is effective in a broad range of chronic pain conditions, including those with a neuropathic element. Whether patients receiving this treatment continue to derive the same level of benefit when the morphine is administered over prolonged periods is more questionable. Often dose escalation is required to maintain effect. Some have suggested that rotation from one strong opioid to another will reduce the rapidity with which analgesic tolerance may develop. Others recommend the use of other therapeutic agents that complement the analgesic effect of the morphine and minimize the dose required to achieve effect.

It is now suggested that single-dose administration of opioids can precipitate a reflex hyperalgesia and allodynia when the serum level of the opioid decreases. This would manifest itself to patients as an increase in pain, which may prompt them to take additional opioids. Therefore, when short-acting opioids are used, analgesia rapidly followed by a reflex exaggeration of pain may complicate use. The logic is that sustained-release preparations should be used to avoid this type of on-off phenomenon, maintaining constant plasma levels, rather than the fluctuating levels found when immediate-release preparations are used. It is suggested, therefore, that when morphine is used in the management of chronic pain conditions, sustained-release preparations be used.

Although the pharmacological mode of action of injected, oral immediate-release, and oral sustained-release morphine are all the same, the clinical effect may be different. Patients often report that injected morphine and oral immediate-release is more efficacious and helpful in a broader range of conditions than oral sustained-release morphine. Presumably with the former modes of administration peak serum levels are higher, and all modes of action attributable to morphine use are operant. With use of sustained-release morphine, these peak levels are not achieved; hence the difference in observable clinical effect. Whether immediate-release morphine should be used in those with chronic painful conditions is therefore debatable.

Currently, morphine is available in a broad range of formulations. Parenteral solutions are used for subcutaneous, intravenous, intramuscular, epidural, and intrathecal use. Immediate-release oral morphine in the form of tablet, suppository, and syrup preparations is available. In addition, sustained-release (12 and 24 hours) preparations are available for oral use. These include tablet and suspension forms. The sustained-release oral forms can be used rectally where the oral route is unavailable, although this use is outside the current product license.

Case report evidence also suggests that morphine can be given in a nebulizer and can also be given through a urinary catheter for specific conditions. These aspects are expanded upon when topical administration is considered.

Diamorphine

A semisynthetic lipid-soluble opioid analgesic that is rapidly deacylated to active metabolites 6-monoacetyl-morphine and morphine, diamorphine has few advantages when compared to morphine. It is reputed to have a greater solubility than morphine and therefore when high doses are required to be dissolved for use as a subcutaneous infusion, diamorphine may offer some advantage.

Hydromorphone

Hydromorphone is a phenanthrene derivative and a structural analogue of morphine. It has strong affinity for the mu opioid receptor.

Quigley (2002) has analyzed all available studies investigating the analgesic effects of hydromorphone. Although many of the studies analyzed were of poor quality or assessed small numbers of patients, the overall conclusions generated by his analysis were that in the context of both acute and chronic pain, hydromorphone appears to be a potent analgesic, but that there is little difference between it and morphine in its analgesic effect or side-effect profile.

Methadone

Methadone is a synthetic mu opioid receptor agonist and antagonist at the NMDA receptor. The pharmacokinetics and pharmacodynamics of methadone are highly variable and hence individualization of dose is necessary. Oral bioavailability varies from 40 to 90 percent, and intestinal metabolism varies to cause wide fluctuations in presystemic inactivation.

Methadone plasma levels follow a biexponential model of decline, and hence the variation between its analgesic action of 6 to 8 hours and its tendency to cumulate. Methadone does not have active metabolites and is excreted in feces and may therefore be a safer analgesic than the other strong opioids in those with renal impairment.

Fentanyl

Fentanyl has a long and established pedigree in postoperative pain management. More recently, the transdermal delivery of fentanyl has become popular in the treatment of chronic pain and that related to terminal illness. The transdermal mode of administration is considered in a later chapter.

Fentanyl possesses intense mu opioid-related analgesic effects. When given intravenously, respiratory depression may complicate use. Fentanyl has a shorter duration of effect than morphine, with peak action diminishing after 20 minutes or so. Consequently, immediate-release fentanyl has little place in the long-term management of chronic pain conditions but may be useful in the acute management of pain of short duration such as may occur with change of wound or burn dressings or when a movement is anticipated in the presence of a movement-related pain condition, such as is seen with fractured ribs.

A number of preparations (apart from the transdermal delivery preparation) are currently available, including a parenteral formulation, a sublingual tablet, and a lozenge-type formulation designed for rapid buccal absorption.

Buprenorphine

Buprenorphine is a kappa agonist with a relatively long half-life, available in oral, sublingual, parenteral, and transdermal formulations. It is associated with dysphoriant side effects.

Oxycodone

Oxycodone is now available in immediate-release and sustained-release oral preparations as well as a parenteral form. Oxycodone undergoes extensive hepatic metabolism and conjugation to inactive metabolites.

Recent studies have shown that oxycodone can be effective in relieving osteoarthritis pain and that caused by diabetic neuropathy and postherpetic neuralgia.

Given that tricyclic antidepressants, antiepileptics, and capsaicin have all been shown to reduce the pain of diabetic neuropathy, the question arises as to which has the best chance of being efficacious. Watson and colleagues (2003) have demonstrated in a randomized controlled trial that controlled-release oxycodone does have an analgesic effect when used in patients with painful diabetic neuropathy. They have calculated the numbers needed to treat (NNT), that is, the number of patients who need to be given the drug for one to obtain a 50 percent reduction in pain, as 2.6. The NNT is 2.3 for carbamazepine, 2.1 for phenytoin, 3.8 for gabapentin, and 3.5 for tricyclic antidepressants. On this basis, oxycodone is at least as good as other treatments conventionally used for painful diabetic neuropathy. Whether it should be used in preference to these other treatments is more debatable.

SIDE EFFECTS OF OPIOID ANALGESICS

It is clear that a substantial body of evidence supports the contention that opioid analgesics have a useful pain-relieving effect in a broad range of conditions. That is still not to say that they are necessarily the best agents for treating these pain conditions, but merely to say that they can be logically considered.

A major influence on the decision to use an opioid is the risk of producing side effects. Some of these side effects are predictable and well known; others are less so. In treating acute pain, immediate side effects are apparent: nausea and respiratory depression are the most obvious. With longer-term use, others such as constipation often become apparent.

Cepeda and colleagues (2003) evaluated 8,855 patients given a variety of strong opioid analgesics. They found that 26 percent had nausea and vomiting while 1.5 percent had respiratory depression. They found that the risk of respiratory depression increased significantly in patients older than 60 years. Side effects were least frequent in the short term with meperidine.

Nausea and Vomiting

If the data supplied by Cepeda and colleagues (2003) are a true reflection of the incidence of nausea and vomiting after strong opioid administration, then prophylactic administration of an antiemetic is warranted. When strong opioids are being initiated for chronic pain conditions, compliance may be reduced if nausea occurs. If it is prevented, then there is a greater chance that opioid treatment will be maintained by the patient. With the use of strong opioids on a chronic basis, antiemetics may only need to be given for the first five days of treatment. A variety of antiemetics is available: 5HT3 antagonists (ondansetron, granisetron, tropisetron), dopamine receptor antagonists (metoclopramide, phenothiazines), muscarinic receptor antagonists (scopolamine), and H1 receptor antagonists (diphenhydramine).

In clinical practice, the following antiemetics may be useful. With acute parenteral use of strong opioids, cyclizine 50 mg or ondansetron 4 mg given with the opioid may be useful. When sustained-release preparations are used, then for the first five days ondansetron 4 mg twice daily or sustained-release metoclopramide 15 mg twice daily can be used.

Constipation

An almost inevitable consequence of long-term opioid use is constipation. As with nausea, prophylactic measures can avoid or minimize this side effect. Fecal softeners are a useful initial therapy, with the use of stimulant laxatives if these prove inadequate.

Pruritus

Puritus is most marked after intrathecal and epidural administration but may also complicate oral and parenteral use. It usually responds to use of antihistamines such as chlorpheniramine given as 4 mg orally or 10 mg parenterally.

Tolerance

Analgesic tolerance, that is, the need to increase the dose of opioid to derive the same level of pain relief, is common with opioids. This issue can be approached in a number of ways. First, opioids can be reserved for short-term use so that there is no risk of analgesic tolerance. Second, adjuvant agents can be given either to minimize the dose of opioid required to produce pain relief or to reduce the risk of tolerance developing. Third, a process of opioid rotation can be instituted where after a defined period of time the initial opioid is changed to another and then to yet another after a similar period of time. Fourth, the dose of opioid can be substantially reduced by changing the route of administration: a fraction of the oral dose administered by the intrathecal route can achieve the same level of analgesia. Fifth, as tolerance occurs, the dose of opioid is increased to maintain the same level of analgesia, with the hope that analgesic tolerance is accompanied by tolerance to the principle side effects of that opioid.

Edwards and Salib (2002) found that 2.8 percent of elderly patients in a group of four practices were taking weak opioids for longer than one year. Using diagnosis criteria for research (DCR-10) for dependence syndrome, they found that 40 percent of elderly patients taking weak opioids on a long-term basis fulfilled the DCR-10 criteria for dependence syndrome.

Effect on Cognitive and Motor Function

Clinical experience suggests that neuropsychological side effects due to opioid therapy usually decrease during the first weeks of therapy. A single dose of morphine has been shown to significantly reduce motor task reaction time. Other known adverse effects include mental clouding, sedation, and confusion. These effects are well known and accepted in patients given a single dose of strong opioid. Since these patients are likely to be under supervision, these effects are less important than the issue of the effects of long-term administration of opioids in patients with pain of a more chronic nature. These patients may already experience cognitive impairment because of the severity of their pain or because of other medications taken for the pain. If medication is rationalized and pain reduced, then the burden of cognitive impairment induced by the opioid may be lessened or even removed because of the pain reduction consequent to its use.

An insight into the consequences of cognitive and motor impairment in elderly patients is given by the work of Ensrud and colleagues (2003). They found that the incidence of nonspine fracture in elderly community-dwelling females was significantly higher in those taking strong opioid drugs.

When considering the effects of opioids on cognitive and motor function, it seems clear that stable use of sustained-release preparations such as controlled-release morphine and transdermal fentanyl are not associated with impairment of cognitive or motor performance. However, impairment of these functions may temporarily complicate the initiation phase of opioid treatment and probably at times when dose is increased. As cognitive and motor function impairment are such major issues in elderly patients, if they require the use of strong opioids, then controlled or sustained-release preparations should be used to achieve a stable serum level of the drug and give less reason why cognitive and motor function should be adversely affected.

Effect on Endocrine Function

Acute administration of opioids increases prolactin, growth hormone, thyroid-stimulating hormone, and adrenocoticotropic hormone while inhibiting luteinizing hormone (LH) release. When administered on a long-term basis, different endocrine results are observed. Abs and colleagues (2000) extensively investigated 73 patients receiving intrathecal opioids for chronic nonmalignant pain. Their average duration of opioid treatment was 26 months. Decreased libido and impotence was present in 23 of the 24 men studied. Nine of the men had a significantly reduced testosterone level and most had a decreased LH level. All of the premenopausal females had either amenorrhea or an irregular cycle, with ovulation in only one patient. All postmenopausal women had decreased LH and follicle-stimulating hormone levels when compared to controls. The 24-hour urinary cortisol excretion was significantly lower than controls in 14 of the 73 patients. Also,

15 percent of all patients developed growth hormone deficiency. Therefore, in patients receiving intrathecal opioids on a long-term basis, the majority of men and all women developed hypogonadotrophic hypogonadism, 15 percent developed central hypocorticism, and about 15 percent developed growth hormone deficiency.

Clearly the results of this study are dramatic, but of course these patients were receiving intrathecal rather than oral opioids. It does, however, raise the question as to whether long-term high-dose oral treatment may produce the same picture or at least upset the endocrine system to a lesser extent.

A single case report highlights a different possible side effect of fentanyl use. Kokko and colleagues (2002) report apparent inappropriate antidiuretic hormone (ADH) release in a patient with a known lung tumor treated with fentanyl. Withdrawal of fentanyl terminated the ADH release, while reinstitution of fentanyl at a later date triggered a further inappropriate ADH release.

Paradoxical Pain

Although the primary aim of using opioid analgesics is pain relief, a strong body of evidence suggests that at times they can actually exacerbate, rather than relieve, pain. In a study in rats, Yaksh and colleagues (1986) implanted intrathecal catheters and infused high concentrations of morphine. These rats exhibited features of pain behaviors that involved intermittent bouts of biting and scratching at the dermatomes innervated by levels of the spinal cord proximal to the catheter tip. In addition, during intervals between bouts of agitation, the animals displayed a clear, marked hyperesthesia where an otherwise innocuous stimulus (brush stroke) evoked significant signs of discomfort and consequent aggressive behavior. These effects were perfectly mimicked by a considerably lower dose of morphine-3-glucuronide.

Yaksh and Harty (1988), again using a rat model, have shown that morphine-3-glucuronide has a high chance of inducing this hyperesthesia, with dihydrocodeine and morphine having a lesser potential. They found that the opioids alfentanil, sufentanil, methadone, meperidine, oxycodone, levorphanol, and codeine, even when given at the highest dose, did not induce pain behavior.

Vanderah and colleagues (2001a) give an insight into the possible causes of this phenomenon. They found that rats implanted with pellets or osmotic minipumps delivering morphine displayed tactile allodynia and thermal hyperalgesia (i.e., opioid-induced pain); placebo pellets or saline minipumps did not change thresholds. Rostral ventromedial medulla (RVM) lidocaine, or bilateral lesions of the dorsolateral funiculus, did not change response thresholds in placebo-pelleted rats but blocked opioid-induced pain. These results suggest that opioids elicit pain through tonic activation of bulbospinal facilitation from the RVM.

In addition to this RVM effect, it is known that spinal dorsal horn dynorphin is increased after opioid administration. Although dynorphin was originally identified as an endogenous kappa-opioid agonist and may act as an endogenous antinociceptive agent under certain conditions, this peptide has significant nonopioid activity. Considerable evidence now supports the conclusion that enhanced expression of spinal dynorphin is pronociceptive and promotes opioid tolerance.

A third possible mechanism that is implicated in opioid-induced pain involves the peptide cholecystokinin (CCK). CCK, originally thought to have effects solely on the gastrointestinal system, is now known to be represented in the central nervous system. CCK has an antiopioid effect and its levels are increased by chronic opioid administration (and by neural injury). Therefore, the long-term use of opioids may lead to an elevation of CCK levels that negates the analgesic effect of the opioid and endogenous enkephalins with an apparent magnification of pain. This mechanism is of importance because both animal and human studies have shown that coadministration of a CCK antagonist may enhance the analgesic effect of the opioid and even reduce the rapidity and extent of analgesic tolerance.

It has been suggested that repeated opioids maintain their efficacy, but the concurrent expression of hyperalgesia counteracts antinociception, producing an impression of tolerance. Opioid-induced hyperalgesia has been hypothesized to result from unmasking of compensatory neuronal hyperactivity, which becomes evident after the opioid is removed or occurring intermittently between injections. Thus opioid-induced hyperalgesia might result from repeated episodes of opioid withdrawal (mini withdrawals).

Hood and colleagues (2003) have shown that in human volunteers with capsaicin-induced hyperalgesia, the ultra-short-acting opioid remifentanil reduces the hyperalgesia and allodynia caused by the capsaicin while being administered. However, some time after the end of administration there is an increase in hyperalgesia and allodynia above that which was apparent prior to remifentanil administration. The clinical implication of this study is that while opioids may have an analgesic effect, as their plasma levels fall there is a paradoxical increase in pain that may encourage further opioid consumption beyond the point required by the original injury.

While the animal experiments investigating this phenomenon use intrathecally or systemically administered opioids at high doses, case reports from the human literature suggest that paradoxical opioid-induced pain may occur with intrathecally and intravenously administered morphine at less substantial doses. In a case report by Parisod and colleagues (2003), allodynia was apparent after a single intrathecal administration of 0.5 mg of morphine. If it appears that morphine, regardless of its mode of administration, is causing an increase in pain, then substitution of the morphine with another strong opioid may end the problem. We have seen that the work by Yaksh and Harty (1988) suggests that opioid-induced pain may occur with morphine and dihydrocodeine, but, in animals, is less likely with meperidine, oxycodone, and codeine.

The implication of the studies discussed is that strong opioids are not always the best option for the treatment of either acute or chronic pain. In some circumstances, they may actually exacerbate rather than relieve pain. Because of the suggestion that this opioid-induced pain may be partially related to mini-withdrawal reactions, if opioids are to be used in the long term, then controlled-release formulations that prevent rapid and frequent changes in plasma concentrations of the opioid, with associated mini-withdrawal reactions, are to be preferred.

CLINICAL USE OF OPIOIDS IN THE ELDERLY

Both the weak and strong opioids have an important place in the management of all varieties of pain in elderly patients. That is not to say that they are always the best form of treatment. For example, if an elderly patient has a small area of postherpetic neuralgia, while opioids may well help, how much better to use a local option such as a lidocaine patch that has an equal chance of helping yet substantially less chance of producing short- and long-term side effects? If it is decided that an opioid is appropriate, then thought needs to be given to whether a weak or strong opioid is needed and to the duration of treatment. If this is likely to be long term, then a sustained/controlled-release preparation will be more appropriate. Side effects will occur, and therefore prophylactic use of laxatives or antiemetics may be advisable. If the pain in question is acute, then normal-release opioids may be appropriate and parenteral titration to achieve effect wise. With acute use, no fixed-dose recommendations for elderly patients can be given, especially as this group of patients varies so widely in size, health, and concomitant drug consumption. The slow intravenous administration of a strong opioid to achieve analgesia will allow an individualization of dose not possible with intramuscular or oral use.

Concomitant use of acetaminophen or a nonsteroidal anti-inflammatory can reduce the dose of weak opioid needed to achieve pain relief. Remember that a proportion of patients will not respond to codeine-containing preparations due to their metabolizer status and there must be a process of assessment of response to opioid treatment.

Before using strong opioids in elderly patients, the following checklist may be used:

1. Is a strong opioid the best form of treatment available for this pain?
2. Will this opioid interact with any concomitantly administered medication?
3. Can other therapeutic agents be added to minimize the dose of opioid required to achieve analgesia?
4. Can other agents be added to minimize the risk of analgesic tolerance?
5. Will other therapeutic agents (e.g., laxatives, antiemetics) be given to reduce the risk of side effects?
6. Which route of administration is most appropriate?
7. At what dose will the opioid be initiated?
8. What is the expected duration of treatment?
9. Will rules be imposed that limit the rate of dose escalation?
10. Will there be a limit to the dose of this opioid used?
11. How will the effect of opioid treatment be measured?

So the evidence suggests that both weak and strong opioids are efficacious for a wide range of pain conditions, although side effects are commonly associated with their use. Are they then good agents to use in elderly patients? To answer this question introduces personal views that are based on past experience. It is my feeling that opioids, both weak and strong, are appropriate treatments for pain in elderly patients that is expected to be of short duration. I am less sure how appropriate they are for pain that is expected to be more long term. Given the wide range of effective alternatives, and given the propensity of opioids to be associated with side effects in the long term (analgesic tolerance, partial efficacy, constipation, endocrine disturbance, paradoxical pain), then the use of strong opioids in elderly patients should be limited and carefully monitored. If a positive response, in terms of improvement in quality of life overall, is produced, then that is all right. However, if the stage is reached where continued use produces less favorable results, then alternatives should be sought.

CONCLUSION

Weak and strong opioids achieve their analgesic effect predominantly by interacting with well-defined opioid receptors, and the strength of an opioid is related to its affinity for the receptor.

Codeine requires an enzyme-dependent metabolic step to become activated. A proportion of the population is deficient in this enzyme and will therefore gain little analgesia from codeine. Dihydrocodeine does not require this process.

Both weak and strong opioids have a proven analgesic effect in a broad range of pain conditions. They have well-recognized side effects including analgesic tolerance, nausea, constipation, mood disturbance, endocrine effects, and, at times, paradoxical pain associated with their use.

A careful process should be carried out before strong opioid therapy is initiated in elderly patients.

BIBLIOGRAPHY

Abs R, Verhelst J, Maeyaert J, Van Buyten J-P, Opsomer F, Adriaensen H, Verlooy J, Van Havenbergh T, Smet M, Van Acker K. Endocrine consequences of long-term intrathecal administration of opioids. *J Clin Endocrinol Metab* 2000; 85: 2215-2222.

Adriaensen H, Vissers K, Noorduin H, Meert T. Opioid tolerance and dependence: An inevitable consequence of chronic treatment? *Acta Anaesthesiol Belg* 2003; 54: 37-47.

Alder L, McDonald C, O'Brien C, Wilson M. A comparison of once daily tramadol with normal release tramadol in treatment of pain in osteoarthritis. *J Rheumatol* 2002; 29: 2196-2199.

Allen GJ, Hartl TL, Duffany S, Smith SF, Van Heest JL, Anderson J, Hoffman JR, Kraemer WJ, Maresh CM. Cognitive and motor function after administration of hydrocodone bitartrate plus ibuprofen, ibuprofen alone, or placebo in healthy subjects with exercise-induced muscle damage: A randomized, repeated dose, placebo controlled study. *Psychopharmacology* 2003; 166: 228-233.

Ammon S, Hofmann U, Griese EU, Gugeler N, Mikus G. Pharmacokinetics of dihydrocodeine and its active metabolites after single and multiple oral dosing. *Br J Clin Pharmacol* 1999; 48: 317-322.

Armstrong SC, Cozza KL. Pharmacokinetic drug interactions of morphine, codeine and their derivates: Theory and clinical reality. *Psychosomatics* 2003; 44: 167-171.

Arora S, Herbert ME. Myth: Codeine is a powerful and effective analgesic. *WJM* 2001; 174: 428.

Attal N, Guirimand F, Brasseur L, Gaude V, Chauvin M, Bouhassira D. Effects of IV morphine in central pain: A randomized, placebo controlled study. *Neurology* 2002; 58: 554-563.

Aubrun F, Bunhe D, Langeron O, Saillant G, Coriat P, Riou B. Postoperative morphine consumption in the elderly patient. *Anesthesiology* 2003; 99: 160-165.

Bolton EA, Tallarida RJ, Pasternak GW. Synergy between mu opioid ligands: Evidence for functional interactions among mu opioid receptor subtypes. *J Pharmacol Exp Ther* 2002; 303: 557-562.

Boureau F, Legallicier P, Kabir-Ahmadi M. Tramadol in post-herpetic neuralgia: A randomized, double-blind, placebo-controlled trial. *Pain* 2003; 104: 323-331.

Bredenberg S, Duberg M, Lennernas B, Lennernas H, Pettersson A, Westerberg M, Nystrom C. In vitro evaluation of a new sublingual tablet system for rapid oromucosal absorption using fentanyl citrate as the active substance. *Eur J Pharmacol Sci* 2003; 20: 327-334.

Caldwell JR, Rapoport RJ, Davis JC, Offenberg HL, Marker HW, Roth SH, Yuan W, Eliot L, Babul N, Lynch PM. Efficacy and safety of a once daily morphine formulation in chronic, moderate to severe osteoarthritis pain: Results from a randomized, placebo controlled, double blind trial and an open label extension trial. *J Pain Symptom Manage* 2002; 23: 278-291.

Cepeda MS, Farrar JT, Baumgarten M, Boston R, Carr DB, Strom I. Side effects of opioids during short term administration: Effect of age, gender and race. *Clin Pharmacol Ther* 2003; 74: 102-112.

Chew M, White JM, Somogyi AA, Bochner F, Irvine RJ. Precipitated withdrawal following codeine administration is dependent on CYP genotype. *Eur J Pharmacol* 2001; 425: 159-164.

Compton P, Athanasos P, Elashoff D. Withdrawal hyperalgesia after acute opioid physical dependency in non addicted humans: A preliminary study. *J Pain* 2003; 4: 511-519.

De Conno F, Caraceni A, Martini C, Spoldi E, Salvetti M, Ventafridda V. Hyperalgesia and myoclonus with intrathecal infusion of high-dose morphine. *Pain* 1991; 47: 337-339.

Dellemijn PL, Vanneste JA. Randomized double blind active placebo controlled crossover trial of intravenous fentanyl in neuropathic pain. *Lancet* 1997; 349: 753-758.

Edwards I, Salib E. Analgesics in the elderly. *Aging Ment Health* 2002; 6: 88-92.

Enggaard TP, Poulsen L, Arendt-Nielsen L, Honore-Hansen S, Bjornsdottir I, Gram LF, Sindrup SH. The analgesic effect of codeine as compared to imipramine in different human experimental pain models. *Pain* 2001; 92: 277-282.

Ensrud KE, Blackwell T, Mangione CM, Bowman PJ, Bauer DC, Schwartz A, Nevitt MC, Whooley MA. Central nervous system active medications and risk for fractures in aged women. *Arch Intern Med* 2003; 163: 949-957.

Gagnon B, Bruera E. Differences in the ratios of morphine to methadone in patients with neuropathic pain versus non-neuropathic pain. *J Pain Symptom Manage* 1999; 18: 120-125.

Gharagozlou P, Demirci H, Clark JD, Lameh J. Activity of opioid ligands in cells expressing cloned mu opioid receptors. *BMC Pharmacol* 2003: 3: 1-8.

Griessinger N, Sittl R, Jost R, Schaefer M, Likar R. The role of opioid analgesics in rheumatoid disease in the elderly population. *Drugs Aging* 2003; 20: 571-583.

Grilo RM, Bertin P, Scotto di Fazano C, Coyral D, Bonnet C, Vergne P, Treves R. Opioid rotation in the treatment of joint pain: A review of 67 cases. *Joint Bone Spine* 2002; 69: 491-494.

Grossman A. Brain opiates and neuroendocrine function. *Clin Endocrinol Metab* 1983; 12: 725-746.

Harati Y, Gooch C, Swenson M, Edelman S, Greene D, Raskin P, Donofrio P, Cornblath D, Sachdeo R, Siu CO, Kamin M. Double-blind randomized trial of tramadol for the treatment of pain of diabetic neuropathy. *Neurology* 1998; 50: 1842-1846.

Heger S, Maier C, Otter K, Helwig U, Suttorp M. Morphine induced allodynia in a child with brain tumor. *BMJ* 319: 627-629.

Hood DD, Curry R, Eisenach JC. Intravenous remifentanil produces withdrawal hyperalgesia in volunteers with capsaicin-induced hyperalgesia. *Anesth Analg* 2003; 97: 810-815.

Inturrisi CE. Clinical pharmacology of opioids for pain. *Clin J Pain* 2002; 18: S3-S13.

Jamison RN, Schein JR, Vallow S, Ascher S, Vorsanger GJ, Katz NP. Neuropsychological effects of long term opioid use in chronic pain patients. *J Pain Symptom Manage* 2003; 26: 913-921.

Jourdan D, Pickering G, Marchand F, Gaulier JM, Alliot J, Eschalier A. Impact of ageing on the antinociceptive effect of reference analgesics in the Lou/c rat. *Br J Pharmacol* 2002; 137: 813-820.

Kalman S, Osterberg A, Sorensen J, Boivie J, Bertler A. Morphine responsiveness in a group of well defined multiple sclerosis patients: A study with IV morphine. *Eur J Pain* 2002; 6: 69-80.

Kokko H, Hall PD, Afrin LB. Fentanyl associated syndrome of inappropriate antidiuretic hormone secretion. *Pharmacotherapy* 2002; 22: 1188-1192.

Maier C, Hildebrandt J, Klinger R, Henrich-Eberl C, Lindena G. Morphine responsiveness, efficacy and tolerability in patients with chronic non-tumor associated pain-results of a double blind placebo controlled trial. *Pain* 2002; 97: 223-233.

McDowell TS. Fentanyl decreases Ca^{2+} currents in a population of capsaicin responsive sensory neurons. *Anesthesiology* 2003; 98: 223-231.

Moore A, Collins S, Carroll D, McQuay H, and Edwards J. Single dose (acetaminophen) with and without postoperative pain. *Cochrane Database Rev* 2000; 2: CD001547.

Mullican WS, Lacy JR. Tramadol/acetaminophen combination tablets and codeine/acetaminophen combination capsules for the management of chronic pain: A comparative trial. *Clin Ther* 2001; 23: 1429-1445.

Narita M, Imai S, Itou Y, Yajima Y, Suzuki T. Possible involvement of mu1-opioid receptors in the fentanyl morphine-induced antinociception at supraspinal and spinal sites. *Life Sci* 2002; 70: 2341-2354.

Ossipov MH, Lai J, Vanderah TW, Porreca F. Induction of pain facilitation by sustained opioid exposure: Relationship to opioid antinociceptive tolerance. *Life Sci* 2003; 73: 783-800.

Paice JA, Penn RD, Ryan WG. Altered sexual function and decreased testosterone in patients receiving intraspinal opioids. *J Pain Symptom Manage* 1994; 9: 126-131.

Parisod E, Siddall PJ, Viney M, McClelland JM, Cousins MJ. Allodynia after acute intrathecal morphine administration in a patient with neuropathic pain after spinal cord injury. *Anesth Analg* 2003; 97: 183-186.

Peloso PM, Bellamy N, Bensen W, Thomson GT, Harsanyi Z, Babul N, Darke AC. Double blind randomized placebo control trial of controlled release codeine in the treatment of osteoarthritis of the hip or knee. *J Rheumatol* 2000; 27: 764-771.

Oral oxycodone: New preparation. No better than oral morphine. *Prescrire Int* 2003; 12: 83-84.

Quigley C. Hydromorphone for acute and chronic pain. *Cochrane Database Syst Rev* 2002; 1: CD003447.

Raffa RB, Friderichs E. The basic science aspect of tramadol hydrochloride. *Pain Rev* 1996; 3: 249-271.

Raja SN, Haythornwaite JA, Pappagallo M, Clark MR, Travison TG, Sabeen S, Max MB. Opioids versus antidepressants in postherpetic neuralgia: a randomized, placebo controlled trial. *Neurology* 2002; 59: 1015-1021.

Roth SH, Fleischmann RM, Burch FX, Dietz F, Bockow B, Rapaport RJ, Rutstein J, Lacouture PG. Around the clock, controlled release oxycodone therapy for osteoarthritis related pain: Placebo controlled trial and long term evaluation. *Arch Int Med* 2000; 160: 853-860.

Rowbotham MC, Reisner-Keller LA, Fields HL. Both intravenous lidocaine and morphine reduce the pain of postherpetic neuralgia. *Neurology* 1991; 41: 1024-1028.

Rowbotham MC, Twilling L, Davies PS, Reisner L, Taylor K, Mohr D. Oral opioid therapy for chronic peripheral and central neuropathic pain. *N Engl J Med* 2003; 348: 1223-1232.

Sabatowski R, Schwalen S, Rettig K, Herberg KW, Kasper SM, Radbruch L. Driving ability under long term fentanyl treatment with transdermal fentanyl. *J Pain Symptom Manage* 2003; 25: 38-47.

Schmidt H, Vormfelde S, Klinder K, Gundert-Remy U, Gleiter CH, Skopp G, Aderjan R, Fuhr U. Affinities of dihydrocodeine and its metabolites to opioid receptors. *Pharmacol Toxicol* 2002; 91: 57-63.

Schmidt H, Vormfelde SV, Walchner-Bonjean M, Klinder K, Freudenthaler S, Gleiter CH, Gundert-Remy U, Skopp G, Aderjan R, Fuhr U. The role of active metabolites in dihydrocodeine effects. *Int J Clin Pharmacol Ther* 2003; 41: 95-106.

Silverfield JC, Kamin M, Wu SC, Rosenthal N. Tramadol/acetaminophen combination tablets for the treatment of osteoarthritis flare pain: A multicenter, outpatient, randomized, double blind, placebo controlled, parallel group, add on study. *Clin Ther* 2002; 24: 282-297.

Sindrup SH, Andersen G, Madsen C, Smith T, Brosen K, Jensen TS. Tramadol relieves pain and allodynia in polyneuropathy: A randomized, double-blind, controlled trial. *Pain* 1999; 83: 85-90.

Sjogren P, Jensen N-K, Jensen TS. Disappearance of morphine induced hyperalgesia after discontinuing or substituting morphine with other opioid analgesics. *Pain* 1994; 59: 313-316.

Sjogren P, Jonsson T, Jensen N-K, Drenck N-E, Jensen TS. Hyperalgesia and myoclonus in terminal cancer patients treated with continuous intravenous morphine. *Pain* 1993; 55: 93-97.

Smith MA, Gray JD. Age-related differences in sensitivity to the antinociceptive effects of opioids in male rats. Influence of nociceptive intensity and intrinsic efficacy at the mu receptor. *Psychopharmacol* 2001; 156: 445-453.

Soares LG, Martins M, Uchoa R. Intravenous fentanyl for cancer pain: A "fast titration" protocol for the emergency room. *J Pain Symptom Manage* 2003; 26: 876-881.

Su CF, Liu MY, Li MT. Intraventricular morphine produces pain relief, hypothermia, hyperglycaemia and increased prolactin and growth hormone levels in patients with cancer pain. *J Neurol* 1987; 235: 105-108.

Tassain V, Attal N, Fletcher D, Brasseur L, Degieux P, Chauvin M, Bouhassira D. Long term effects of oral sustained release morphine on neuropsychological performance in patients with chronic non-cancer pain. *Pain* 2003; 104: 389-400.

Vanderah TW, Gardell LR, Burgess SE, Ibrahim M, Dogrul A, Zhong C-M, Zhang E-T, Malan TP, Ossipov MH, Lai J, Porreca F. Dynorphin promotes abnormal pain and spinal opioid antinociceptive tolerance. *J Neurosci* 2000; 20: 7074-7079.

Vanderah TW, Ossipov MH, Lai J, Malan TP, Porreca F. Mechanisms of opioid induced pain and antinociceptive tolerance: Descending facilitation and spinal dynorphin. *Pain* 2001; 92: 5-9.

Vanderah TW, Suenaga NM, Ossipov MH, Malan TP, Lai J, Porreca F. Tonic descending facilitation from the rostral ventromedial medulla mediates opioid induced abnormal pain and antinociceptive tolerance. *J Neurosci* 2001; 21: 279-2286.

Vigano A, Bruera E, Suarez-Almazor ME. Age, pain intensity, and opioid dose in patients with advanced cancer. *Cancer* 1998; 83: 1244-1250.

Walsh D, Tropiano PS. Long-term rectal administration of high dose sustained release morphine tablets. *Support Care Cancer* 2002; 10: 653-655.

Watson CP, Babul N. Efficacy of oxycodone in neuropathic pain: A randomized trial in postherpetic neuralgia. *Neurology* 1998; 50: 1837-1841.

Watson CP, Moulin D, Watt-Watson J, Gordon A, Eisenhoffer J. Controlled release oxycodone relieves neuropathic pain: A randomized controlled trial in painful diabetic neuropathy. *Pain* 2003; 105: 71-8.

Webb JA, Rostami-Hodjegan A, Abdul-Manap R, Hofmann U, Miku, Kamali F. Contribution of dihydrocodeine and dihydromorphine to analgesia following dihydrocodeine administration in man: A PK-PD modeling analysis. *Br J Clin Pharmacol* 2001; 52: 35-43.

Wilder-Smith CH, Hill L, Spargo K, Kalla A. Treatment of severe pain from osteoarthritis with slow-release tramadol or dihydrocodeine in combination with NSAIDs: A randomized study comparing analgesia, antinociception and gastrointestinal effects. *Pain* 2001; 91: 23-31.

Wilkinson TJ, Robinson BA, Begg EJ, Duffull SB, Ravenscroft PJ, Schneider JJ. Pharmacokinetics and efficacy of rectal versus oral sustained release morphine in cancer patients. *Chemother Pharmacol* 1992; 31: 251-254.

Williams DG, Patel A, Howard RF. Pharmacogenetics of codeine metabolism in an urban population of children and its implications for analgesic reliability. *Br J Anaesth* 2002; 89: 839-845.

Wolf CJ. Intrathecal high dose morphine produces hyperalgesia in the rat. *Brain Res* 1981; 209: 491-495.

Yaksh TL, Harty GJ. Pharmacology of the allodynia in rats evoked by high dose intrathecal morphine. *J Pharmacol Exp Ther* 1988; 244: 501-507.

Yaksh TL, Harty GJ, Onofrio BM. High doses of spinal morphine produce a non-opiate receptor mediated hyperaesthesia: Clinical and theoretical implications. *Anesthesiology* 1986; 64: 590-597.

Yamakura T, Sakimura K, Shimoji K. Direct inhibition of the N-methyl-D-aspartate receptor channel by high concentrations of opioids. *Anesthesiology* 1999; 91: 1053-1063.

Yu A, Kneller BM, Rettie AE, Haining RL. Expression, purification, biochemical characterization, and comparative function of human cytochrome P450 2D6.1, 2D6.2, 2D6.10 and 2D6.17 allelic isoforms. *J Pharmacol Exp Ther* 2002; 303: 1291-1300.

Chapter 6

NSAIDs and the Elderly

Jennifer A. Elliott

Nonsteroidal anti-inflammatory drugs (NSAIDs) are among the most commonly used drugs in the world. Many of us will use NSAIDs on at least an occasional basis during our lifetimes. As the population ages and arthritic conditions become more prevalent, the use of NSAIDs will likely continue to increase. Unfortunately, though they are often perceived as very safe drugs, especially since some forms are available over-the-counter, NSAIDs have been associated with significant morbidity and mortality. Many elderly patients suffer from concomitant illnesses that may increase their risk for morbid events when using NSAIDs. Such conditions may include congestive heart failure, renal dysfunction, hypertension, and use of various pharmacological agents that may negatively interact with NSAIDs. Adverse events related to NSAID use that may be of clinical concern in the elderly include gastrointestinal bleeding, acute renal failure, precipitation of congestive heart failure, cognitive impairment, and hypertension. In this chapter, the potential benefits and drawbacks of NSAID use as well as appropriate precautions for their use in the elderly population are explored.

MECHANISM OF ACTION
AND PHYSIOLOGICAL EFFECTS OF NSAIDs

NSAIDs act via inhibition of cyclooxygenase, an enzyme required for prostaglandin synthesis. Prostaglandins are active in many tissues and have also been associated with the production of fever, inflammation, and pain. Two forms of the cyclooxygenase enzyme have been identified. Cyclooxygenase-1 is constitutively expressed in many tissues and plays an important role in the regulation of several important physiological processes, such as regulation of renal blood flow, maintenance of gastrointestinal mucosal integrity, and platelet aggregation. Cyclo-oxygenase-2 (COX-2)

Clinical Management of the Elderly Patient in Pain
© 2006 by The Haworth Press, Inc. All rights reserved.
doi:10.1300/5356_06

appears to be an inducible enzyme that becomes upregulated in the setting of inflammation. Most traditional NSAIDs lack selectivity in their inhibition of cyclooxygenase isoenzymes. In the past few years, a new generation of NSAIDs with COX-2 selectivity has become available for clinical use. These newer agents may provide some advantage over the nonselective NSAIDs with regard to potential undesired effects. However, some adverse effects seen with the use of traditional NSAIDs have not been eliminated through the use of COX-2 inhibitors. NSAIDs undergo hepatic metabolism and are renally excreted. Age-related declines in renal function or hepatic impairment associated with such conditions as congestive heart failure may result in drug accumulation and thereby increase the risk of development of a variety of adverse effects from these agents in the elderly.

Gastrointestinal Effects of NSAIDs

Prostaglandins play an important role in maintenance of gastrointestinal (GI) mucosal integrity. When NSAIDs are administered, homeostatic mechanisms in the GI mucosa may be disrupted, resulting in the development of ulcerations or frank perforations in some patients. A significant number of people suffer fatal GI hemorrhage every year as a consequence. Unfortunately, many significant GI bleeding episodes occur in the absence of premonitory warning signs of abdominal pain or dyspepsia, making prediction of such events difficult. The elderly may have lower baseline levels of prostaglandins in the GI mucosa and are at higher risk for GI bleeding compared with younger populations in general, making them potentially more susceptible to adverse GI effects of NSAIDs. Other factors that may increase the risk of GI hemorrhage in the elderly using NSAIDs include concurrent use of aspirin (commonly used for prophylaxis against acute coronary events in the elderly) and concomitant anticoagulant therapy, which might exacerbate GI hemorrhage. Some of these effects may be mitigated by the use of gastroprotective agents in conjunction with NSAID therapy. Such treatments might include the use of misoprostol, proton pump inhibitors, and H_2 receptor antagonists. Use of COX-2 inhibitors may result in a lower incidence of significant adverse GI effects as compared with traditional NSAIDs. That said, concern regarding the long-term cardiovascular safety of some COX-2 inhibitors has caused their withdrawal from the market and cautions have been issued with the use of others. How far these concerns extend to more conventional NSAIDs that alos possess COX-2 effects is unclear.

Renal Effects of NSAIDs

NSAIDs may cause a variety of changes in renal physiology. This is an important consideration when NSAIDs are selected for use in elderly patients, as many elderly patients suffer from comorbid conditions that can increase the risk of adverse renal effects from NSAIDs or may experience exacerbation of underlying disease states as a result of the renal effects of NSAIDs. Prostaglandins play a role in the regulation of renal blood flow. In patients with such diseases as congestive heart failure, significant hepatic dysfunction, renal insufficiency, and intravascular volume depletion, use of NSAIDs may precipitate acute renal failure due to changes in renal blood flow related to prostaglandin inhibition. Renal prostaglandins also play an important role in the regulation of sodium reabsorption in Henle's loop. Inhibition of these prostaglandins by NSAIDs may result in increased sodium reabsorption, which consequently may cause excess fluid retention. This may be of particular importance when NSAIDs are administered to patients with preexisting heart failure, renal insufficiency, or hypertension, which may be worsened under these circumstances. Such effects may be seen relatively quickly after NSAID therapy is initiated. Another important consideration with regard to NSAID use in the elderly hypertensive patient is the decreased efficacy of several antihypertensives when used in conjunction with NSAIDs. In particular, the activity beta-blockers, angiotensin-converting enzyme inhibitors, and diuretics may be affected. Therefore, NSAIDs should be employed with caution in patients on these drugs, especially since congestive heart failure may be precipitated. It should be noted that while the incidence of adverse GI events appears to be lower when COX-2 inhibitors are used (compared with traditional NSAIDs), the incidence of adverse renal and cardiovascular events remains significant even when COX-2 inhibitors are chosen.

Platelet Effects of NSAIDs

Many NSAIDs affect platelet aggregation and may thereby increase the potential for bleeding complications in patients taking NSAIDs. Aspirin is particularly well known for this effect and is used for this very property in the management of patients at risk for myocardial infarction or stroke. Aspirin permanently acetylates platelets, causing platelet dysfunction that lasts the lifespan of the platelet, typically 7 to 14 days. Most nonselective NSAIDs also create platelet dysfunction, but this effect is reversible and platelet aggregation will return to normal within four to five drug half-lives after these drugs are discontinued. COX-2-specific inhibitors do not impact platelet aggregation in doses used in clinical practice. NSAID use in elderly patients may lead to bleeding complications, particularly when combined with coumadin. Coumadin is utilized more frequently in the elderly population than among other demographic groups, creating a potential area of concern when NSAID therapy is considered in these patients. This drug combination may increase the risk of bleeding due to both the antiplatelet effects of NSAIDs and the anticoagulant effects of coumadin, resulting in impairment of the two primary clotting mechanisms of the body. In addition, displacement of coumadin from serum protein-binding sites by some NSAIDs may enhance the effective anticoagulant activity of coumadin. Therefore, caution and monitoring are warranted when these classes of drugs are to be coprescribed.

Central Nervous System Effects of NSAIDs

Central nervous system (CNS) side effects are commonly seen with analgesics such as opioids and are not widely appreciated as a potential consequence of NSAID use. However, NSAIDs are not devoid of CNS effects. Elderly patients taking NSAIDs may manifest CNS toxicity with sedation, confusion, cognitive dysfunction, psychosis, and personality changes. Such side effects may be construed as signs of developing dementia in the elderly, but will abate with discontinuation of the drug. Dizziness and tinnitus have also been described with NSAID use.

Other NSAID-Associated Effects

NSAIDs have potentially beneficial effects in the prevention of cancer and Alzheimer's disease. Currently, COX-2 inhibitors (particularly celecoxib) are being used in treatment of patients with familial adenomatous polyposis, a genetic condition that predisposes individuals to the development of colon cancer. It appears that the development of polyps in these patients can be substantially diminished when COX-2 inhibitors are used. This finding may have relevance to other forms of cancer as well, although thus far COX-2 inhibitors are not being used for prophylaxis against cancer at this point. Further studies may help to elucidate a potential role for chronic COX-2 inhibitor therapy in individuals who are at risk for the development of cancer. If a clear benefit can be established for the use of COX-2 inhibitors for this purpose, there will undoubtedly be a large population of individuals taking these drugs for prolonged periods of time. This population will likely include a large number of elderly patients, especially as life expectancies continue to get longer. With regard to Alzheimer's disease, it has been speculated that NSAIDs may delay the onset of dementia. It has been theorized that Alzheimer's disease may involve an inflammatory process in the brain that leads to the development of dementia. Thus far, there are no recommendations for the use of NSAIDs in the prevention of Alzheimer's disease, but with continued research this may change.

CLASSIFICATION OF NSAIDs AND INDIVIDUAL AGENTS OF PARTICULAR CONCERN IN THE ELDERLY

NSAIDs are classified according to their chemical structure into various groups. The following is a breakdown of NSAIDs in current clinical use:

I. Salicylates
  A. Aspirin
  B. Nonacetylated salicylates
    1. Choline magnesium trisalicylate (Trilisate)
    2. Diflunisal (Dolobid)
II. Propionic acid derivatives
  A. Naproxen (Naprosyn, Aleve, Anaprox)
  B. Ketorolac (Toradol)
  C. Oxaprozin (Daypro)
  D. Ketoprofen (Orudis, Oruvail)
  E. Ibuprofen (Advil, Motrin)
  F. Flurbiprofen (Ansaid)
III. Indoleacetic acids
  A. Etodolac (Lodine)
  B. Indomethacin (Indocin)
  C. Sulindac (Clinoril)
IV. Phenylacetic acids
  A. Diclofenac (Cataflam, Voltaren, Arthrotec [diclofenac in combination with misoprostol])
V. Naphthylalkanone
  A. Nabumetone (Relafen)
VI. Oxicam
  A. Piroxicam (Feldene)
  B. Meloxicam (Mobic)
VII. Pyrroleacetic acid
  A. Tolmetin (Tolectin)
VIII. COX-2 selective inhibitors
  A. Celecoxib (Celebrex)
  B. Valdecoxib (Bextra)

With regard to selection of a particular agent for any particular patient, duration of action, the potential for organ-specific side effects, comorbid conditions, and potential for drug interactions may play a role in the choice of NSAID to be used. Specific areas of concern will be addressed as certain individual NSAIDs are further described in the following sections.

Aspirin

Aspirin is the prototypical NSAID and has been used clinically for well over a century. It is widely used as it is available over-the-counter and is present in many combination analgesic preparations. For this reason, many elderly patients may be unaware that they are consuming substantial amounts of aspirin on a regular basis and may not consider it important to inform their physicians about the use of such products. This situation can lead to problems, as physicians may prescribe NSAID therapy, unaware of concurrent aspirin therapy, which could increase the potential for adverse effects. Many elderly patients may be taking aspirin as a preventive therapy for myocardial infarction and stroke, which should also be taken into consideration. Gastrointestinal toxicity is a concern when aspirin is used, and selection of an enteric-coated aspirin product may be advisable. A single dose of aspirin can irreversibly acetylate platelets, rendering them permanently dysfunctional. This property may be of significant concern in patients on anticoagulant therapy.

Nonacetylated Salicylates

Nonacetylated salicylates in clinical use for arthritic conditions include choline magnesium trisalicylate (Trilisate) and diflunisal (Dolobid). Trilisate is usually dosed between 2000 and 3000 mg daily while diflunisal is usually given in doses of 500-1000 mg daily. These agents are typically dosed two to three times per day and appear to have lower potential for gastrointestinal toxicity than aspirin. Antiplatelet effects are less intense as well, which may make these agents more desirable than other NSAIDs in certain populations. These agents may also be less expensive compared to the more selective COX-2 inhibitors, which can be of particular importance to many elderly patients who lack prescription drug benefits with their health insurance.

Propionic Acid Derivatives

Commonly used propionic acid derivative NSAIDs include naproxen (Naprosyn, Aleve, Anaprox), ketorolac (Toradol), oxaprozin (Daypro), ketoprofen (Orudis, Oruvail), ibuprofen (Advil, Motrin), and flurbiprofen (Ansaid). Typical daily doses for naproxen are 500-1000 mg. Ketorolac is given in doses of up to 120 mg per day parenterally and 40 mg per day orally. Oxaprozin dosing is usually 1200 mg daily, while ketoprofen is dosed at 200-300 mg daily. Ibuprofen is given in a dose range of 1200-3200 mg daily and flurbiprofen in a dose of 200-300 mg per day. These drugs are typically administered two to four times per day, but oxaprozin may be administered once daily. Naprosyn and ibuprofen are available over-the-counter and are generally inexpensive compared with other NSAIDs. Ketorolac is unique in that it is available for parenteral use. However, it also has significant potential for toxicity, and it is therefore recommended that its use (both parenteral and enteral) be limited to a total of five days. It is typically used in acute settings, especially those in which a patient has restriction of oral intake, such as the perioperative period. Dose reduction is recommended in the elderly (where doses of 10 mg or even less may provide analgesia).

Indoleacetic Acid Derivatives

Sulindac (Clinoril) is a prodrug that is converted in the liver to its active metabolite. It may affect renal prostaglandins to a lesser extent than other NSAIDs, potentially making it more desirable in patients at risk for renal complications compared with other NSAIDs (however, evidence has not demonstrated a difference). It is dosed in the range of 300-400 mg daily. It should be dose reduced in the elderly and in the presence of significant renal or hepatic disease. Indomethacin (Indocin) is unique among NSAIDs in its ability to penetrate the blood-brain barrier to a significant extent. This property has made indomethacin useful in the management of certain headache syndromes (ironically, headache is also a frequently occurring side effect of indomethacin that may result in termination of its use). It may also explain a relatively higher incidence of adverse CNS effects with this drug compared with other NSAIDs, particularly in patients with preexisting CNS disorders such as depression, psychosis, and Parkinsonism. Indomethacin is also available in suppository form for patients incapable of taking the drug orally. Its utility is limited, however, due to significant GI toxicity with relatively high potential for ulcer formation with repeated use. Dosing of indomethacin is typically 150-200 mg daily. Etodolac (Lodine) is more COX-2 selective than most traditional NSAIDs and accordingly appears to have a lower incidence of adverse GI side effects than many other NSAIDs. An extended-release preparation is available that allows for once-a-day dosing. Etodolac is dosed at 400-1200 mg daily with dosage varying depending upon the formulation chosen (Lodine versus Lodine XL). Dosage adjustment of etodolac is generally unnecessary in the elderly.

Phenylacetic Acid

Diclofenac is available in an immediate-release (Cataflam), a delayed-release enteric-coated (Voltaren), and an extended-release (Voltaren-XR) formulation. It is also available in combination with misoprostol (a prostaglandin E_1 analog) for enhanced GI protection (Arthrotec). The typical adult daily dose of diclofenac is 100-200 mg daily. This may be administered in divided doses or as a single dose when the Voltaren XR formulation is chosen. No dosage adjustment appears to be necessary in the elderly.

Naphthylalkanone

Nabumetone (Relafen), like sulindac, is a prodrug that is converted to its active metabolite in the liver. This property may decrease the risk of GI ulceration as the GI mucosa is not directly exposed to active drug. Nabumetone is typically dosed between 1000 and 2000 mg daily in single or divided doses. Dose reduction may be advisable in the elderly.

Oxicam

Piroxicam (Feldene) is a long-acting NSAID that can be dosed once daily. The recommended daily dose of piroxicam is 20 mg, which may be divided. Concurrent attempts at GI mucosal protection should be considered. Steady-state blood levels of piroxicam may not be achieved for 1-2 weeks after initiation of therapy due to its prolonged half-life. Meloxicam (Mobic) may have relative COX-2 selectivity when used in low doses (7.5 mg per day). Typical daily dosing of meloxicam is in the range of 7.5-15 mg. No dosage adjustment is necessary in the elderly with either of these agents.

Pyrroleacetic Acid

Tolmetin (Tolectin) is usually dosed between 600 and 1800 mg daily, with typical adult dosing being 400 mg three times daily. Concurrent attempts at GI mucosal protection should be considered. No dose reduction is necessary in the elderly.

COX-2 Selective Inhibitors

These drugs are relatively new among the NSAIDs. They have become widely used due to their lower levels of GI toxicity compared with traditional NSAIDs. These agents also do not exhibit significant antiplatelet effects, making them attractive for use in patients on anticoagulant therapy who need to use anti-inflammatory medication. Unfortunately, there still does appear to be potential for adverse renal effects with use of these drugs, so at-risk patients with renal disease may still be prohibited from using them. The COX-2 selective inhibitor celecoxib (Celebrex) is currently marketed in the United States. Use of celecoxib is contraindicated in patients with sulfonamide allergy due to the presence of a sulfa moiety on these compounds. Celecoxib is typically dosed at 100-400 mg daily in single or twice-daily doses. Dose reduction is not necessary in the elderly. These agents are generally quite expensive, which may be of significant concern to elderly patients, who often live on fixed incomes and may lack prescription drug benefits.

POTENTIAL ADVERSE DRUG INTERACTIONS WITH NSAIDs IN THE ELDERLY

As previously mentioned, many elderly patients may be taking medications for concomitant diseases in conjunction with NSAIDs. This may lead to potential complications as interactions between these drugs may render them more or less effective, or may increase the potential for NSAID-associated toxicity. The following sections review classes of drugs that may adversely interact with NSAIDs.

Antihypertensives

NSAIDs may interact with beta-blockers, calcium channel blockers, and angiotensin-converting enzyme inhibitors, resulting in diminished antihypertensive effects of these agents. This is possibly related to antagonism of synthesis of vasodilatory prostaglandins by NSAIDs as well as fluid and salt retention.

Diuretics

NSAIDs may disrupt the natriuretic and diuretic effects of thiazides and furosemide via inhibition of formation of prostaglandin E_2, which affects sodium resorption in the kidney and acts to antagonize the antidiuretic effect of vasopressin. This may lead to fluid and salt retention with edema formation and hypertension, and possibly congestive heart failure in susceptible individuals. It has also been reported that there may be a significant risk for the development of frank renal failure when indomethacin is used in combination with triamterene, and therefore combined use of these drugs is contraindicated.

Digoxin

The half-life of digoxin may be increased in the presence of NSAIDs. This could result in the accumulation of digoxin and subsequent digoxin toxicity. Caution is warranted when NSAIDs are used in patients on digoxin therapy.

Anticoagulants

NSAIDs may cause displacement of anticoagulants such as warfarin from protein-binding sites, resulting in increased effective serum anticoagulant concentration and subsequent over-anticoagulation. This is of particular concern with the potential for development of gastrointestinal bleeding from NSAID-associated gastropathy, which could be complicated in the presence of anticoagulation. In addition, antiplatelet effects that many traditional NSAIDs exhibit may enhance the risk of bleeding when added to anticoagulants.

Lithium

NSAIDs can cause decreased renal clearance of lithium and thereby increase serum lithium levels in patients taking this drug, potentially increasing the risk for lithium toxicity.

Oral Hypoglycemics

Hyper- or hypoglycemia may result when NSAIDs are used in combination with oral hypoglycemic agents. Careful monitoring of blood glucose levels is warranted when diabetics taking these drugs are prescribed concurrent NSAID therapy.

Immunosuppressants

The clearance of methotrexate may be decreased in the presence of NSAIDs, increasing the potential for methotrexate toxicity. Likewise, there may be increased potential for cyclosporine nephrotoxicity when combined with NSAIDs. Caution is warranted when these agents are given simultaneously, as each agent may produce renal toxicity, which can be compounded when they are coadministered.

CONCLUSION

NSAIDs are effective in the management of painful conditions such as osteoarthritis and rheumatoid arthritis and may significantly improve the quality of life of patients suffering from these disease entities. As these conditions commonly afflict the elderly, NSAIDs may be widely used in this population. It is important for clinicians employing these drugs in the treatment of the elderly to keep in mind the potential for serious adverse effects that may be associated with these drugs. These adverse effects may include effects on the gastrointestinal system, the kidneys, the central nervous system, and platelet aggregation. Also, hypertension and congestive heart failure may occur when NSAIDs are administered to patients taking antihypertensives or diuretics. Other potential drug interactions of concern may occur with anticoagulants, oral hypoglycemics, lithium, digoxin and immunosuppressants. An appreciation for the potential adverse effects as well as the benefits of NSAIDs is necessary when these drugs are used in the elderly population.

BIBLIOGRAPHY

Bell GM, Schnitzer TJ. COX-2 inhibitors and other nonsteroidal anti-inflammatory drugs in the treatment of pain in the elderly. *Clinics Ger Med* 2001; 17: 489-502.

Buffum M, Buffum JC. Nonsteroidal anti-inflammatory drugs in the elderly. *Pain Manage Nur* 2000; 1: 40-50.

Heerdinnk ER, Leufkens HG, Herings RM, et al. NSAIDS Associated with increased risk of congestive heart failure in elderly patients taking diuretics. *Arch Intern Med* 1998; 158: 1108-1112.

Johnson AG. NSAIDS and blood pressure: Clinical importance for older patients. *Drugs Aging* 1998; 12: 17-27.

Mamdani M, Rochon PA, Juurlink DN, et al. Observational study of upper gastrointestinal hemorrhage in elderly patients given selective cyclo-oxygenase-2 inhibitors or conventional non-steroidal anti-inflammatory drugs. *BMJ* 2002; 325: 624-627.

Mulkerrin EC, Clark BA, Epstein FH. Increased salt retention and hypertension from non-steroidal agents in the elderly. *Q J Med* 1997; 90: 411-415.

Page J, Henry D. Consumption of NSAIDS and the development of congestive heart failure in elderly patients: An underrecognized public health problem. *Arch Intern Med* 2000; 160: 777-784.

Pertusi RM, Godwin KS, House JK, et al. Gastropathy induced by nonsteroidal anti-inflammatory drugs: Prescribing patterns among geriatric practitioners. *JAOA* 1999; 99: 305-310.

Phillips AC, Polisson RP, Simon LS. NSAIDS and the elderly: Toxicity and economic implications. *Drugs Aging* 1997; 10: 119-130.

Pilotto A, Franceschi M, Leandro G, et al. NSAID and aspirin use by the elderly in general practice. *Drugs Aging* 2003; 20: 701-710.

Roberts LJ, Morrow JD. Analgesic-antipyretic and anti-inflammatory agents and drugs employed in the treatment of gout. In: Hardman JG, Limbird LE, eds. *Goodman and Gilman's The Pharmacological Basis of Therapeutics,* 10th ed. (pp. 695-720). New York: McGraw-Hill, 2001.

Samad T, Abdi S. A basic science aspect of COX-2 inhibitors. In: Smith HS, ed. *Drugs for Pain.* Philadelphia: Hanley & Belfus, 2003.

Simon LS. Nonsteroidal anti-inflammatory drugs and cyclooxygenase-2 selective inhibitors. In: Smith HS. *Drugs for Pain.* Philadelphia: Hanley & Belfus, 2003.

Smith HS. Nonsteroidal anti-inflammatory drugs: Bedside. In: Smith HS, ed. *Drugs for Pain.* Philadelphia: Hanley & Belfus, 2003.

Whelton A, Fort JG, Puma JA, et al. Cyclooxygenase-2-specific inhibitors and cardiorenal function: A randomized, controlled trial of celecoxib and rofecoxib in older hypertensive osteoarthritis patients. *Am J Therap* 2001; 8: 85-95.

Chapter 7

Tramadol for the Elderly

Pradeep Chopra
Howard Smith

Tramadol is considered a centrally acting synthetic analgesic. The chemical name is (±) *cis*-2-[(dimethylamino)methyl]-1-(3-methoxyphenyl)cyclohexanol hydrochloride (see Figure 7.1). It has a molecular weight of 299.8 and a pKa of 9.41. It is white, bitter, odorless, crystalline powder that is readily soluble in water and ethanol.

CLINICAL PHARMACOLOGY

Tramadol's mechanism of action is not fully understood. Its analgesic action appears to be derived from two complementary mechanisms: as a weak mu-opioid agonist and inhibition of reuptake of norepinephrine and serotonin.

Tramadol may have dual opioid activities. The mono-*O*-desmethyl tramadol metabolite is known as M1. The M1 metabolite has a higher affinity for the mu-receptor and is six times more potent than the parent compound. Studies have shown that only 30 percent of the analgesic effect of tramadol could be reversed with naloxone, an opioid antagonist.

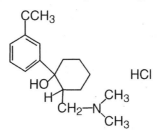

FIGURE 7.1. Tramadol molecule.

Clinical Management of the Elderly Patient in Pain
© 2006 by The Haworth Press, Inc. All rights reserved.
doi:10.1300/5356_07

The analgesic effects of tramadol can also be explained by its inhibition of norepinephrine reuptake. Presynaptic membranes have a norepinephrine transporter (NET) function. NETs regulate neurotransmission by taking up norepinephrine into the synaptic cleft.

Tramadol is almost completely absorbed easily when taken orally. The mean peak plasma concentration for tramadol after oral administration is 2 hours and that of its active metabolite is 3 hours. Only 20 percent of the drug is bound to plasma proteins. Its bioavailability is 75 percent. Tramadol's half-life is 6.3 hours and that of its M1 metabolite is 7.4 hours. It is metabolized by the CYP2D6 and the CYP3A4 pathways. The parent drug and its metabolite are both conjugated.

Tramadol and its metabolites are excreted through the urine. Up to 60 percent of the administered drug is excreted in the urine as its metabolites.

ADVERSE EVENTS

The most common adverse effects were dizziness, nausea, and constipation. These effects were especially seen in patients over 65 years of age. Most adverse effects are dose related and transient. Other adverse effects that maybe seen in the elderly are headaches, lethargy, pruritus, and dry mouth. Although tramadol may lower the seizure threshold, it is unlikely to cause seizures by itself. It enhances the risk of seizures in patients prone to seizures or epilepsy. It may increase the risk of seizures when taken concomitantly with the following classes of drugs:

- Tricyclic compounds: antidepressants, cyclobenzaprine (Flexeril), promethazine.
- Selective serotonin reuptake inhibitor (SSRI): it may precipitate serotonin syndrome.
- Opioids.
- Monoamine oxidase inhibitor (MAOI): tramadol should be avoided with MAOIs.
- Neuroleptics.
- Other drugs that reduce seizure threshold.

Overdose

There is potentially a risk of respiratory depression and seizures with overdosage. Other risks are coma, cardiac arrest, and death. Naloxone may reverse some of the respiratory depression but not all. Unfortunately, naloxone may increase the risk of seizures. Seizures following an overdose of tramadol have been treated with barbiturates and benzodiazepines in animal models.

Drug Abuse and Dependence

Tramadol can induce a mu-opioid-type psychological and physical dependence (withdrawal symptoms may occur if it is discontinued abruptly) even in the absence of a history of substance abuse. Dependence and abuse, including drug-seeking behavior and taking illicit actions to obtain the drug, are not strictly limited to those patients with prior history of opioid dependence. Tramadol is not recommended for patients with a prior history of drug abuse and drug dependence. Rates of tramadol abuse or dependence have been less than 0.75 per 100,000 patients.

The true incidence of psychological dependence or addiction to tramadol without a history of drug or alcohol abuse, although unknown, is low, and physicians should not be concerned about writing appropriate prescriptions for patients as long as they continue to monitor their patients using sound medical doctrines and judgment.

DOSAGE AND ADMINISTRATION

Tramadol is indicated for treating moderate to severe chronic pain. If the dose is titrated slowly, its adverse effects may be minimized. A suggested titration guide is as follows. Start tramadol at 25 mg/day in the morning. Increase by 25 mg every three days as separate doses of 25 mg every six hours (100 mg/day). If a further increase in the dose is needed, then it is increased by 50 mg every three days. Tramadol maybe administered at 50-100 mg as needed for pain relief every four to six hours. The total dose must not exceed 400 mg per day.

Tramadol and Acetaminophen Combinations

Using a combination of analgesic drugs provides an enhanced analgesic effect, reduced dose-dependent side effects, greater compliance, and reduced side effects. A tramadol and acetaminophen combination (Ultracet) is now available in the United States. It consists of tramadol 37.5 mg and acetaminophen 325 mg. Both tramadol and acetaminophen have complementary pharmacokinetics with respect to absorption, distribution, and elimination half-life. Each compound is metabolized along separate pathways.

A randomized, double-blind, placebo-controlled, multicenter study performed in 308 patients with osteoarthritis showed that two tablets of tramadol/acetaminophen combination resulted in higher pain relief scores than treatment with placebo as early as two hours after the drug was administered.

The combination of tramadol and acetaminophen has 25 percent less tramadol per tablet and provides significantly greater pain relief than the same dose of tramadol, with a faster onset of action (17 versus 31 minutes) and a longer duration of action (5 hours 26 minutes versus 2 hours 4 minutes) compared with tramadol alone.

GUIDELINES FOR USING TRAMADOL IN THE ELDERLY

- Start tramadol at a lower dose and titrate up slowly, given their decreased hepatic, cardiac, and renal function.
- In patients over 75 years, do not exceed a maximum dose of 300 mg per day.
- Nausea and constipation are more common in patients over 75 years of age than in patients under 65 years.
- Tramadol should be used with caution when taken in conjunction with tranquilizers, hypnotics, and opioids.
- It appears that tramadol exhibits less respiratory depression in the elderly than opioids.
- Postmarketing surveillance of tramadol has revealed rare reports of digoxin toxicity.
- The dose may need to be doubled in patients taking concurrent carbamazepine.
- In patients with impaired renal function with a creatinine clearance less than 30 ml/min, the dosing interval should be increased to 12 hours with a maximum of 200 mg per day.
- The dose of tramadol should be decreased to 100 mg per day in patients with significant hepatic insufficiency.
- The combination of tramadol 37.5 mg and acetaminophen 325 mg is safe, moderately effective, and well tolerated by the elderly.

BIBLIOGRAPHY

Adler L. A comparison of once-daily tramadol with normal release tramadol in the treatment of osteoarthritis. *J Rheumatol* 2002; 29(10):2196-2199.

American College of Rheumatology Subcommittee on Osteoarthritis. Recommendations for the medical management of osteoarthritis of the hip and knee. *Arthritis Rheum* 2000; 43:1905-1915.

Bamigbade TA, Lanford RM. The clinical use of tramadol hydrochloride . *Pain Rev* 1998; 5:155-182.

Collart L, Luthy C, Dayer P. Multimodal analgesic effect of tramadol. *Clin Pharmacol Ther* 1993; 53:223.

Collart L, Luthy C, Dayer P. Partial inhibition of tramadol antinociceptive effect by naloxone in man. *Br J Clin Pharmacol* 1993; 35:73P.

Dayer P, Collart L, Desmenles J. The pharmacology of tramadol. *Drugs* 1994; 47 (suppl):3-7.

Desmules JA, Piguet V, Collart L, Dayer P. Contribution of monoaminergic modulation to the analgesic effect of tramadol. *Br J Clin Pharmacol* 1996; 41:7-12.

Lewis KS, Han NH. Tramadol: a new centrally acting analgesic. *Am J Health Syst Pharm* 1997; 54:643-652.

Medve R, Wang J, Karim R. Tramadol and acetaminophen tablets for dental pain. *Anesth Prog.* 2001; 48:79-81.

Mullican WS, Lacy JR, for the TRAMAP-ANAG-006 Study Group. Tramadol/ acetaminophen combination tablets and codeine/acetaminophen combination capsules for the management of chronic pain: A comparative trial. *Clin Ther* 2001; 23:1429-1445.

Radbruch L, Grond S, Lehmann KA. A risk-benefit assessment of tramadol in the management of pain. *Drug Saf* 1996; 15:8–29.

Raffa RB. Exploring the mechanisms of action of tramadol. *J Am Pharm Assoc.* 1999; 39:276.

Raffa BB, Friderichs E, Reimann W, Shank RP, Codd EE, Vaught JL. Opioid and nonopioid components independently contribute to the mechanism of action of tramadol, an "atypical" opioid analgesic. *J Pharmacol Exp Ther* 1992; 260: 276-285.

Rauck RL, Ruoff GE, McMillen JI. Comparison of tramadol and acetaminophen with codeine for long-term pain management in elderly patients. *Curr Ther Res* 1994; 55:417-431.

Stubhaug A, Grimstad J, Breivik H. Lack of analgesic effect of 50 and 100 mg oral tramadol after orthopaedic surgery: a randomized, double-blind, placebo and standard active drug comparison. *Pain* 1995; 62:111-118.

Chapter 8

Topical Local Anesthetics

Charles Argoff

The treatment of chronic pain in the elderly remains a significant public health issue. Special issues regarding the treatment of pain in the elderly include the appropriate assessment of pain given the possibility of cognitive impairment in this population as well as the special pharmacotherapeutic issues in the elderly, including age-affected changes in pharmacokinetics, the need to utilize polypharmacy as the result of other medical conditions that are being treated, and the resulting drug-drug interactions and systemic toxicities that can occur with such treatment. Topical analgesics may be ideal for the elderly since they exert their analgesic benefit locally and without significant systemic absorption. The mechanism of the topical analgesic is unique to the specific medication. Key differences between topical and transdermal analgesics need to be appreciated by the health care provider. Topical analgesics have been studied in an increasing number of painful clinical conditions—the results of many of these studies are summarized here. Recent data suggest that at least one topical analgesic, although applied peripherally, may result in central nervous system alterations of pain activity.

The undertreatment of chronic pain in general remains a significant public health issue worldwide. Specifically, however, the treatment of pain in the elderly is associated with special issues. Despite the fact that guidelines have been established for the treatment of chronic pain in the geriatric population, suboptimal assessment and treatment of chronic pain in the elderly persist (Cohen-Mansfield and Upson, 2002). The purpose of this chapter is to review the use of topical analgesics in the elderly.

Age alone does not by itself result in impairment of pain sensitivity. Age alone does not alter the quality of the pain experience for an individual. Pain in fact may be a source of or an exacerbating factor for depression in the elderly. Not being able to perform basic activities of daily living as the result of pain can be quite disturbing and depressing to the older person with

Clinical Management of the Elderly Patient in Pain
© 2006 by The Haworth Press, Inc. All rights reserved.
doi:10.1300/5356_08

chronic pain. Cognitive impairment in the geriatric population may limit the full assessment of pain as well as impair the ability to fully treat the condition due to suboptimal assessment of treatment response. The elderly are likely to experience other diseases or illnesses that may contribute to their frailty or at the very least complicate the treatment approaches. As a result, it is especially important when prescribing analgesic medications for elderly patients that specific attention is paid to choosing regimens that are least likely to cause organ toxicities and are least likely to have significant drug-drug interactions or have other adverse effects such as somnolence or ataxia that would severely limit their use and safety in this population (Harkins and Scott, 1996). Especially for these reasons, the use of a topical analgesic for elderly persons may be an ideal approach if otherwise appropriate to the management of their chronic pain.

The pharmacological treatment of pain in the elderly has some unique aspects. No single dose of analgesic is appropriate for all patients with chronic pain. The elderly may metabolize certain medicines more slowly than a younger patient would. It is therefore recommended in general that starting treatment with a low dose of medication and slowly titrating the dose upward is the best way to achieve satisfactory analgesia and minimize side effects. In general, using the least invasive route of administration and reassessing the patient's complaint of pain frequently is advisable. The scope of this chapter does not permit a detailed description of each of the currently available pharmacological therapies for elderly, patients with chronic pain. Instead the chapter focuses on the use of topical analgesics for this population of patients with chronic pain. Although nonopioid analgesics including acetaminophen and nonsteroidal anti-inflammatory drugs (NSAIDs) are commonly used to treat pain in the elderly, and while the tolerability of acetaminophen may make it appear to be an ideal choice as an analgesic for mild to moderate pain, long-term use of acetaminophen must be very carefully monitored because of the potential for hepatic and renal toxicities—even with use of the recommended doses. In particular in managing pain in the elderly, care must be taken to maximize benefit and minimize harm; therefore, ideal analgesic choices might include topical therapies.

One can be certain that there is no such thing as pain without a brain. Certain painful conditions such as central poststroke pain exist in which the mechanisms of the pain lie almost entirely within the brain; however, for most commonly encountered pain syndromes, including postherpetic neuralgia (PHN), chronic low back pain, and osteoarthritis, the pain results from peripheral as well as likely central nervous system mechanisms as well. The term *topical analgesic* has been used to describe analgesics that are applied locally and directly to painful areas and whose site of action is local to the site of application. The term *topical analgesic* not only suggests the primary site of action of an analgesic but also helps to distinguish it from a transdermal analgesic. Unlike a topical analgesic, whose primary site of action lies directly underneath where the analgesic is applied, a transdermal analgesic requires a systemic concentration to be effective (Argoff, 2000).

Assuming acceptable efficacy, a review of the subject has suggested that topical analgesics have several potential advantages compared with systemic analgesic agents (Argoff, 2002). Although not formally studied, this may be especially relevant in the management of pain in the elderly. In contrast to systemic analgesics (oral or transdermal) such as opiates, anticonvulsants, alpha-adrenergic receptor agonists, and antidepressants, topical peripheral analgesics, whatever their mechanism of action, direct their primary pharmacological action at peripheral as opposed to central sites of pain generation. These agents work through topical rather than systemic means, therefore reducing the risk of adverse effects compared to a systemic analgesic. Localized reactions such as rash are experienced by some but not most patients (Galer, 2001). Using a topical analgesic will not result in a significant systemic concentration of the analgesic; however, use of oral analgesics or a transdermal preparation such as the fentanyl patch will certainly result in such. Regular use of a topical analgesic is possible therefore without the development of significant systemic accumulation. To emphasize this point, consider the following. In a study designed to evaluate the tolerability and safety of continuous 24 hour per day use of four lidocaine 5 percent patches, measured plasma lidocaine levels remained below those associated with interference with cardiac activity, and no significant systemic side effects were experienced. Regardless of whether the subject changed the patches every 24 hours or every 12 hours, the same acceptable safety and tolerability was demonstrated in this study (Gammaitoni and Alvarez, 2002). Consider also that in a separate study, patients with chronic low back pain were treated safely with four lidocaine 5 percent patches every 24 hours for extended periods of time (Argoff, 2002). In each study, extended use of the lidocaine 5 percent patch did not lead to any significant dermal sensitivity reactions (Gammaitoni and Alvarez, 2002; Argoff et al., 2002). Keep in mind that different topical analgesics have potential adverse reactions that are unique to the topical agent itself. For example, while it is true that the use of topical capsaicin, is not associated with notable systemic adverse effects, upon application of topical capsaicin, severe burning of the skin at the site of application has been reported to occur in almost 80 percent of treated patients. This particular side effect is not associated with any life-threatening outcome and its incidence may decrease with repeated use; however, the frequent occurrence of this side effect of capsaicin severely impairs patient compliance and as a result, may hinder the patient's ability to benefit from it (Watson, 1994).

The risk of any drug-drug interaction is minimized with a topical analgesic compared with a systemic analgesic. This characteristic of topical analgesics may be of key importance for a patient who is using other medications for other medical conditions, for example, the elderly patient who is using a variety of medications for various chronic medical conditions such as diabetes or hypertension, who is also in need of treatment for a chronic pain problem, perhaps PHN or osteoarthritis (Gammaitoni and Davis, 2002).

Dose titration of a topical analgesic is less likely to be required (almost never) compared to a systemic agent and therefore again makes it an easier-to-use analgesic type. It is certainly true that not all of the topical analgesics currently in use are commercially available products and for years many health care providers have utilized compounding pharmacies to obtain such agents through other means. For example, in a survey of members of the American Society of Regional Anesthesia and Pain Medicine, 27 percent of survey responders indicated that they prescribed such an agent. Perhaps even more important and quite interesting was that 47 percent of the responders indicated that they felt that their patients benefited from the agent prescribed (Ness, Jones, and Smith, 2002).

Great interest abounds in the development of potential compounds as topical analgesics. In a review of this topic, the following agents have been considered as new potential topical analgesics: NSAIDs, opioids, capsaicin, local anesthetics, antidepressants, glutamate receptor antagonists, alpha-adrenergic receptor agonists, adenosine, cannabinoids, cholinergic receptor agonists, GABA-agonists, prostanoids, bradykinin, ATP, biogenic amines, and nerve growth factor (Sawynok, 2003). Although some of these agents, including capsaicin as well as local anesthetics, are currently commercially available in a topical form, newer formulations of these agents are also being considered as well.

The mechanism of action of a topical analgesic is unique to the specific agent considered. For example, capsaicin-containing topical analgesics appear to achieve their action through their interaction with the VR1 receptor on C and A-delta fibers (Robbins, 2000). This in turn leads to the release of substance P as well as calcitonin gene-related peptide. Repeated topical application of capsaicin is generally required over several weeks to achieve a therapeutic response. The depletion of substance P in C fibers has been hypothesized to lead to diminished peripheral as well as central excitability with resulting less pain through reduced afferent input (Watson, 1994; Robbins, 2000). Data from human nerve biopsies and animal studies have suggested that application of capsaicin may lead to the degeneration of nerve fibers in the skin underlying the application site. A neurodegenerative effect of capsaicin has been hypothesized to be one of its mechanisms of analgesia (Rowbotham, 1994).

For NSAIDs, inhibition of prostaglandin synthesis and the resulting reduction of inflammation have been considered important mechanisms of action; however, because the extent of anti-inflammatory effect does not always correlate with the degree of analgesia experienced, other potential mechanisms of action are under investigation (Cashman, 1996). An animal study has demonstrated that a topical cannabinoid may enhance the antinociceptive effects of topical morphine (Yesilyurt et al., 2003).

The mechanism of the analgesic action of local anesthetic agents appears to be related to the ability of these agents to reduce the activity of peripheral sodium channels within sensory afferents, with a subsequent reduction of ectopic, paroxysmal discharges and ultimate reduction of pain transmission. The use of local anesthetic agents as analgesic agents in fact has been associated with reduced expression of mRNA for certain types of sodium channels (Argoff, 2000; Galer, 2001). A separate mechanism of action of the lidocaine 5 percent patch may be that the patch itself may serve to protect allodynic skin (Argoff, 2000).

Different local anesthetic preparations may have different effects with respect to the manner in which they create analgesia. For example, the lidocaine 5 percent patch produces its analgesic effect without causing anesthesia; in contrast, the use of EMLA cream (eutectic mixture of local anesthetics, 2.5 percent lidocaine and 2.5 percent prilocaine) may result in a clearly demonstrable anesthetic effect on the skin where it is applied. Consequently, these differences might lead one to use EMLA cream for acute painful states such as venipuncture, lumbar puncture, intramuscular injections, and circumcision (Galer, 2001). However, at least two professional sports teams in the United States have reported successfully using the lidocaine 5 percent patch for the management of acute sports injury-related pain. Antidepressants are commonly used for the management of various chronic pain states and the need to cautiously use certain of these, especially the tricyclics, in the elderly is well documented; however, their potential as topical analgesics is just being investigated. Of the many mechanisms of action that these agents are known to have, their effect as sodium channel antagonists is being widely investigated (Sawynok, Esser, and Reid, 2001; Gerner et al., 2003). Zonalon (doxepin hydrochloride) is indicated for use by the Food and Drug Administration (FDA) for the treatment of eczema-associated pruritus. It has been used by some clinicians in an off-label manner as a topical analgesic (*Physicians Desk Reference*, 2002). Even though no FDA-approved product currently exists for agents containing, among others, opioids, glutamate receptor antagonists, and cannabinoids, there is great interest among basic and clinical scientists in their potential as topical analgesics.

THE USE OF TOPICAL LOCAL ANALGESICS FOR NEUROPATHIC PAIN

Topical analgesics have been used in the treatment of neuropathic pain. The lidocaine 5 percent patch is FDA approved for the treatment of PHN. Two important clinical trials involving patients with PHN are associated with this approval, and each demonstrated that the lidocaine 5 percent patch is well-tolerated and efficacious in the management of this condition (Rowbotham et al., 1996; Galer et al., 1999). Subsequent to the studies that led to its FDA approval, a more recent study has demonstrated that use of the patch by patients with PHN is frequently associated with improvement in quality of life measures. Using several measures of the Brief Pain Inventory, a validated assessment tool, this study of 332 patients with PHN using up to three lidocaine 5 percent patches for 12 hours each day measured certain quality of life indicators over a four-week period. Some 66 percent of the study population (n = 204) reported reduced pain intensity with repeated patch application by the seventh day of the study. Even for those patients who did not experience this effect by the seventh day of patch use, 43 percent (n = 46) of the remaining patients experienced reduced pain intensity by the 14th day of patch use. By the end of the study, approximately 70 percent of patients experienced notable improvement (Katz, Davis, and Dworkin, 2001). The reader should be reminded that PHN most commonly occurs in the elderly.

The lidocaine 5 percent patch has also been studied in neuropathic pain states other than PHN. A randomized, double-blind, placebo-controlled study completed in Europe examining the efficacy of the lidocaine 5 percent patch in the treatment of focal neuropathic pain syndromes such as PHN, mononeuropathies, intercostal neuralgia, and ilioinguinal neuralgia, has suggested that as an add-on treatment, the patch was effective in reducing ongoing pain as well as allodynia, not only during the first eight hours of use but also over a period of seven days (Meier et al., 2003).

In an earlier, open-label study of 16 patients with severe, refractory, chronic neuropathic pain (postthoracotomy pain, complex regional pain syndrome, postamputation pain, painful diabetic neuropathy, meralgia paresthetica, postmastectomy pain, neuroma pain), 81 percent of the patients experienced notable pain relief from the patch without any significant side effects (Devers and Galer, 2000). Of particular interest, again because of the special issues associated with the pharmacotherapeutic management of pain in the elderly, the term *refractory* was used to describe patients who had experienced, prior to the study, inadequate pain relief and/or intolerable side effects with the use of opiate analgesics, anticonvulsants, antidepressants, or antiarrythmic agents. Thus, in this small study, a topical analgesic was able to help patients where systemic analgesics, with their increased risk of systemic side effects, were not.

Several other studies involving patients with painful diabetic neuropathy and treatment with the lidocaine 5 percent patch have been completed. Interim analysis of an ongoing study of the use of the lidocaine 5 percent patch in patients with painful diabetic neuropathy with or without allodynia has yielded evidence of efficacy as well. In this study, patients with painful diabetic neuropathy were able to use up to four lidocaine 5 percent patches for 18 consecutive hours of each 24-hour day. Three main groups of patients have been studied in this trial. The first group consists of patients with either type 1 or type 2 diabetes mellitus who have a painful distal symmetric diabetic polyneuropathy but who do not experience significant allodynia. The second group of patients also have either type 1 or type 2 diabetes mellitus and a painful distal symmetric diabetic polyneuropathy. In contrast to patients in group 1, patients in group 2 experience allodynia. The third group is comprised of patients with an idiopathic painful sensory neuropathy (Endo Pharmaceuticals, n.d.). Initial data regarding groups 1 and 2 were presented at the most recent World Congress on Pain. Pain relief was reported in the majority of patients studied regardless of whether or not allodynia was present (Hart-Gouleau et al., 2002). Treatment benefit in this study was also measured by favorable changes noted in the Neuropathic Pain Scale (NPS) with treatment (Galer and Jensen, 1997).

In a separate multicenter open-label study involving patients with painful diabetic neuropathy with or without allodynia, patients experienced less pain and improvements in quality of life with use of up to four lidocaine 5 percent patches for up to 18 hours each day (Barbano et al., 2004).

In a multicenter, randomized, vehicle-controlled study of 150 patients with PHN who were treated with either active or placebo lidocaine 5 percent patches (up to three lidocaine 5 percent or vehicle patches for 12 hours each day), the lidocaine 5 percent patch but not the vehicle patch was found to reduce the intensity of all common neuropathic pain qualities. This study is of particular interest because the results suggested that this topical analgesic was able to diminish qualities of neuropathic pain (dull, deep, sharp, and burning) that had previously been assumed not to be related to peripheral but to central mechanisms, suggesting that in fact, peripheral mechanisms may indeed play a role in the development of these neuropathic pain qualities (Galer et al., 2002). Of course, this is only a hypothesis at this point.

EMLA cream is not FDA approved for any neuropathic pain disorder; however, several studies of the use of EMLA cream in the treatment of PHN have been completed with mixed results. In a randomized, controlled study of PHN patients, EMLA was found to have efficacy similar to a placebo (Lycka et al., 1996). Two uncontrolled studies have suggested that EMLA cream may be an effective agent for patients with PHN (Attal et al., 1999; Litman, Vitkun, and Poppers, 1996). EMLA may from a practical viewpoint be difficult to use at this point as the result of manufacturing issues. Besides the local anesthetics, other topical therapies are being explored as well. In an open-label study assessing the potential benefit of a combination of topical amitriptyline and ketamine for neuropathic pain, encouraging results have been reported (Lynch, Clark, and Sawynok, 2003). Two other noncontrolled studies, one in patients with PHN and one in patients with complex regional pain syndrome type 1, have suggested that topical ketamine may be an effective topical analgesic; however, in neither study were serum levels of ketamine measured, making it therefore uncertain if the effect was truly topical or systemic (Quan, Wellish, and Gilden, 2003). This has particular relevance in the treatment of pain in the elderly, since systemic ketamine is far more likely to result in adverse effects than topical ketamine (Quan, Wellish, and Gilden, 2003). One report has suggested that the topical application of geranium oil may be helpful in providing temporary relief from PHN (Greenway et al., 2003).

There has been great interest in using capsaicin for the pain associated with a number of neuropathic pain disorders such as diabetic neuropathy, PHN, and postmastectomy pain. Currently available strengths of capsaicin (.025 percent and .075 percent) have unfortunately been associated with poor patient compliance due to side effects and short duration of benefit (Rains and Bryson, 1995). Significant analgesia was experienced by patients with painful HIV neuropathy receiving a 7.5 percent topical capsaicin cream; however, concurrent anesthesia was required for these patients so that they could tolerate the medication (Robbins et al., 1998). A study comparing the analgesic effect of a topical preparation containing either 3.3 percent doxepin alone or 3.3 percent doxepin combined with 0.075 percent capsaicin to placebo in patients with various different chronic neuropathic pain problems demonstrated that each treatment resulted in equal degrees of analgesia and each was superior to placebo (McCleane, 2000).

THE USE OF TARGETED PERIPHERAL ANALGESICS FOR PAIN ASSOCIATED WITH SOFT TISSUE INJURY AND OSTEOARTHRITIS

Soft tissue injuries are common for all populations, including the elderly. Although systemic analgesics are often considered in this setting, one must again consider the risk of systemic side effects with any of these agents. Injection therapies are certainly commonly utilized; however, the regular use of corticosteroids or even local anesthetics through injections can weaken tendons and ligaments, causing scarring and other adverse effects. Assuming acceptable efficacy, a topical analgesic may offer a more favorable side effect profile than a systemic agent and therefore may be a more ideal choice of analgesic.

Different topical NSAIDs have been evaluated in soft tissue pain. In one open-label study of patients described as experiencing soft tissue pain, topical flurbiprofen was found to reduce pain more effectively than oral diclofenac, with fewer reported side effects (Marten, 1997). In both an open-label study and subsequently a separate multicenter, randomized, controlled two-week study of acute sports injury, a diclofenac patch was found to be an effective analgesic. In the open-label study, the magnitude of pain relief was 60 percent (Galer et al., 2000; Jenoure, 1993). A double-blind randomized controlled study assessing the safety and efficacy of a topical diclofenac patch in patients with osteoarthritis of the knee has demonstrated that this patch may be effective for this condition (Bruhlmann and Michel, 2003). A controlled study of the use of topical ibuprofen cream in the management of acute ankle sprains found this cream to be superior to placebo (Campbell and Dunn, 1994). The treatment of acute soft tissue pain with a topical analgesic was also assessed in a controlled study of the use of ketoprofen gel, which was found to be more effective than placebo (Airaksinen, Venalainen, and Pietilainen, 1993).

A randomized study of the efficacy of a different, proprietary topical formulation of ibuprofen 5 percent gel in patients with soft tissue injuries has been completed. Patients received either the ibuprofen 5 percent gel ($n = 40$) or placebo gel ($n = 41$) for a maximum of seven days. Pain as well as limitations of physical activity caused by the pain were assessed daily using visual analogue and other scales. There was a significant difference ($p < .001$) in pain reduction as well as for improvement in physical activities for those patients who received the active gel compared to placebo recipients (Machen and Whitefield, 2002). In a second similar study performed by the same group of investigators, a greater number of patients was studied (50) with similar outcomes seen (Whitefield, O'Kane, and Anderson, 2002).

The efficacy and safety of the use of another NSAID, eltenac, in the treatment of osteoarthritis of the knee has been confirmed as well in a randomized controlled study involving 237 patients (Ottillinger et al., 2001). In a comparative study of different topical NSAIDs, topical eltenac gel was compared to oral diclofenac and placebo in patients with osteoarthritis of the knee. Both the oral and topical therapies were found to be superior to placebo with respect to analgesia, yet the incidence of gastrointestinal side effects was much lower in the group treated with topical eltenac gel compared to those treated with oral diclofenac (Sandelin et al., 1997). This finding is especially important for elderly patients who require treatment.

The results of three additional studies have demonstrated that topical diclofenac may be effective in reducing the pain associated with various types of degenerative joint disease (Dreiser and Tisne-Camus, 1993; Galeazzi and Marcolongo, 1993; Gallachia and Marcolongo, 1993). Controlled clinical trials evaluating the use of the lidocaine 5 percent patch in the treatment of osteoarthritis are planned, but to date only open-label (but positive) reports of its use in osteoarthritis are available. Thirty patients with pain in the temporomandibular joint were treated with either 0.025 percent capsaicin cream or vehicle cream in a randomized controlled study. No benefit of the capsaicin cream over placebo was demonstrated (Winocur et al., 2000). A topical cream containing glucosamine sulfate, chondroitin sulfate, and camphor for osteoarthritis of the knee showed a significant reduction of pain in the treatment group after eight weeks compared to the placebo group in a randomized controlled study (Cohen et al., 2003).

Two anecdotal reports of the use of the lidocaine 5 percent patch for an acute sports injury are noted. One should not underestimate the activities of today's elderly. A professional basketball player with a ligamentous strain in his left fifth toe was advised by the team doctor to use the lidocaine 5 percent patch for pain relief with a good outcome, and a professional football player with chronic acromioclavicular joint pain due to a dislocation was anecdotally reported to experience pain relief with use of the lidocaine 5 percent patch as well.

THE USE OF TARGETED PERIPHERAL ANALGESICS FOR THE TREATMENT OF LOW BACK PAIN AND MYOFASCIAL PAIN

Very few studies of topical analgesics in chronic low back or myofascial pain have been published. A double-blind study comparing topical capsaicin to placebo in 154 patients with chronic low back pain demonstrated that 60.8 percent of capsaicin-treated patients compared with 42.1 percent of placebo patients experienced 30 percent pain relief after three weeks of treatment ($p < 0.02$). Fifteen of the capsaicin-treated and nine of the placebo-treated patients experienced adverse effects, none of which were believed to be harmful (Keitel et al., 2001).

In another study involving the lidocaine 5 percent patch, 120 patients with acute (<6 weeks), subacute (<3 months), short-term chronic (3-12 months), or long-term chronic (>12 months) low back pain were tested at eight sites in the United States. During the six-week study period, participants applied four lidocaine 5 percent patches to areas of maximal low back pain every 24 hours. Initial analysis of the first two weeks of data was presented at the 10th World Congress on Pain. Initial evaluation suggests that the majority of patients experience moderate or greater degree of pain relief. Significant positive changes in quality of life indicators on this scale have been noted as well as demonstrated by the use of the NPS in this study. A more complete analysis of these data as well as additional studies are expected soon (Argoff et al., 2002; Argoff, 2004). Although this was a nonrandomized study, it was in fact a multicenter study. Sixteen patients with chronic myofascial pain were treated with the lidocaine 5 percent patch and the results of this open-label study presented at the 2003 Scientific Meeting of the American Pain Society. Utilizing the Brief Pain Inventory as one of the outcome measures, after 28 days of treatment, statistically significant improvements were noted for average pain, general activity level, ability to walk, ability to work, relationships, sleep, and overall enjoyment of life in approximately 50 percent of the patients studied (Lipman, Dalpiaz, and London, 2002).

OTHER USES OF TOPICAL ANALGESICS

The use of a topical analgesic of various types including topical opiates may help to reduce pain associated with pressure ulcers or dressing changes (Briggs and Nelson, 2003; Flock, 2003; Zeppetella and Ribeiro, 2003). Controlled studies have already been completed showing the benefit of EMLA cream in the reduction of pain associated with venipuncture as well as for the pain associated with breast cancer surgery (Galer, 2001; Fassoulaki et al., 2000). According to several studies, ketamine or morphine may be used topically for mucositis-associated pain following chemotherapy or radiation therapy in patients with head and neck carcinomas (Cerchietti et al., 2002; Slatkin and Rhiner, 2003). A report suggests that the analgesic effect of menthol, an ingredient common to many over-the-counter analgesic preparations, may be partially related to the activation of kappa-opioid receptors (Galeotti et al., 2002).

SUMMARY

Topical analgesics may provide significant pain relief in a variety of acute and chronic pain disorders with fewer side effects and in general better tolerability than that seen with analgesics administered orally, transdermally, parenterally, or via a spinal route. Although there is a need for additional controlled studies to further explore the role of topical analgesics in the management of acute and chronic pain, initial studies do suggest great potential for this category of analgesic therapy. For the elderly, in whom the need for polypharmacy is quite common and who require pharmacological approaches that minimize organ toxicities, cognitive dysfunction, and drug-drug interactions, development of existing as well as new topical analgesics may be especially relevant and helpful.

REFERENCES

AGS Panel on Persisten Pain in Older Persons. Guidelines for Treatment of Pain in the Elderly. *J Am Geriatric Soc* 2002; 50(6 Suppl):S205-S224.

Airaksinen O, Venalainen J, Pietilainen T. Ketoprofen 2.5% gel versus placebo gel in the treatment of acute soft tissue injuries. *Int J Clin Pharmacol Ther Toxicol* 1993; 31:561-563.

Argoff C. Chronic pain studies of lidocaine 5% using the neuropathic pain scale. *Current Med Res Opinion* 2004; 52: 29-31.

Argoff CE. New analgesics for neuropathic pain: The lidocaine patch. *Clin J Pain* 2000; Suppl 16(2):S62-S65.

Argoff CE. Targeted topical peripheral analgesics in the management of pain. *Curr Pain Headache Rep* 2002; 7:34-38.

Argoff C, Nicholson B, Moskowitz M, et al. Effectiveness of lidocaine patch 5% (Lidoderm®) in the treatment of low back pain. Presented at the 10th World Congress on Pain, August 17-22, 2002, San Diego, CA.

Attal N, Brasseur L, Chauvin M, et al. Effects of single and repeated applications of a eutectic mixture of local anesthetics (EMLA®) cream on spontaneous and evoked pain in post-herpetic neuralgia. *Pain* 1999; 81:203-209.

Barbano RL, Herrmann DN, Hart-Gouleau S, et al. Effectiveness, tolerability and impact on quality of life of lidocaine patch 5% in diabetic polyneuropathy. Accepted for publication in *Archives of Neurology* 2004; 63: 879-885.

Briggs M, Nelson EA. Topical agents or dressings for pain in venous leg ulcers. *Cochrane Database Syst Rev* 2003; (1):CD001177.

Bruhlmann P, Michel BA. Topical diclofenac patch in patients with knee osteoarthritis: A randomized, double-blind, controlled clinical trial. *Clin Exp Rheumatol* 2003; 21:193-198.

Campbell J, Dunn T. Evaluation of topical ibuprofen cream in the treatment of acute ankle sprains. *J Accident Emerg Med* 1994; 11:178-182.

Cashman JN. The mechanism of action of NSAIDs in analgesia. *Drugs* 1996; 52(suppl 5):13-23.

Cerchietti LC, Navigante AH, Bonomi MR, et al. Effect of topical morphine for mucositis-associated pain following concomitant chemoradiotherapy for head and neck carcinoma. *Cancer* 2002; 15; 95:2230-2236.

Cohen M, Wolfe R, Mai T, et al. A randomized, double blind placebo-controlled trial of a topical crème containing glucosamine sulfate, chondroitin sulfate and camphor for osteoarthritis of the knee. *J Rheumatol* 2003; 30:523-528.

Cohen-Mansfield J and Upson S. *J Am Geriatric Soc* 2002; 50: 1039.

Devers A, Galer BS. Topical lidocaine patch relieves a variety of neuropathic pain conditions: An open-label study. *Clin J Pain* 2000; 16:205-208.

Dreiser RL, Tisne-Camus M. DHEP plasters as a topical treatment of knee osteo-arthritis: A double-blind placebo-controlled study. *Drugs Exp Clin Res* 1993; 19:107-115.

Endo Pharmaceuticals, Inc. Data on file. Chadds Ford, PA. n.d.

Fassoulaki A, Sarantopoulos C, Melemeni A, et al. EMLA reduces acute and chronic pain after breast surgery for cancer. *Reg Anesth Pain Med* 2000; 25:35-355.

Flock P. Pilot study to determine the effectiveness of diamorphine gel to control pressure ulcer pain. *J Pain Symptom Manage* 2003; 25(6):547-554.

Galeazzi M, Marcolongo R. A placebo-controlled study of the efficacy and toler-ability of a nonsteroidal anti-inflammatory drug, DHEP plaster in inflammatory peri- and extra-articular rheumatological diseases. *Drugs Exp Clin Res* 1993; 19: 107-115.

Galeotti N, DeCesare Mannelli L, Mazzanti G, et al. Menthol: A Natural analgesic compound. *Neurosci Lett* 2002; 12(322):145-148.

Galer BS. Topical medications. In: Loeser JD, ed. *Bonica's Management of Pain.* Philadelphia: Lippincott-Williams & Wilkins, 2001:1736-1741.

Galer BS, Jensen MP. Development and preliminary validation of a pain measure specific to neuropathic pain: The Neuropathic Pain Scale. *Neurology* 1997; 48:332-338.

Galer BS, Jensen MP, Ma T, et al. The lidocaine patch 5% effectively treats all neuropathic pain qualities: Results of a randomized, double-blind, vehicle-controlled, 3-week efficacy study with use of the Neuropathic Pain Scale. *Clin J Pain* 2002; 18:297-301.

Galer BS, Rowbotham MC, Perander J, et al. Topical diclofenac patch significantly reduces pain associated with minor sports injuries: Results of a randomized, double-blind, placebo-controlled, multicenter study. *J Pain Symptom Manage* 2000; 19:287-294.

Galer BS, Rowbotham MC, Perander J, et al. Topical lidocaine patch relieves post-herpetic neuralgia more effectively than vehicle patch: Results of an enriched enrollment study. *Pain* 1999; 80:533-538.

Gallachia G, Marcolongo R. Pharmacokinetics of diclofenac hydroxyethylpyr-rolidine (DHEP) plasters in patients with monolateral knee joint effusion. *Drugs Exp Clin Res* 1993; 19:95-97.

Gammaitoni AR, Alvarez NA. 24-hour application of the lidocaine patch 5% for 3 consecutive days is safe and well tolerated in healthy adult men and women. Abstract PO6.20. Presented at the 54th Annual American Academy of Neurology Meeting, April 13-20, 2002, Denver, CO.

Gammaitoni AR, Davis MW. Pharmacokinetics and tolerability of lidocaine 5% patch with extended dosing. *Ann Pharmacother* 2002; 36:236-240.

Gerner P, Kao G, Srinivasa V, et al. Topical amitriptyline in health volunteers. *Reg Anesth Pain Med* 2003; 28:289-293.

Greenway FL, Frome BM, Engels TM, et al. Temporary relief of postherpetic neuralgia pain with topical geranium oil. *Am J Med* 2003; 115:586-587.

Harkins SW, Scott RB. Pain and prebyalgos. In: Birren J, ed. *Encyclopedia of gerontology*. San Diego: Academic Press, 1996:247-260.

Hart-Gouleau S, Gammaitoni A, Galer BS, et al. Open-label study of the effectiveness and safety of the lidocaine patch 5% (Lidoderm®) in patients with painful diabetic neuropathy. Presented at the 10th World Congress on Pain, August 17-22, 2002, San Diego, CA.

Jenoure P, Segesser B, Luhti U, et al. A trial with diclofenac HEP plaster as topical treatment in minor sports injuries. *Drugs Exp Clin Res* 1993; 19:125-131.

Katz NP, Davis MW, Dworkin RH. Topical lidocaine patch produces a significant improvement in mean pain scores and pain relief in treated PHN patients: results of a multicenter open-label trial. *J Pain* 2001; 2:9-18.

Keitel W, Frerick H, Kuhn U, et al. Capsicum pain plaster in chronic non-specific low back pain. *Arzneimittelforschung* 2001; 51:896-903.

Lipman AG, Dalpiaz AS, London SP. Topical lidocaine patch therapy for myofascial pain. Abstract 782. Presented at the Annual Scientific Meeting of the American Pain Society, March 14-17, 2002, Baltimore, MD.

Litman SJ, Vitkun SA, Poppers PJ. Use of EMLA® cream in the treatment of postherpetic neuralgia. *J Clin Anesth* 1996; 8:54-57.

Lycka BA, Watson CP, Nevin K, et al. EMLA® cream for the treatment of pain caused by post-herpetic neuralgia: a double-blind, placebo-controlled study. In: *Proceedings of the annual meeting of the American Pain Society*. Glenview, IL: American Pain Society, 1996:A111 (abstract).

Lynch ME, Clark AJ, Sawynok J. A pilot study examining topical amitriptyline, ketamine, and a combination of both in the treatment of neuropathic pain. *Clin J Pain* 2003; 19:323-328.

Machen J, Whitefield M. Efficacy of a proprietary ibuprofen gel in soft tissue injuries: A randomized, double-blind, placebo-controlled study. *Intl J Clin Prac* 2002; 56:102-106.

Marten M. Efficacy and tolerability of a topical NSAID patch (local action transcutaneous flurbiprofen) and oral diclofenac in the treatment of soft-tissue rheumatism. *Clin Rheumatol* 1997; 16:25-31.

McCleane G. Topical application of doxepin hydrochloride, capsaicin and a combination of both produces analgesia in chronic neuropathic pain: A randomized, double-blind, placebo-controlled study. *Br J Clin Pharmacol* 2000; 49:574-579.

Meier T, Wasner G, Faust M, et al. Efficacy of lidocaine patch 5% in the treatment of focal peripheral neuropathic pain syndromes: A randomized, double- blind, placebo-controlled study. *Pain* 2003; 106:151-158.

Ness TJ, Jones L, Smith H. Use of compounded topical analgesics: Results of an Internet survey. *Reg Anesth Pain Med* 2002; 27:309-312.

Ottillinger B, Gomor B, Michel BA, et al. Efficacy and safety of eltenac gel in the treatment of knee osteoarthritis. *Osteoarthritis Cartilage* 2001; 9:273-280.

Physicians Desk Reference, 55th ed. Montvale, NJ: Medical Economics Company, 2002.

Quan D, Wellish M, Gilden DH. Topical ketamine treatment of postherpetic neuralgia. *Neurology* 2003; 22; 60:1391-1392.

Rains C, Bryson HM. Topical capsaicin: A review of its pharmacological properties and therapeutic potential in post-herpetic neuralgia, diabetic neuropathy, and osteoarthritis. *Drugs Aging* 1995; 7:317-328.

Robbins W. Clinical applications of capsaicinoids. *Clin J Pain* 2000; Suppl 16: S86-S89.

Robbins WR, Staats PS, Levine J, et al. Treatment of intractable pain with topical large-dose capsaicin: Preliminary report. *Anesth Analg* 1998; 86:579-583.

Rowbotham MC. Topical analgesic agents. In Fields HL, Liebeskind JC, eds. *Pharmacologic Approaches to the Treatment of Chronic Pain: New Concepts and Critical Issues.* Seattle: IASP Press, 1994:211-227.

Rowbotham MC, Davies PS, Verkempinck, et al. Lidocaine patch: double-blind controlled study of a new treatment method for post-herpetic neuralgia. *Pain* 1996; 65:39-44.

Sandelin J, Harilainen A, Crone H, et al. Local NSAID gel (eltenac) in the treatment of osteoarthritis of the knee: A double-blind study comparing eltenac with oral diclofenac and placebo gel. *Scand J Rheumatol* 1997; 26:287-292.

Sawynok J. Topical and peripherally acting analgesics. *Pharmacol Rev* 2003; 55:1-20.

Sawynok J, Esser MJ, Reid AR. Antidepressants as analgesics: an overview of central and peripheral mechanisms of action. *J Psychiatry Neurosci* 2001; 26:21-29.

Slatkin NE, Rhiner M. Topical ketamine in the treatment of mucositis pain. *Pain Med* 2003; 4:298-303.

Watson CPN. Topical capsaicin as an adjuvant analgesic. *J Pain Symptom Manage* 1994; 9:425-433.

Whitefield M, O'Kane CJ, Anderson S. Comparative efficacy of a proprietary topical ibuprofen gel and oral ibuprofen in acute soft tissue injuries: A randomized, double-blind study. *J Clin Pharm Ther* 2002; 27:409-417.

Winocur E, Gavish A, Halachmi M, et al. Topical application of capsaicin for the treatment of localized pain in the temporomandibular joint area. *J Orofac Pain* 2000; 14:31-36.

Yesilyurt O, Dogrul A, Gul H, et al. Topical cannabinoid enhances topical morphine antinociception. *Pain* 2003; 105:303-308.

Zeppetella G, Ribeiro PJ. Analgesic efficacy of morphine applied topically to painful ulcers. *J Pain Symptom Manage* 2003; 25:555-558.

Chapter 9

Nitrates, Capsaicin, and Tricyclic Antidepressants

Gary McCleane

NITRATES

It would be hard to argue against the contention that the nonsteroidal anti-inflammatory drugs (NSAIDs) are effective at reducing both inflammation and pain. Yet with their well-defined side-effect profiles that include gastric erosion and ulceration, salt and water retention, and interaction with a broad range of other drugs, their use in elderly patients should be the result of considered thought rather than a reflex action. So often they are given for a localized pain condition, such as monoarticular arthritis where a local effect is desired but where a risk of systemic side effects exists. Although much medical skepticism has existed in relation to the topical, local use of NSAIDs, their level of use by patients suggests that this skepticism is not shared by patients. Indeed, consideration of available controlled studies does confirm an analgesic effect of topically applied NSAIDs, but also that significant systemic absorption can follow topical use and hence even topical application is not without the risk of systemic side effects. Given the fact that patient acceptability is high, then the topical use of an NSAID in those who lack contraindications is not unreasonable. However, the sequential use of a number of different topical NSAIDs in the face of failure of one is illogical and unlikely to be associated with therapeutic success. This leaves us with the dilemma of what to do if a patient has localized pain or inflammation and the use of a topical NSAID is unsuccessful. It is suggested that a topical nitrate may be an alternative.

Mode of Action of Topical Nitrates

It is known that exogenous nitrates stimulate the release of nitric oxide (NO). This substance is known to be a potent mediator in a wide variety of

Clinical Management of the Elderly Patient in Pain
© 2006 by The Haworth Press, Inc. All rights reserved.
doi:10.1300/5356_09

different cellular systems such as the endothelium and both the central and peripheral nervous system. It is released from the endothelium and from neutrophils and macrophages, all known to be intimately involved in the inflammatory process. It appears that NO exerts its effect by stimulating increases in guanylate cyclase, thereby increasing the levels of 3'5'cyclic guanidine monophosphate (cGMP). Cholinergic drugs, such as acetylcholine, produce analgesia in a similar fashion by releasing NO and increasing NO at the nociceptor level.

In addition to this action, NO may activate adenosine triphosphate (ATP) sensitive potassium channels and activate peripheral antinociception. Endogenous NO levels may be increased if glutamate levels are raised. Glutamate is known to be an excitatory amino acid activating N-methyl-D-aspartate (NMDA) receptors, thereby initiating sensitization and protracting the pain process.

But of course, while these actions may produce analgesia, the most well-known consequence is vascular smooth muscle relaxation—hence the use of nitrates as vasodilators. Although this effect is extensively utilized in the management of patients with ischemic heart disease, it also produces the most troublesome side effect of the nitrates, headache. Currently, nitrates are presented in ointment formulations, transdermal patches, sprays, and oral and parenteral formulations. To date, work examining the analgesic effect has been predominantly carried out using the ointment and transdermal formulations. The issue of using a measured dose is more difficult when utilizing an ointment preparation. Furthermore, the transdermal patches are designed to administer a dose at one site, and there are currently no lower-dose patches that would allow use at more than one site.

Clinical Use of Topical Nitrates

There is a risk of some confusion when we talk about the effect of nitrates in particular clinical scenarios. All the currently available descriptions in the literature refer to the same substance but use differing names: it appears as glyceryl trinitrate (GTN), nitroglycerin, and even as nitroglycerine in one study. Since the majority of studies refer to glyceryl trinitrate, this nomenclature is used here.

Anal Fissure

The condition for which the greatest number of clinical studies have been done examining the effect of topical nitrates is the treatment of anal fissure. This painful condition is associated with spasm of the internal anal sphincter. Surgical management may involve internal anal sphincter-otomy or manual anal stretch. The need for a general or regional anesthetic for these procedures means that they require hospital admission and submit the sufferer to the risks of the anesthetic techniques mentioned. Particularly in older patients, anal fissures are more predominant in those with the chronic constipation associated with general debility. In no other individu-als would the prospect of an anesthetic be less attractive, and yet the pain as-sociated with an anal fissure may be of a level to require the use of strong opioids, which only exacerbate the precipitating constipation.

Many of the studies have suggested that the effect of the nitrate, almost always GTN, is that of a smooth muscle relaxant. However, since we know that GTN also has analgesic and anti-inflammatory properties, it may be that its beneficial effect is related to its analgesic action, or more likely a combination of its relaxant and analgesic effect. The normal concentration of GTN in the majority of these studies is 0.2 percent (as an ointment). The overriding impression is that the use of a topical nitrate can prevent the need for operative intervention.

Posthemorrhoidectomy Pain

Isolated reports suggest that GTN may reduce pain after surgical hemor-rhoidectomy. Not only may pain be reduced, but healing rates may also be improved, and consequently the duration of pain after the procedure may be less. Unfortunately, the results of some studies are of less value because of the small number of trial subjects.

It is interesting to speculate on the effect of topical nitrate on hemorrhoid pain prior to operative intervention. Although the nitrate may reduce sphinc-ter spasm and have some analgesic effect, this may well be negated by the vasodilatation and further engorgement of these already distended veins.

Vulval Pain

An isolated report suggests that 0.2 percent GTN ointment can signifi-cantly reduce vulvodynia.

Vertebral Collapse Fracture Pain and Pathological Fracture

Whether it be vertebral collapse fracture consequent to osteoporosis or as a result of secondary tumor infiltration, spinal pain is universal and per-sistent pain not uncommon. Such vertebral collapse fractures give rise to a number of types of pain. For example, they can give rise to localized pain over the vertebra concerned, impinge on exiting nerve roots and give neuropathic pain, or give rise to referred pain around the dermatome involved. The localized pain often seen over the fracture site is often amenable to use of a GTN patch. Similarly, any pathological fracture producing localized pain can be palliated with topical nitrate use allowing for transfer for operative intervention, radiotherapy, or more definitive treatment.

Thrombophlebitis, Varicose Veins, and Venous Cannulation

Intravenous infusion of a variety of solutions is associated with inflammation and pain at the infusion site. Even dilute glucose solutions may precipitate pain, while more irritant solutions may cause thrombosis in the vein itself. Not uncommonly, veins suitable for insertion of cannulas are at a premium, and therefore anything that can maintain the useful life of an infusion site may be useful. A 2 percent GTN ointment has been shown to fulfill this need, although the use of a GTN patch may be more practical and less messy.

Similarly, inflammation and pain are common after sclerotherapy for varicose veins. GTN reduces the pain, swelling, and redness after this procedure. It would be reasonable to suggest on the basis of studies that have generated these conclusions that GTN may have an effect on any vein- related pain, including thrombophlebitis, and the pain produced by deep venous thrombosis (ensuring, of course, that adequate treatment for that venous thrombosis has been instituted).

Quite apart from their analgesic and anti-inflammatory effects, topical nitrates also enlarge peripheral veins and make them potentially easier to cannulate.

Musculoskeletal Pain

With advancing age, the occurrence of minor aches and pains seems to increase. Degenerative changes restrict mobility and bring on pain that precludes further movement. If conventional analgesics are taken, their side effects may impede activity even while they have the desired effect of reducing pain. The concept of placing a topical preparation over the site that is causing pain on a particular day and have a degree of reassurance that it will reduce pain is appealing. Topical GTN has been shown to be effective at reducing the pain of osteoarthritis, supraspinatus tendonitis, and less well-defined musculoskeletal pain. In the studies examining osteoarthritis the 2 percent ointment was used, while the study examining supraspinatus tendonitis utilized a patch version. Unfortunately, one is restricted as to the number of locations where a GTN patch may be applied, as use at multiple sites will almost inevitably produce a nitrate headache, given the relatively large dose contained in currently available patch preparations.

Topical Nitrates to Enhance Systemic Analgesics

I have suggested that nitrates act by increasing NO levels and that, conversely, levels of NO can be increased by activation of glutamate and subsequently NMDA receptors and therefore have, at least, an influence on pain-processing mechanisms. So far I have concentrated on the local effects seen when nitrates are used in topical formulations. Yet it is clear that even topical administration can be associated with systemic effects, as evidenced by the occurrence of nitrate headaches. Indeed, nitrate patches are traditionally used to cause coronary vasodilation, and yet they are applied at a site some distance from the heart. If NO has a role in nociception, then topical administration may influence pain that is not localized. Several workers have examined this hypothesis and have shown that topical nitrates used in a patch version can augment the analgesic efficacy of oral morphine and even reduce requests for rescue analgesia in patients with cancer-related pain already taking oral morphine. In another study, topical nitrate was used in subjects receiving the short-acting opioid analgesic sufentanil given intrathecally as an analgesic after orthopedic surgery. It showed that topical nitrate in this situation had no analgesic effect when used alone. However, it significantly increased the duration of analgesia observed when sufentanil was given intrathecally as compared to sufentanil alone.

Although much work needs to be done, there is at least the suggestion that topically applied nitrate can augment the systemic effect of opioid analgesics. This also raises the question of whether this effect is replicated by oral and parenteral nitrates and other NO generators.

CAPSAICIN

The knowledge that capsaicin, an active constituent of the chili pepper, has pain-relieving properties is not new, with reports dating back to the mid-19th century of chili pepper extract being used to treat pain.

We know that the effect of capsaicin is dependent on the concentration of capsaicin actually used. In low concentrations it can reduce pain, while at higher concentrations it has a neurotoxic effect. Only with the availability of low-concentration preparations of capsaicin has its use become more widespread.

Mode of Action

Capsaicin is thought to achieve analgesia by a number of mechanisms. Immunohistochemical studies have shown that repeated application of capsaicin is associated with a decrease in epidermal nerve fibers. The concentration of these fibers returns to normal when treatment is discontinued. It is also known that substance P (SP) acts as a neurotransmitter in both peripheral nerves and in those neurons on the superficial lamina of the spinal cord expressing receptors for SP, the neurokinin 1 (NK1) expressing neurons. By binding to vanilloid receptors, capsaicin reversibly depletes nerve endings of SP, thereby interfering with the transmission of pain signals. Again, this depletion is reversible, so that on discontinuation of treatment, SP-mediated transmission returns toward normal. The nerve pathways involved are not responsible for touch, so that even with desensitization of a painful area, numbness or alteration in awareness of tactile sensation does not occur.

Capsaicin may also reduce the flare or vasodilation that occurs around the site of an injury. Whether this is a consistent effect is not yet elucidated, as the study suggesting this response, while performed on human subjects, utilized a 1 percent capsaicin preparation that is much more concentrated than that currently used in the clinical environment.

The principle of treatment with capsaicin, therefore, is the repeated application of a low concentration of capsaicin to interfere with SP-mediated neurotransmission and to reduce the concentration of epidermal nerve fibers in a reversible manner, with the aim of reducing pain but not sensation.

Capsaicin Formulations

If we accept that a low concentration of capsaicin is required to achieve analgesia, the issue of which exact concentration will give optimal pain relief arises. In Europe, two concentrations of capsaicin in cream form are marketed. A 0.075 percent concentration is marketed for the treatment of the pain associated with postherpetic neuralgia and painful diabetic neuropathy, while a 0.025 percent concentration is licensed for the treatment of pain with osteoarthritis. However, no human clinical studies have verified that these concentrations are optimal for these pain conditions. In reality we do not have firm evidence about which concentration is best in terms of quality of pain relief in individual pain conditions or in minimizing the time to effect.

A number of practitioners still use capsicum ointment rather than capsaicin cream. Although it is often cheaper, it tends to be messy and, given the color and consistency of the ointment, staining of clothes around the site of application can occur.

Clinical Use

The evidence confirming an analgesic effect from the repeated application of capsaicin is extensive. Numerous controlled studies evidence its effect in a broad range of neuropathic and musculoskeletal pain conditions. It
can reduce the pain associated with postherpetic neuralgia, painful diabetic
neuropathy, and neuropathic pain associated with surgery, cancer, and
Guillain-Barre syndrome. In terms of musculoskeletal pain, osteoarthritis
and chronic neck pain may respond. Isolated reports suggest that it may be
effective for rheumatoid arthritis pain as well, but in this circumstance it is
possibly better reserved for patients whose disease is in remission, rather
than those with active joint inflammation.

Perhaps the major problem associated with the use of capsaicin is the occurrence of a burning, tingling discomfort associated with application of the
cream. This usually, but not always, lessens with time, but may be severe
enough to discourage the patient from continuing its use. In the case of
neuropathic pain where allodynia (that is, pain arising from a normally nonpainful stimulus) may be a feature, the act of cream application may induce
allodynic pain and again discourage use. That said, capsaicin is more effective at reducing allodynia than any of the other component symptoms or
signs of neuropathic pain (burning, numbness, paresthesia/dysesthesia,
shooting or lancinating pain) so encouragement to continue use in those
with allodynia may be worthwhile.

Some patients find the burning discomfort associated with application to
be helpful, and in these circumstances it may act as a counterirritant. However, to achieve its reversible effect on nerve function, several weeks of application three to four times daily may be necessary before maximal benefit
is apparent. If relief is then apparent, then it may be maintained by less frequent application. Given this, if patients have discomfort at a number of different sites, then they can concentrate on one, hopefully achieve a degree of
relief, maintain that relief with less frequent application, and move on to
target other sites.

When it comes to quality of relief, capsaicin is similar to many of the
other preparations we use. Many patients get no relief, some get partial relief, and only a few get complete relief. Therefore, when explaining this
treatment, we need to put the chances of success with its use in context.

Recent work suggests that the use of a high-dose capsaicin patch that is
applied once for a period of one hour can give pain relief that is of better

quality than conventional capsaicin and of significantly longer duration. Indeed, weeks to months of relief may be achieved, and while the area of application of the patch requires pretreatment with a local anesthetic preparation prior to capsaicin use, the inconvenience of this is more than offset by the quality and duration of relief produced.

Recent evidence suggests that capsaicin may have uses beyond its analgesic actions. Reports suggest that 0.05 percent capsaicin linament may reduce hemodialysis-related pruritus, while 0.006 percent capsaicin ointment can significantly palliate idiopathic pruritus ani.

Side Effects

As mentioned, discomfort of application is the most frequently encountered side effect. This seems to be worse if the cream is applied to a moist area, so mucous membranes and the periocular regions should be avoided. Hands should be washed after application to avoid transferring the capsaicin to moist areas elsewhere (although this tends to be a mistake patients make only once). In those with impaired mobility or sight, assistance in applying the capsaicin may be required, and the caution suggested when patients apply the cream obviously extends to third parties applying the cream on a patient's behalf.

Bouts of sneezing occasionally occur after application. If the cream is applied in larger quantities, then instead of being absorbed it dries on the skin, and the dust from this dried capsaicin is an intense nasal stimulant.

Clearly, careful explanation to the patient is required before treatment with capsaicin is instituted. One often tries to give simple explanations to clarify the aim and rationale of treatment. Some care is needed, however. Many elderly patients have rather conservative tastes when it comes to their diet. If one explains that the use of a chili pepper cream is suggested for their ailment, then they expect a substance that they associate with highly spiced food, with intense tastes and smells that would often not be to their liking. Reassurance that the preparation is odorless, white, and nonstaining may remove some of these understandable worries.

Strategies to Reduce the Discomfort of Application of Capsaicin

Reassurance that the discomfort lessens with time is important and usually, but not always, true. Bathing and drying before application is wiser than the converse. Restricting application to a defined site also helps. Several pharmacological options exist.

Pretreatment with local anesthetic cream may augment the analgesia from the capsaicin and reduce the discomfort of application. However, the need to apply a local anesthetic cream four times daily as well as capsaicin four times daily complicates use.

We have seen already that nitrates have an analgesic effect. It also appears that GTN can reduce the burning discomfort of application and the thermal allodynia induced by application of capsaicin and can also augment its analgesic effect (see Table 9.1).

TRICYCLIC ANTIDEPRESSANTS

It is universally accepted that the tricyclic antidepressants (TCAs) can have an analgesic effect that is independent of their antidepressant actions. This analgesia may be obtained by virtue of a number of actions of TCAs. They can augment the descending serotinergic and noradrenergic inhibitory pathways, effect opioid and NMDA receptors, and have a sodium-channel and adenosine receptor-blocking effect. Sodium channels and adenosine receptors, while represented in the central nervous system, also have peripheral representation and on the basis of these actions it could be proposed that TCAs may have an analgesic effect when applied topically.

TABLE 9.1. Analgesic efficacy and tolerability of capsaicin, glyceryl trinitrate, and a combination of both in osteoarthritis pain ($n = 200$).

	Mean change in joint pain score	Mean application discomfort
Placebo	−0.05	0.90
1.33 percent GTN	−0.39	2.41
0.025 percent capsaicin	−0.48	1.03
1.33 percent GTN & 0.025 percent capsaicin	−0.81	1.69

Source: Reprinted from *Eur J Pain,* 4, McCleane, G.J., The analgesic efficacy of topical capsaicin is enhanced by glyceryl trinitrate in painful osteoarthritis: a randomized, double blind, placebo controlled study, 355-360. Copyright (2000), with permission from European Federation of Chapters of the International Association for the Study of Pain.
Note: This table is a comparison of mean baseline scores and those after four weeks treatment (0 to 10 cm linear visual analog score).

Although we could speculate on the potential peripheral effects of TCAs, use in this fashion is only of value if it confers an advantage. The oral use of TCAs, while associated with analgesia on some occasions, is also associated with side effects such as urinary retention, somnolence, weight gain, blurring of vision, and tachycardia. We know that the analgesic effect of TCAs is dose related, but then so is the incidence of side effects. If we were able to harness some of the analgesic effects of the TCAs and yet avoid the unacceptable systemic side effects, this would be a significant advantage.

A number of placebo-controlled clinical studies have verified an analgesic effect of the topical application of a TCA preparation, 5 percent doxepin cream. When applied repeatedly in subjects with neuropathic pain, a proportion derive analgesia in the virtual absence of side effects. This analgesia without side effects (unless excessive quantities of the cream are applied when systemic side effects are more commonly seen) suggests that the effect is local rather than systemic. Clearly such use is only of value where the area over which the neuropathic pain is felt is relatively small. It would be appropriate, therefore, for the likes of postherpetic neuralgia, painful diabetic neuralgia, supraorbital neuralgia, complex regional pain syndrome, and the like. The time to effect is measured in weeks, and therefore a trial for one month is suggested. The clinical studies suggest that topical doxepin can reduce the perception of pain rather than the component symptoms and signs. In other words, pain may be reduced while paresthesia/dysesthesia, shooting/lancing pain, allodynia, and burning pain are unaltered.

Another clinical problem is oral mucous membrane pain, seen, for example, in subjects who have received chemotherapy. Oral rinse with doxepin has been shown to significantly palliate this symptom, again with few notable side effects.

One other interesting use of topical doxepin is in the management of the urinary frequency and dysuria associated with intermittent self-catheterization of the urethra. In those with bladder dysfunction, self-catheterization is undertaken to empty the bladder to prevent urinary stasis. The trauma of catheterization can induce urethral and trigonal sensitivity, which manifests itself as urinary frequency and dysuria. Application of a small quantity of doxepin cream to the catheter tip can reduce these unpleasant symptoms.

The contention would be, therefore, that in the elderly patient with neuropathic pain experienced over a relatively small area, a trial of topical TCA would be considerably safer than the use of an oral TCA. Of course an oral TCA could still be tried if the topical version fails, as systemic administration is associated with additional potential effects on the pain pathways, but then, of course, the potential for additional side effects exists.

TABLE 9.2. Suggested formulations and uses of topical nitrates, capsaicin, and TCAs.

Drug	Formulation	Concentration/ dose	Time to effect	Clinical uses
Glyceryl trinitrate	Ointment	0.2%	Hours	Anal fissure
	Ointment	2%	Hours	Osteoarthritis
	Patch	5mg/24 hours		Tendonitis
				Thrombophlebitis
				Post-op pain
				Vertebral-collapse pain
				Pathological fracture
Capsaicin	Cream	0.025% and 0.075%	2-4 weeks	Neuropathic pain
				Osteoarthritis
				Pruritus ani
				Pruritus
Doxepin	Cream	5%	2-4 weeks	Neuropathic pain
				Urethral and trigonal irritation
				Oral mucous membrane pain

CONCLUSION

In general, agents that have a topical mode of administration and peripheral mode of action tend to be complicated by a lower incidence of adverse effects when compared to oral agents with styemic effects. Therefore, consideration should be given to their use before these oral agents are utilized. The lower incidence of side effects is, however, dependent on the correct use of these agents, being mindful of the concentration of agent used and their time to effect (Table 9.2).

BIBLIOGRAPHY

Altman RD, Aven A, Holmburg CE, Pfeifer LM, Sack M, Young GT. Capsaicin cream 0.025 percent as monotherapy for osteoarthritis: A double-blind study. *Sem Arth Rheum* 1994; 23(S): 25-33.

Andrew M, Barker D, Laing R. The use of glyceryl trinitrate ointment with EMLA cream for cannulation in children undergoing routine surgery. *Anaesth Intensive Care* 2002; 30: 321-325.

Bacher H, Mischinger H-J, Werkgartner G, Cerwenka H, El-Shabrawi A, Pfeifer J, Schweiger W. Local nitroglycerin for treatment of anal fissures: An alternative to lateral sphincterotomy? *Dis Colon Rectum* 1997; 40: 840-845.

Banerjee AK. Treating anal fissure. *BMJ* 1997; 314: 1637-1638.

Bernstein JE, Korman NJ, Bickers DR, Dahl MV, Millikan LE. Topical capsaicin treatment of chronic postherpetic neuralgia. *J Am Acad Dermatol* 1989; 21: 265-270.

Berrazueta JR, Fleitas M, Salas E, Amado JA, Poveda JJ, Ochoteco A, Sanchez de Vega MJ, Ruiz de Celis G. Local transdermal glyceryl trinitrate has an anti-inflammatory action on thrombophlebitis induced by sclerosis of leg varicose veins. *Angiology* 1994; 45: 347-351.

Berrazueta JR, Losada A, Poveda J, Ochoteco A, Riestra A, Salas E, Amado JA. Successful treatment of shoulder pain syndrome due to supraspinatus tendonitis with transdermal nitroglycerin. A double blind study. *Pain* 1996; 66: 63-67.

Berrazueta JR, Poveda JJ, Ochoteco JA, Amado JA, Puebla F, Salas E, Sarabia M. The anti-inflammatory and analgesic action of transdermal glyceryl trinitrate in the treatment of infusion related thrombophlebitis. *Postgrad Med J* 1993; 69: 37-40.

Capsaicin Study Group. Effect of treatment with capsaicin on daily activities of patients with painful diabetic neuropathy. *Diabetes Care* 1992; 15: 159-165.

Capsaicin Study Group. Treatment of painful diabetic neuropathy with topical capsaicin. *Arch Intern Med* 1991; 151: 2225-2229.

Carpenter SE, Lynn B. Vascular and sensory responses of human skin to mild injury after topical treatment with capsaicin. *Br J Pharmacol* 1981; 73: 755-758.

Chad DA, Aronin N, Lundstrom R, McKeon P, Ross D, Molitch M, Schipper HM, Stall G, Dyess E, Tarsy D. Does capsaicin relieve the pain of diabetic neuropathy? *Pain* 1990; 42: 387-388.

Deal CL. The use of topical capsaicin in managing arthritis pain: A clinician's perspective. *Sem Arth Rheum* 1994; 6(S): 48-52.

Deal CL, Schnitzer TJ, Seibold JR, Stevens RM, Levy MD, Albert D, Renold F. Treatment of arthritis with topical capsaicin: A double-blind trial. *Clin Therapeutics* 1991; 13: 383-395.

Devulder JE. Could nitric oxide be an important mediator in opioid tolerance and morphine side effects? *J Clin Anaesth* 2002; 14: 81-82.

Duarte ID, Lorenzetti BB, Ferreira SH. Acetylcholine induces peripheral analgesia by the release of nitric oxide. In: Moncada S, Higgs A (Eds.), *Nitric oxide from L-arginine. A bioregulatory system.* Amsterdam: Elsevier, 1990; 165-170.

Ellis N, Loprinzi CL, Kugler J, Hatfield AK, Miser A, Sloan JA, Wender DB, Rowland KM, Molina R, Cascino TL, et al. Phase III placebo-controlled trial of capsaicin cream in the management of surgical neuropathic pain in cancer patients. *J Clin Oncol* 1997; 15: 2974-2980.

Elton C, Sen P, Montgomery AC. Initial study to assess the effects of topical glyceryl trinitrate on pain after haemorrhoidectomy. *Int J Surg Inves* 2001; 2: 353-357.

Epstein JB, Marcoe JH. Topical application of capsaicin for treatment of oral neuropathic pain and trigeminal neuralgia. *Oral Surg Oral Med Oral Pathol* 1994; 77: 135-140.

Epstein JB, Truelove EL, Oien H, Allison C, Le ND, Epstein MS. Oral topical doxepin rinse: Analgesic effect in patients with oral mucosal pain due to cancer or cancer therapy. *Oral Oncol* 2001; 37: 632-637.

Esser MJ, Chase T, Allen GV, Sawynok J. Chronic administration of amitriptyline and caffeine in a rat model of neuropathic pain: Multiple interactions. *Eur J Pharmacol* 2001; 430: 211-218.

Esser MJ, Sawynok J. Acute amitriptyline in a rat model of neuropathic pain: Differential symptom and route effects. *Pain* 1999; 80: 643-653.

Esser MJ, Sawynok J. Caffeine blockade of the thermal antihyperalgesic effect of acute amitriptyline in a rat model of neuropathic pain. *Eur J Pharmacol* 2000; 399: 131-139.

Feelisch M, Noack EA. Correlation between nitric oxide formation during degradation of organic nitrates and activation of guanylate cyclase. *Eur J Pharmacol* 1987; 139: 19-30.

Fitzgerald M. Capsaicin and sensory neurones—A review. *Pain* 1983; 15: 109-130.

Haderer A, Gerner P, Kao G, Srinivasa V, Wang GK. Cutaneous analgesia after transdermal application of amitriptyline versus lidocaine in rats. *Anesth Analg* 2003; 96: 1707-1710.

Heughan CE, Allen GV, Chase TD, Sawynok J. Peripheral amitriptyline suppresses formalin-induced Fos expression in the rat spinal cord. *Anesth Analg* 2002; 94: 427-431.

Hwang Do Y, Yoon SG, Kim HS, Lee JK, Kim KY. Effect of 0.2 percent glyceryl trinitrate ointment on wound healing after hemorrhoidectomy: Results of a randomized, prospective, double-blind, placebo-controlled trial. *Dis Colon Rectum* 2003; 46: 950-954.

Kennedy ML, Sowter S, Nguyen H, Lubowski DZ. Glyceryl trinitrate ointment for the treatment of chronic anal fissure: Results of a placebo-controlled trial and long-term follow-up. *Dis Colon Rectum* 1999; 42: 1000-1006.

Knowles RG, Palacios M, Palmer RM, Moncada S. Formation of nitric oxide from L-arginine in the central nervous system: A transduction mechanism for stimulation of the soluble guanylate cyclase. *Proc Natl Acad Sci USA* 1989; 86: 5159-5162.

Kocher HM, Steward M, Leather AJ, Cullen PT. Randomized clinical trial assessing the side-effects of glyceryl trinitrate and diltiazem hydrochloride in the treatment of chronic anal fissure. *Br J Surg* 2002; 89: 413-417.

Lauretti GR, de Oliveira R, Reis MP, Mattos AL, Pereira NL. Transdermal nitroglycerine enhances spinal sufentanil postoperative analgesia following orthopaedic surgery. *Anesthesiology* 1999; 90: 734-739.

Lauretti GR, Lima IC, Reis MP, Prado WA, Pereira NL. Oral ketamine and transdermal nitroglycerin as analgesic adjuvant to oral morphine therapy for cancer pain management. *Anesthesiology* 1999; 90: 1528-1533.

Lauretti GR, Perez MV, Reis MP, Pereira NL. Double-blind evaluation of transdermal nitroglycerine as adjuvant to oral morphine for cancer pain management. *J Clin Anesth* 2002; 14: 83-86.

Loder PB, Kamm MA, Nichols RJ, Phillips RK. Reversible chemical sphincterotomy by local application of glyceryl trinitrate. *Br J Surg* 1994; 81: 1386-1389.

Low PA, Opfer-Gehrking TL, Dyck PJ, Litchy WJ, O'Brien PC. Double-blind, pla-cebo-controlled study of the application of capsaicin cream in chronic distal painful polyneuropathy. *Pain* 1995; 62: 163-168.

Lund JN, Armitage NC, Scholefield JH. Use of glyceryl trinitrate ointment in the treatment of anal fissure. *Br J Surg* 1996; 83: 776-777.

Lund JN, Scholefield JH. Glyceryl trinitrate is an effective treatment of anal fissure. *Dis Colon Rectum* 1997; 40: 468-470.

Lund JN, Scholefield JH. A randomised, prospective, double-blind, placebo-controlled trial of glyceryl trinitrate ointment in the treatment of anal fissure. *Lancet* 1997; 349: 11-13.

Lynch ME, Clark AJ, Sawynok J. A pilot study examining topical amitriptyline, ketamine, and a combination of both in the treatment of neuropathic pain. *Clin J Pain* 2003; 19: 323-328.

Lysy J, Sistiery-Ittah M, Israelit Y, Shmueli A, Strauss-Liviatan N, Mindrul V, Keret D, Goldin E. Topical capsaicin—A novel and effective treatment for idio-pathic intractable pruritis ani: A randomised, placebo controlled, crossover study. *Gut* 2003; 52: 1323-1326.

Mathias BJ, Dillingham TR, Zeigler DN, Chang AS, Belandres PV. Topical cap-saicin for chronic neck pain. *Am J Phys Med Rehab* 1995; 74: 39-44.

McCarthy GM, McCarty DJ. Effect of topical capsaicin in the therapy of painful osteoarthritis of the hands. *J Rheumatol* 1992; 19: 604-607.

McCleane GJ. The addition of piroxicam to topically applied glyceryl trinitrate en-hances its analgesic effect in musculoskeletal pain: A randomised, double-blind, placebo-controlled study. *Pain Clinic* 2000; 12: 113-116.

McCleane GJ. The analgesic efficacy of topical capsaicin is enhanced by glyceryl trinitrate in painful osteoarthritis: A randomized, double-blind, placebo con-trolled study. *Eur J Pain* 2000; 4: 355-360.

McCleane GJ. Topical application of doxepin hydrochloride can reduce the symp-toms of complex regional pain syndrome: A case report. *Injury* 2002; 33: 88-89.

McCleane GJ. Topical application of doxepin hydrochloride, capsaicin and a com-bination of both produces analgesia in chronic human neuropathic pain: A ran-domized, double-blind, placebo-controlled study. *Br J Clin Pharmacol* 2000; 49: 574-579.

McCleane GJ. Topical application of the tricyclic antidepressant doxepin can re-duce dysuria and frequency. *Scan J Urol Nephrol* 2003; 38:88-89.

McCleane GJ. Topical doxepin hydrochloride reduces neuropathic pain: a random-ized, double-blind, placebo controlled study. *Pain Clinic* 1999; 12: 47-50.

McCleane GJ, McLaughlin M. The addition of GTN to capsaicin cream reduces the discomfort associated with application of capsaicin alone: A volunteer study. *Pain* 1998; 78: 149-151.

Morgenlander JC, Hurwitz BJ, Massey EW. Capsaicin for the treatment of pain in Guillain-Barre syndrome. *Ann Neurol* 1990; 28: 199.

Nolano M, Simone DA, Wendelschafer-Crabb G, Johnson T, Hazen E, Kennedy WR. Topical capsaicin in humans: Parallel loss of epidermal nerve fibers and pain sensation. *Pain* 1999; 81: 135-145.

Oatway M, Reid A, Sawynok J. Peripheral antihyperalgesic and analgesic actions of ketamine and amitriptyline in a model of mild thermal injury in the rat. *Anesth Analg* 2003; 97: 168-173.

Okuda K, Sakurada C, Takahashi M, Yamada T, Sakurada T. Characterization of nociceptive responses and spinal releases of nitric oxide metabolites and glutamate evoked by different concentrations of formalin in rats. *Pain* 2001; 92: 107-115.

Perkins P, Morgan S, Closs SP, Olwen T. Topical capsaicin for saphenous neuralgia. *J Pain Symptom Manage* 2003; 26: 785-786.

Rains C, Bryson HM. Topical capsaicin: A review of its pharmacological properties and therapeutic potential in post-herpetic neuralgia, diabetic neuropathy and osteoarthritis. *Drugs Ageing* 1995; 7: 317-328.

Rashid MH, Inoue M, Kondo S, Kawashima T, Bakoshi S, Ueda H. Novel expression of vanilloid receptor 1 on capsaicin-insensitive fibers accounts for the analgesic effect of capsaicin cream in neuropathic pain. *J Pharmacol Exp Ther* 2003; 304: 940-948.

Sawynok J. Adenosine receptor activation and nociception. *Eur J Pharmacol* 1998; 317: 1-11.

Sawynok J. Antidepressants as analgesics: an overview of central and peripheral mechanisms of action. *J Psy Neurosci* 2001; 26: 21-29.

Sawynok J, Esser MJ, Reid AR. Peripheral antinociceptive actions of desipramine and fluoxetine in an inflammatory and neuropathic pain test in the rat. *Pain* 1999; 82: 149-158.

Sawynok J, Reid A. Peripheral interactions between dextromethorphan, ketamine and amitriptyline on formalin-evoked behaviours and paw edema in rats. *Pain* 2003; 102: 179-186.

Sawynok J, Reid AR, Esser M. Peripheral antinociceptive action of amitriptyline in the rat formalin test: Involvement of adenosine. *Pain* 1999; 80: 45-55.

Schnitzer T, Morton C, Coker S. Topical capsaicin therapy for osteoarthritis pain: Achieving a maintenance regimen. *Sem Arth Rheum* 1994; 23(S): 34-40.

Scholefield JH, Bock JU, Marla B, Richter HJ, Athanasiadis S, Prols Herold A. A dose finding study with 0.1%, 0.2%, and 0.4% glyceryl trinitrate ointment in patients with chronic anal fissures. *Gut* 2003; 52: 264-269.

Soares A, Leite R, Tatsuo M, Duarte I. Activation of ATP sensitive K channels: Mechanisms of peripheral antinociceptive action of the nitric oxide donor, sodium nitroprusside. *Eur J Pharmacol* 2000; 14: 67-71.

Su X, Gebhart GF. Effects of tricyclic antidepressants on mechanosensitive pelvic nerve afferent fibers innervating the rat colon. *Pain* 1998; 76: 105-114.

Sudoh Y, Cahoon EE, Gerner P, Wang GK. Tricyclic antidepressants as long-acting local anesthetics. *Pain* 2003; 103: 49-55.

Svendsen CB, Matzen P. Treatment of chronic anal fissure with topically applied nitroglycerin ointment: A systematic review of evidence-based results. *Ugeskr Laeger* 2002; 164: 3845-3849.

Tandan R, Lewis GA, Krusinski PB, Badger GB, Fries TJ. Topical capsaicin in painful diabetic neuropathy. *Diabetes Care* 1992; 15: 8-13.

Turnbull A. Tincture of capsicum as a remedy for chillblains and toothache. *Dublin Med Press* 1850; 95: 6.

Walker RA, McCleane GJ. The addition of gylceryltrinitrate to capsaicin cream reduces the thermal allodynia associated with the application of capsaicin alone in humans. *Neurosci Lett* 2002; 323: 78-80.

Walsh KE, Berman JR, Berman LA, Vierregger K. Safety and efficacy of topical nitroglycerin for treatment of vulvar pain in women with vulvodynia: A pilot study. *J Gend Specif Med* 2002; 5: 21-27.

Wasvary HJ, Hain J, Mosed-Vogel M, Bendick P, Barkel DC, Klein S. Randomized, prospective, double-blind, placebo-controlled trial of effect of nitroglycerin ointment on pain after hemorrhoidectomy. *Dis Colon Rectum* 2001; 44: 1069-1073.

Watson CP, Evans RJ, Watt VR. Post-herpetic neuralgia and topical capsaicin. *Pain* 1988; 33: 333-340.

Watson CP, Tyler KL, Bickers DR, Millikan LE, Smith S, Coleman E. A randomized vehicle-controlled trial of topical capsaicin in the treatment of postherpetic neuralgia. *Clin Ther* 1993; 15: 510-526.

Weisshaar E, Dunker N, Gollnick H. Topical capsaicin therapy in humans with hemodialysis-related pruritis. *Neurosci Lett* 2003; 345: 192-194.

Yosipovitch G, Maibach HI, Rowbotham MC. Effect of EMLA pre-treatment on capsaicin-induced burning and hyperalgesia. *Acta Derm Venereol* (Stockh) 1999; 79: 118-121.

Zuberi BF, Rajput MR, Abro H, Shaikh SA. A randomized trial of glyceryl trinitrate ointment and nitroglycerin patch in healing of anal fissures. *Int J Colorectal Dis* 2000; 15: 243-245.

Chapter 10

Topical Opioids

Gary McCleane

At first sight, topical application of an opioid would seem to be an alternative method of administration of a drug that may be of advantage when the oral route is unavailable, rather than a technique with any specific advantage. But there may be more to this use of opioids than is initially apparent. We know that opioids have a principal action on opioid receptors and that these have a significant spinal cord representation. However, it is now becoming evident that opioid receptors also exist in the periphery. Therefore, the topical application of an opioid at a site close to where pain arises may have the additional benefit of ensuring a high local concentration of opioid, which can interact with local peripheral opioid receptors as well as providing enough opioid to allow interaction with central opioid receptors.

PERIPHERAL OPIOID RECEPTORS

Hassan and colleagues (1993) studied peripheral opioid receptors using autoradiographic techniques in a rat model. When the sciatic nerve of these animals was ligated, opioid receptors were seen to accumulate proximally and distally to the ligature in a time-dependent manner, indicating bidirectional axonal transport. Some opioid receptors were observed in non-inflamed paw tissue in these animals. When inflammation was induced by the application of Freund's adjuvant in one paw, the density of opioid receptors on both sides of the ligature and on the inflamed paw increased massively. In the inflamed paw, opioid receptors were observed in the cutaneous nerves and in immune cells infiltrating the surrounding tissue.

Also studying the effect of inflammation on peripheral opioid receptors, Czlonkowski and colleagues (1993) investigated the effect of cytokines on opioid-mediated antinociception. When the rat paw was inflamed after the administration of Freund's adjuvant, local injection of tumor necrosis factor

Clinical Management of the Elderly Patient in Pain
© 2006 by The Haworth Press, Inc. All rights reserved.
doi:10.1300/5356_10

or interleukin into the paw caused a dose-dependent increase in paw pressure threshold—in other words, a reduction in pain.

This increase was prevented by local injection of the opioid antagonist naloxone and by the mu-opioid-specific antagonist CTOP (D-Phe-Cys-Tyr-D-Trp-Arg-Thr-Pen-Tr-NH$_2$). In animals pre-treated with cyclosporin to suppress the immune system, the antinociceptive effect of tumor necrosis factor was completely removed. These results suggest that cytokines release opioid peptides from immune cells of inflamed tissue, which act on opioid receptors present on sensory nerve terminals, resulting in antinociception.

When DAMGO ([d-Ala(2), NMePhe(4), Gly(01)(S)], enrephalin) a mu-opioid ligand, is injected into tissue, the nociceptive effects of local irritant injection are reduced. In contrast, when DPDPE, a delta-opioid ligand, is applied in a similar fashion, no change in nociception is observed. This suggests that peripheral mu-opioid receptors, and not delta-opioid receptors, are actively involved in nociceptive processing.

In contrast to the central effect of opioids, there is a relative lack of antinociceptive tolerance to the effects of opioids on peripheral opioid receptors in inflamed tissue.

EFFECT OF PERIPHERAL APPLICATION OF OPIOIDS FOR ACUTE PAIN

Two systematic reviews have examined the effect of peripheral application of opioids in acute pain. In that performed by Picard and colleagues (1997), they examined studies that investigated the peripheral application of opioids when compared to placebo, local anesthetics, or systemic opioids. They found no evidence of a clinically relevant peripheral analgesic effect of opioids in acute pain.

In the systematic review of Gupta and colleagues (2001) examining the peripheral analgesic effect of intra-articular morphine when given after arthroscopy, they found that intra-articular morphine had a definite analgesic effect, but the extent to which a systemic effect contributed was impossible to define.

Why then is there a disparity between these reviews? We have seen from the animal literature that opioid receptors are present in uninjured tissue, but at relatively low concentrations. It is only after sciatic nerve ligation or paw inflammation that opioid receptors migrate to the site of injury. Could it therefore be that in the case of patients with acute pain, the increases in density of peripheral opioid receptors have not yet occurred and consequently insignificant extra pain relief occurs when the opioid is administered peripherally? In the case of patients undergoing arthroscopy, preexisting pain and inflammation are often present and are an indication for arthroscopy, and hence the density of peripheral opioid receptors in the knee joint will already have been increased by this inflammation. Thus pain relief is more evident.

TRANSDERMAL FENTANYL

Because of its short half-life, oral and parenteral use of fentanyl is of little value in the treatment of most pain conditions apart from those of expected short duration or where it is used as a stopgap before more long-term treatment becomes effective. It is, however, an effective strong opioid analgesic with a short time to effect. In nonanesthesiological practice, this quick time to effect is utilized in fentanyl lozenges, which are particularly effective for the management of breakthrough pain in patients with terminal illnesses. Their use is less appropriate when conditions associated with chronic pain are considered.

As well as parenteral and lozenge formulations, fentanyl is available in a transdermal preparation, currently available in 25, 50, and 75 μg/hr strengths, with larger doses requiring the use of a combination of these patches to achieve the dosage. Each patch supplies drug for a three-day period and in opioid-naive patients, therapeutic levels of fentanyl and clinical effect are usually achieved within 12 to 18 hours.

The potential value of fentanyl patches includes the known strong opioid effect of fentanyl, the need to replace patches only once every three days (which may improve compliance), and the clinical impression of a slightly more favorable side effect profile than other strong opioid analgesics. In addition, their use continues to be appropriate even if the oral route of administration is unavailable because of, for example, intractable nausea or vomiting.

Menten and colleagues (2002) studied over 600 elderly patients using transdermal fentanyl for cancer-related pain. The fentanyl doses ranged from 25 to 950 μg/hr and patient acceptance was found to be high. Constipation was recorded in 40 percent of patients, although this seemed to be related to the use of rescue doses of morphine. In those studies where transdermal fentanyl is compared to another strong opioid, pain relief is as good with fentanyl and yet the incidence of opioid-related side effects is less.

Ringe and colleagues (2002) have studied patients using transdermal fentanyl for back pain caused by vertebral osteoporosis. Their results give an indication of what might be expected from the use of transdermal fentanyl. They looked at 64 patients with at least one osteoporotic vertebral fracture that required the use of strong opioid analgesics. Pain and quality of life were recorded at baseline and after four weeks of treatment. Of the 64 patients enrolled, 12 withdrew because of opioid-related side effects. In those who remained on treatment with fentanyl, pain at rest and on movement fell significantly (both by around 4 points on a 0-10 pain score) and quality of life also improved. Overall, 61 percent of patients were satisfied with their treatment.

Larsen and colleagues (2003) have examined dermal penetration of fentanyl in an in vitro model and found an intraindividual difference in absorption rates of around 18 percent. That said, when treatment is initiated, a process of gradual dose escalation to an effective dose is used, and this gradual process of dose increase will prevent an unexpectedly high dose from being delivered in isolated individuals whose absorption characteristics are different from the majority. Larsen and colleagues also report that they found no difference in penetration of the drug when the patch was applied to either breast or abdominal skin.

Transdermal fentanyl therefore represents a useful method of administration of a strong opioid, and its use is probably associated with slightly fewer side effects than other strong opioids.

TOPICAL MORPHINE

Although no commercial transdermal preparation containing morphine is currently available, a number of studies demonstrate an analgesic effect when morphine is applied peripherally.

Painful mucositis is a common occurrence following chemotherapy for head and neck carcinoma. This may be severe enough to prevent the oral intake of food and fluid. Cerchietti and colleagues (2002) examined patients with this condition treated with mouth rinses containing morphine and a local anesthetic. They compared their relief with patients receiving local anesthetic alone. The duration of severe pain following chemotherapy was 3.5 days shorter and overall pain less severe in the morphine-treated group. Cerchietti and colleagues (2003) have gone on to show that the response to morphine oral rinses is dose related, with a 2 percent solution being more efficacious than a 1 percent solution. The average duration of relief after an oral wash was 216 minutes. The time elapsed before consumption of an adequate oral diet was also reduced in morphine-treated patients. When systemic morphine levels were measured, even in those obtaining good pain relief, they were found to be insignificant.

A further use is in the case of painful ulcers. In a small randomized placebo-controlled crossover study, Zeppetella and colleagues (2003) found that all patients obtained relief when their ulcers were washed out with 10 mg morphine and that their relief was significantly greater during the morphine as compared to placebo treatment phases. No local or systemic side effects were observed.

It has already been mentioned that the density of peripheral opioid receptors is increased in the presence of inflammation. The clinical relevance of this has been highlighted in the case of pain following dental surgery. Likar and colleagues (2001) studied dental patients who received an injection of local anesthetic alone or in combination with 1 mg of morphine around noninflamed, inflamed, and perineural tissue. There were no differences in pain scores between the morphine and control group when the injection was perineural or around noninflamed tissue, but differences appeared when the injection was made into inflamed tissue.

So although transdermal preparations of morphine are not currently available, a number of studies suggest a potential utility for the peripheral application of morphine, particularly where the pain has an inflammatory component.

TRANSDERMAL BUPRENORPHINE

Buprenorphine is a lipophilic opioid analgesic previously available only in a sublingual and parenteral formulation, but now also available as a 35, 52.5, and 70 µg/hr transdermal matrix patch formulation. These patches deliver the drug over a 72-hour period. Because of the relatively long half-life of buprenorphine, time to effect after initial patch application can be prolonged; conversely, after patch removal, pain relief (or side effects) can persist for many hours. Side effects are those found with any opioid analgesic, with nausea and constipation both being predictable, and therefore partially amenable to prophylaxis.

OTHER MODES OF ADMINISTRATION OF STRONG OPIOIDS

Traditionally, breakthrough pain is treated with immediate-release oral opioids. However, the oral route may not be optimal, as conventional morphine preparations are not rapidly absorbed and have a significant first-pass effect, resulting in a relatively low bioavailability. Time to onset of pain relief, according to Sawe and colleagues (1983), can be 45 to 120 minutes. Fitzgibbon and colleagues (2003) have looked at the effect of morphine when administered nasally in cancer patients requiring breakthrough pain treatment. In all patients examined, therapeutic plasma morphine levels were achieved after nasal administration, and perceptible pain relief was apparent after an average time of 2.4 minutes, with meaningful pain relief being apparent at an average of 6.8 minutes. Nasal administration of morphine may therefore represent a useful method of providing quick pain relief when time is not available to wait for the effect of an oral analogue.

Fentanyl has a rapid analgesic effect and is currently available in parenteral, lozenge, and transdermal formulations. Bartfield and colleagues (2003) have shown that nebulized fentanyl, using the parenteral formulation, has a rapidity of onset comparable to intravenous use. What particular advantage such nebulized use has is debatable, but again indicates that novel modes of administration can be achieved when conventional routes are unavailable for whatever reason.

Bladder pain and spasm may complicate urological surgery or pathology. Anticholinergics are often used for bladder spasm, although their effect is sometimes not great. Several reports suggest that intravesical instillation of morphine or diamorphine can reduce both bladder pain and spasm without the production of significant side effects.

CONCLUSION

Peripheral application of opioids confers a number of potential advantages over oral administration. In general, transdermal preparations use controlled-release technology, and therefore the serum peaks and troughs seen with oral immediate-release preparations are avoided. In the presence of inflammation, there may be an increased density of opioid receptors, which are actively involved in nociceptive processing at the site of inflammation, and so application of the opioid adjacent to this site can produce higher opioid levels at these receptors. A further advantage is the prolonged delivery of opioid from the transdermal preparations (three days in the case of both fentanyl and buprenorphine patches), which may improve compliance. The topical application may also allow continued use of a strong opioid when the oral route is no longer available, as when, for example, the patient has intractable nausea or vomiting.

Although application of an opioid patch close to a site of inflammation may infer additional analgesic benefit, if no inflammation exists, then the site of application seems to have little influence on absorption. Therefore a site that is accessible and cosmetically acceptable can be used.

Transdermal application of opioids is therefore a useful method of opioid administration with some potential advantage over the oral route.

BIBLIOGRAPHY

Ackerman SJ, Mordin M, Reblando J, Xu X, Schein J, Vallow S, Brennan M. Patient reported utilization patterns of fentanyl transdermal system and oxycodone hydrochloride controlled release among patients with chronic non malignant pain. *J Manag Care Pharm* 2003; 9: 223-231.

Bartfield JM, Flint RD, McErlean M, Broderick J. Nebulized fentanyl for the relief of abdominal pain. *Acad Emerg Med* 2003; 10: 215-218.

Bohme K. Buprenorphine in a transdermal therapeutic system—A new option. *Clin Rheumatol* 2002; 21: S13-S16.

Caplan RA, Ready LB, Oden RV, Matsen FA, Nessly ML, Olsson GL. Transdermal fentanyl for postoperative pain management. A double-blind, placebo study. *JAMA* 1989; 261: 1036-1039.

Cerchietti LC, Navigante AH, Bonomi MR, Zaderajko MA, Menendez PR, Pogany CE, Roth BM. Effect of topical morphine for mucositis associated pain following concomitant chemo radiotherapy for head and neck carcinoma. *Cancer* 2002; 95: 2230-2236.

Cerchietti LC, Navigante AH, Korte MW, Cohen AM, Quiroga PN, Villaamil EC, Bonomi MR, Roth BM. Potential utility of the peripheral analgesic properties of morphine in stomatitis related pain: A pilot study. *Pain* 2003; 105: 265-273.

Coggeshall RE, Zhou S, Carlton SM. Opioid receptors on peripheral sensory axons. *Brain Res* 1997; 764: 126-132.

Czlonkowski A, Stedin C, Herz A. Peripheral mechanisms of opioid antinociception in inflammation: Involvement of cytokines. *Eur J Pharmacol* 1993; 242: 229-235.

Dale O, Hjortkjaer R, Kharasch ED. Nasal administration of opioids for pain management in adults. *Acta Anaesthesiologica Scand* 2002; 46: 759-770.

Duckett JW, Cangiano T, Cubina M, Howe C, Cohen D. Intravesical morphine analgesia after bladder surgery. *J Urol* 1997; 157: 1407-1409.

Evans HC, Eastope SE. Transdermal buprenorphine. *Drugs* 2003; 63: 1999-2010.

Fitzgibbon D, Morgan D, Dockter D, Barry C, Kharasch ED. Initial pharmacokinetic, safety and efficacy evaluation of nasal morphine gluconate for breakthrough pain in cancer patients. *Pain* 2003; 106: 309-315.

Gupta A, Bodin L, Holmstrom B, Berggren L. A systematic review of the peripheral analgesic effects of intra articular morphine. *Anesth Analg* 2001; 93: 761-770.

Hassan AH, Ableitner A, Stein C, Herz A. Inflammation of the rat paw enhances axonal transport of opioid receptors in the sciatic nerve and increases their density in the inflamed tissue. *Neuroscience* 1993; 55: 185-195.

Kornick CA, Santiago-Palma J, Moryl N, Payne R, Obbens EA. Benefit risk assessment of transdermal fentanyl for the treatment of chronic pain. *Drug Saf* 2003; 26: 951-973.

Krajnik M, Zylicz Z, Finlay I, Luczak J, van Sorge AA. Potential uses of topical opioids in palliative care—Report of 6 cases. *Pain* 1999; 80: 121-125.

Larsen RH, Nieslen F, Sorensen JA, Nielsen JB. Dermal penetration of fentanyl: inter and intraindividual variations. *Pharmacol Toxicol* 2003; 93: 244-248.

Likar R, Koppert W, Blatnig H, Chiari F, Sittl R, Stein C, Schafer M. Efficacy of peripheral morphine analgesia in inflamed, non-inflamed and perineural tissue of dental surgery patients. *J Pain Symptom Manage* 2001; 21: 330-337.

Likar R, Sittl R, Gragger K, Pipam W, Blatnig H, Breschan C, Schalk HV, Stein C, Schafer M. Peripheral morphine analgesia in dental surgery. *Pain* 1998; 76: 145-150.

McCoubrie R, Jeffrey D. Intravesical diamorphine for bladder spasm. *J Pain Symptom Manage* 2003; 25: 1-2.

Menten J, Desmedt M, Lossignol D, Mullie A. Longitudinal follow up of TTS fentanyl use in patients with cancer related pain: Results of a compassionate use study with special focus on elderly patients. *Curr Med Res Opin* 2002; 18: 488-498.

Milligan K, Lanteri-Minet M, Borchert K, Helmers H, Donald R, Adriansen H, Moulin D, Haazen L. Evaluation of long term efficacy and safety of transdermal fentanyl in the treatment of chronic non cancer pain. *J Pain* 2001; 2: 197-204.

Moore UJ, Seymour RA, Gilroy J, Rawlins MD. The efficacy of locally applied morphine in post-operative pain after bilateral third molar surgery. *Br J Clin Pharmacol* 1994; 37: 227-230.

Mystakidou K, Parpa E, Tsilika E, Mavromati A, Smyrniotis V, Georgaki S, Vlahos L. Long term management of non cancer pain with transdermal therapeutic system fentanyl. *J Pain* 2003; 4: 298-306.

Mystakidou K, Tsilika E, Parpa E, Kouloulias V, Kouvaris I, Georgaki S, Vlahos I. Long term cancer pain management in morphine pretreated and opioid naïve patients with transdermal fentanyl. *Int J Cancer* 2003; 107: 486-492.

Picard PR, Tramer MR, McQuay HJ, Moore RA. Analgesic efficacy of peripheral opioids (all except intra-articular): a qualitative systematic review of randomized controlled trials. *Pain* 1997; 72: 309-318.

Ringe JD, Faber H, Bock O, Valentine S, Felsenberg D, Pfeifer M, Schwallen S. Transdermal fentanyl for the treatment of back pain caused by vertebral osteoporosis. *Rheumatol Int* 2002; 22: 199-203.

Sawe J, Dahlstrom B, Rane A. Steady state kinetics and analgesic effect of oral morphine in cancer patients. *Eur J Clin Pharmacol* 1983; 24: 537-542.

Sittl R, Griessinger N, Likar R. Analgesic efficacy and tolerability of transdermal buprenorphine in patients with inadequately controlled chronic pain related to cancer and other disorders: A multicenter, randomized, double-blind, placebo controlled trial. *Clin Ther* 2003; 25: 150-168.

Stein C, Machelska H, Binder W, Schafer M. Peripheral opioid analgesia. *Curr Opin Pharmacol* 2001; 1: 62-65.

Stein C, Machelska H, Schafer M. Peripheral analgesic and anti-inflammatory effects of opioids. *Z Rheumatol* 2001; 60: 416-424.

Stein C, Schafer M, Hassan AH. Peripheral opioid receptors. *Ann Med* 1995: 27: 19-21.

Twillman RK, Long TD, Cathers TA, Mueller DW. Treatment of painful skin ulcers with topical opioids. *J Pain Symptom Manage* 1999; 17: 288-292.

Van Seventer R, Smit JM, Schipper RM, Wicks MA, Zuurmond WW. Comparison of TTS fentanyl with sustained release oral morphine in the treatment of patients not using opioids for mild to moderate pain. *Curr Med Res Opin* 2003; 19: 457-469.

Zeppetella G, Paul J, Ribeiro MD. Analgesic efficacy of morphine applied topically to painful ulcers. *J Pain Symptom Manage* 2003; 25: 555-558.

Zhou L, Zhang Q, Stein C, Schafer M. Contribution of opioid receptors on primary afferent versus sympathetic neurons to peripheral opioid analgesia. *J Pharmacol Exp Ther* 1998; 286: 1000-1006.

Chapter 11

Tricyclic Antidepressants
As Analgesics in the Elderly

Mary E. Lynch
Jana Sawynok

The prevalence of chronic pain increases with advancing age up to the seventh decade, plateaus, and then may decline slightly after age 75. Increasing age may influence pain through changes in neural substrates, modification of emotional responses, or developmental and sociocultural effects on cognition (Farrell and Gibson, 2004). Growing evidence indicates that aging is associated with differences in the appraisal of pain; older people expect to experience pain as they age, and the presence of mild symptoms does not affect self-rated health (Ebrahim, Brittis, and Wu, 1991; Bezchlibnyk-Butler and Jeffries, 2003). Comorbidity is an important consideration due to the overall burden of illness on the human system and the need for increased resources to manage pain.

A significant body of work has documented a high degree of comorbidity of chronic pain and depression, and age does not appear to influence this relationship (Farrell and Gibson, 2004). The incidence of depression among persons with chronic pain is higher than with other chronic medical illnesses (Gallagher and Verma, 2004), and comorbidity increases the probability of depression in older people (Farrell and Gibson, 2004). Rates of major depression range from 11 to 30 percent in elderly clinical populations (Lyness et al., 1995; Rapp, Parisi, and Wallace, 1991). The likelihood of a diagnosis of depression and the general level of depressive symptomatology peak in late middle age and then decline thereafter (Gibson, 1997; Henderson et al., 1998; Jorm, 2000). Thus, it becomes increasingly important to assess both pain and depression as individuals enter late middle age.

As in treating patients with chronic pain of all ages, the use of pharmacotherapy should take place within an overall interdisciplinary management plan that includes an active participatory approach to overall health. Additional treatments might include therapeutic exercise, modalities such as

Clinical Management of the Elderly Patient in Pain
© 2006 by The Haworth Press, Inc. All rights reserved.
doi:10.1300/5356_11

transcutaneous electrical nerve stimulation, use of heat or ice, and the use of cognitive and relaxation strategies. The goals of treatment include pain reduction and optimization of daily living.

Before discussing antidepressants as analgesics, it is important to clarify that antidepressants are analgesic in their own right. Patients do not need to exhibit comorbid depression in order to benefit from a trial of an antidepressant for treatment of pain (Dworkin et al., 2003; Lynch, 2001; Max, 1994, 1995; McQuay et al., 1996).

SYSTEMIC TRICYCLIC ANTIDEPRESSANTS AS ANALGESICS

Considerable evidence supports the notion that tricyclic antidepressants (TCAs) are analgesic when taken orally. Several reviews of randomized controlled trials have concluded that TCAs exhibit clear analgesic efficacy in a number of chronic pain conditions (Dworkin et al., 2003; Lynch, 2001; Max, 1994, 1995; McQuay et al., 1996). Specifically, TCAs have demonstrated analgesia in pain caused by diabetic neuropathy, postherpetic neuralgia (for which there is a solid body of evidence to support efficacy), tension headache, migraine, atypical facial pain, fibromyalgia, and low back pain. However, TCAs do not appear efficacious in painful HIV sensory neuropathy (Kieburtz et al., 1998), spinal cord injury (Cardenas et al., 2002), and cisplatin-induced neuropathy (Hammack et al., 2002). In neuropathic pain, TCAs relieve brief lancinating pain, constant dysesthetic pain, allodynia, and spontaneous pain. Specific TCAs that have been well studied include amitriptyline, imipramine, doxepin, clomipramine, desipramine, and nortriptyline. The pain relief from TCAs is generally moderate in degree and accompanied by side effects such as sedation, postural hypotension, and anticholinergic side effects such as dry mouth and constipation. The analgesic effect is independent of the effect on mood. TCAs with a balanced inhibition of serotonin (5-hydroxytryptamine, 5-HT) and noradrenaline (NA) reuptake, such as amitriptyline, imipramine, and clomipramine, as well as agents with greater NA reuptake inhibition such as desipramine, appear to be effective analgesics.

Clinical Guidelines

The main drawback of the TCAs is their adverse side effect profile (see Table 11.1). This is related to the fact that TCAs exhibit activity on a number of neurotransmitter receptors with resultant anticholinergic, sedating,

TABLE 11.1. Analgesic antidepressants.

Drug	Common trade name	Therapeutic range (mg/24 h)	Half-life (H)	Receptor profile		Most common side effects (percent)					
				NA	5-HT	Sedation	Orthostatic hypotension	Weight gain	Dry mouth	Consti-pation	GI distress, nausea, diarrhea
Tricyclics											
Amitriptyline	Elavil	10-300	10-46	+++	+++	>30	>10	>30	>30	>10	>2
Doxepin	Sinequan	10-300	8-36	+++	++	>30	>10	>10	>30	>10	<2
Trimipramine	Surmontil	10-300	7-30	++	+	>30	>10	>10	>10	>10	<2
Imipramine	Tofranil	10-300	4-34	+++	+++	>10	>30	>10	>30	>10	>10
Clomipramine	Anafranil	10-300	17-37	+++	++++	>2	>10	>10	>30	>10	>10
Desipramine	Norpramin	10-300	12-76	+++++	++	>2	>2	>2	>10	>2	>2
Nortriptyline	Aventyl	10-200	13-88	++++	++	>2	>2	>2	>10	>10	<2
Serotonin/noradrenaline reuptake inhibitors											
Venlafaxine	Effexor	37.5-225	3-7 (parent), 9-13 (metabolite)	++	++++	>10	>10	<2	>10	>10	>30

Source: Adapted from Bezchlibnyk-Butler and Jeffries, 2003.

autonomic, and cardiovascular effects. For this reason, TCAs must be used with caution in patients with a history of cardiovascular disease, glaucoma, urinary retention, and autonomic neuropathy, and with extreme caution in the elderly (Dworkin et al., 2003). The main contraindications to the use of the antidepressants are significant cardiac arrythmias, prostatic hyper-trophy, and narrow-angle glaucoma. A study of depressed patients with ischemic heart disease found that 20 percent of patients treated with nortriptyline after a myocardial infarction developed adverse cardiac events (Roose et al., 1998). The faculty of the Fourth International Conference on the Mechanisms and Treatment of Neuropathic Pain (Dworkin et al., 2003) have therefore recommended a screening cardiogram to check for cardiac conduction abnormalities before beginning treatment with TCAs, espe-cially in patients older than 40 years. Caution is also recommended when there is a risk of suicide or accidental death by overdose.

There is some variation among the TCAs with regard to side effect pro-files. Most are sedating, cause anticholinergic side effects such as dry mouth and constipation, and can cause postural hypotension and weight gain. In the elderly, the risk of postural hypotension is increased. Nortrip-tyline and desipramine have fewer adverse effects and are generally the better tolerated of these agents (Dworkin et al., 2003).

Potential drug interactions of importance include interference with the antihypertensive effect of guanethidine, clonidine, and similarly acting compounds, a risk of paralytic ileus when used in combination with anti-cholinergic drugs, enhanced response to alcohol, barbiturates, and other central nervous system (CNS) depressants, decreased insulin sensitivity with amitriptyline, and a possible serotonin syndrome when used with other serotonergic agents (e.g., selective serotonin reuptake inhibitors or SSRIs, sumatriptan, and other triptans that are serotonin agonists). When used with opioids, TCAs may enhance the analgesic effect, but may also lead to additive sedation. When used with opioids, plasma levels of desipramine are increased; there is also marked inhibition of conversion of codeine to morphine with most of the TCAs (Bezchlibnyk-Butler and Jeffries, 2003). Avoid using the TCAs with irreversible monoamine oxidase inhibitors (phenelzine, tranylcypromine).

Because most patients with chronic pain experience poor sleep and be-cause a number of the antidepressants have sedative qualities that can bene-fit sleep, a TCA with some sedation is generally chosen as a first-line ther-apy. If patients find these agents too sedating, a less sedating agent is chosen. All agents are comparable with regard to efficacy, and the main is-sue governing choice of TCA is the side effect profile. Table 11.1 presents details that should aid clinicians in choosing an appropriate agent.

Doses less than those used for depression generally have been used in analgesic regimens. Unfortunately, there is little data regarding dose-response relationships with the analgesic actions of antidepressants (Lynch, 2001). Usual guidelines are to start patients at a dose of 10-25 mg given at bedtime (unless one of the more activating agents is chosen). In the elderly, the dose can then be titrated gradually every five to seven days until a therapeutic response is achieved or persistent bothersome side effects occur. There is a broad dose range within which analgesic effects can occur, but for most TCAs, a therapeutic response will occur between 10 and 150 mg with most patients.

One study examining imipramine for treatment of diabetic neuropathy found that most patients appeared to obtain optimum relief at or below 400 nm/L, a plasma concentration that required imipramine doses of 125-350 mg day (Sindrup, Gram, Skjold, et al., 1990). These investigators caution that because of variability in pharmacokinetics and plasma TCA concentrations needed to obtain an optimum response, one should not discontinue treatment because of inadequate response at standard doses such as 100 mg per day. It is reasonable to increase the dose to levels that are normally used for depression as long as limiting side effects do not occur. Blood levels for TCAs can be performed to ensure adequate dosing. Special caution should be used in elderly populations who may require the lower range of dosing and conservative titration schedules. Pain relief approaches maximum values after four days of treatment at the therapeutic level. If a patient does not experience a therapeutic response, or if bothersome side effects occur, it is reasonable to try another agent.

Special Issues When Treating Elderly Patients

Elderly patients are at higher risk of decreased cardiovascular function, less efficient renal perfusion, and greater challenges to cognitive function. This leaves elderly patients at higher risk of developing side effects. In addition, many elderly patients are already on a number of other medications for various health conditions and there is the risk of drug interactions and additive side effects. Thus, one must exercise extreme caution in this population with regard to the use of oral TCAs. The best approach is to use the old clinical guideline "start low and go slow." Thus a start dose of 10 mg once daily, usually at bedtime, is recommended, with a dose titration schedule involving 10 mg incremental increases every seven days to an analgesic response or limiting side effects. Amitriptyline is contraindicated in the elderly due to the high risk of postural hypotension, with risk of falls and hip fractures.

OTHER ANTIDEPRESSANTS AS ANALGESICS

Serotonin and Noradrenaline Reuptake Inhibitors

Venlafaxine, a serotonin and noradrenaline reuptake inhibitor (SNRI), is an effective antidepressant with strong inhibition of 5-HT and NA reuptake and minimal muscarinic, histaminergic, and adrenergic activity, and does not have the undesirable side-effect profile of the TCAs. This agent is of particular interest because of its balanced neurotransmitter profile (making it similar to TCAs) and its similar structure to tramadol, an analgesic with both opioid agonist and monoaminergic activity (Markowitz and Patrick, 1998). A number of uncontrolled reports indicate that venlafaxine is effective in postherpetic neuralgia, painful polyneuropathy, headache, neuropathic pain, atypical facial pain, and radicular back pain (Galer, 1995; Songer and Schule, 1996; Sumpton and Moulin, 2001; Taylor and Rowbotham, 1996).

A randomized controlled trial examined venlafaxine compared to imipramine and placebo in treating painful polyneuropathy (Sindrup et al., 2003) and demonstrated that venlafaxine 225 mg per day was superior to placebo and comparable to imipramine 150 mg per day in reducing constant, paroxysmal, and pressure-evoked pain. Venlafaxine was not superior to imipramine with respect to tolerability, as a higher number of patients withdrew because of side effects with venlafaxine than with imipramine, and the severity of side effects in patients completing the trial was similar with the two drugs. There was a higher incidence of dry mouth and sweating with imipramine and tiredness with venlafaxine. A small lower-dose placebo-controlled trial using venlafaxine 37.5-75 mg per day found no difference from placebo on average daily pain intensity, but better pain relief in the treatment of neuropathic pain following treatment of breast cancer (Tasmuth, Hartel, and Kalso, 2002). Thus, some evidence indicates that venlafaxine may be analgesic and that it exhibits a different and nonanticholinergic side effect profile compared to TCAs.

The recommended starting dose for venlafaxine is half of a 37.5 mg tablet titrated every three to seven days to a maximum daily dose of 150 mg given as two divided doses. The most common side effect is nausea. In the elderly, an increase in blood pressure is possible.

Selective Serotonin Reuptake Inhibitors

The SSRI antidepressants are generally used as the first line in the treatment of depression due to equivalent efficacy and a better side effect profile (most common side effects include agitation, anxiety, sleep disturbance, tremor, sexual dysfunction, and headache). SSRIs are also safer in cases of overdose. The literature regarding their potential as analgesics has been conflicting (Lynch, 2001). Of 10 controlled trials examining SSRIs in treatment of chronic headache, 3 found SSRIs to be no better than placebo and 2 marginally superior to placebo. In the remainder, there was some improvement but the analgesic effect was not superior to the comparison drug (Jung, Staiger, and Sullivan, 1997). Three placebo-controlled trials have used SSRIs for diabetic neuropathy; the larger study ($N = 46$) found no difference between fluoxetine and placebo (Max et al., 1992), while the two smaller studies found that paroxetine (Sindrup, Gram, Brosen, et al., 1990) and citalopram (Sindrup et al., 1992) exhibited some analgesic effect compared to placebo. In studies comparing SSRIs to TCAs (Bendtsen, Jensen, and Olesen, 1996; Max et al., 1992; Sindrup, Gram, Brosen, et al., 1990), analgesia with TCAs was superior in every case (Lynch, 2001).

In a review of placebo-controlled trials involving painful polyneuropathy, the NNT value (number needed to treat, the number of patients one needs to treat in order to obtain one patient with greater than 50 percent pain relief) for TCAs was 2.6 and for SSRIs was 6.7; values for other agents were 2.5 for sodium channel-blocking anticonvulsants, 4.1 for calcium channel-blocking anticonvulsants such as gabapentin, and 3.4 for tramadol (Sindrup and Jensen, 2000). A further systematic review of antidepressants for diabetic neuropathy and postherpetic neuralgia reported similar NNT values for TCAs (NNT 2.1-3.5); much less benefit was observed with SSRIs, which did not differ from placebo (Collins et al., 2000).

Thus, the literature indicates that the SSRIs are less likely to exhibit efficacy as analgesics. In the case of comorbid depression where treatment of the depression is the priority, TCAs are contraindicated, and venlafaxine has either failed or is too costly for the patient, then one may make the decision to use an SSRI as a first-line agent. When using SSRIs, it is important to be aware of the metabolism in liver by cytochrome P450 (CYP) isoenzymes and potential interactions. Citalopram and escitalopram are the least affected by the CYP isoenzymes (Gallagher and Verma, 2004). In the elderly, fluoxetine should be avoided due to its extensive half life (two to three days with active metabolites for seven to nine days).

Other Antidepressants

A single trial has examined the dopamine and norepinephrine reuptake inhibitor bupropion in neuropathic pain, and it demonstrated an analgesic effect at a dose of 150-300 mg (Semenchuk, Sherman, and Davis, 2001).

However, the side-effect profile (related to the dopaminergic system, delusions, hallucinations, seizure risk) argues against the use of this agent in elderly populations. The serotonin-2 antagonist/reuptake inhibitors include trazodone and nefazodone. Three of four placebo-controlled trials regarding trazodone were negative, and there have been no controlled trials regarding nefazodone. There have been no randomized controlled trials examining the monoamine oxidase inhibitors in nondepressed patients with pain (Lynch, 2001).

In conclusion, in elderly patients TCAs other than amitriptyline and the SNRI venlafaxine are reasonable options to consider in the treatment of pain. There is significantly more evidence from randomized controlled trials indicating that TCAs are analgesic, but the side-effect profile obliges clinicians to use caution in elderly populations. In situations where TCAs are relatively contraindicated, then venlafaxine or analgesic agents other than the antidepressants are recommended as first-line agents. Further controlled trials are needed.

COMORBID PAIN AND DEPRESSION

How does one choose the best antidepressant for elderly patients suffering with comorbid pain and depression? No single antidepressant drug has proved more efficacious than any other for treatment of depression (Mulrow et al., 2000). However, evidence indicates that the dual-action antidepressants may exhibit increased efficacy in treatment of depression alone. A meta-analysis of eight randomized controlled trials comparing SSRIs versus venlafaxine found that at high doses, 45 percent of patients achieved remission on venlafaxine, 35 percent on SSRIs, and 25 percent on placebo (Thase, 2003). This observation, together with evidence reviewed above indicating that SNRIs are analgesic, provides good support for using an SNRI such as venlafaxine as the first line in treating comorbid pain and depression.

MECHANISMS OF ACTION OF ANTIDEPRESSANTS AS ANALGESICS

The analgesic properties of antidepressants are observed in the absence of depression in humans (discussed previously) and can be observed directly in preclinical models of pain (includes acute and chronic administration in nociceptive, inflammatory and neuropathic models), indicating that their efficacy is a direct effect on nociception rather than a secondary effect due to the relief of depression. Antidepressants exhibit a wide range of acute pharmacological actions (discussed later), and a number of these may contribute to their analgesic properties (Eschalier, Ardid, and Dubray, 1999; Sawynok, Esser, and Reid, 2001; Sindrup, 1997). Actions on neuronal plasticity, stress, and neurogenesis, which are observed following chronic administration of antidepressants and are implicated in antidepressant efficacy (Duman, Malberg, and Thome, 1999; Skolnick, 1999), may further contribute to efficacy in chronic pain where central sensitization and plasticity are known to occur, but these mechanisms are still largely unexplored in preclinical models of chronic pain.

Antidepressants were first understood to act centrally at supraspinal and spinal sites, and direct administration to these compartments by intracerebroventricular and intrathecal routes has been shown to produce analgesia in various rodent pain models (Eschalier, Ardid, and Dubray, 1999; Sawynok, Esser, and Reid, 2001). More recently, it has been demonstrated that peripheral administration of antidepressants can produce antinociception in models of acute nociception (Gerner et al., 2001; Khan, Gerner, and Want, 2002), persistent pain (Sawynok, Reid, and Esser, 1999a,b) and neuropathic pain (Esser and Sawynok, 2000; Ulugol et al., 2002). These observations have led to the suggestion that antidepressants may also be effective as topical analgesics (Sawynok, 2003).

Monoamines

Descending monoamine pathways containing NA and 5-HT originate from various brainstem nuclei and project to the dorsal horn of the spinal cord, and are well recognized to be important contributors to the modulation of nociceptive input as it enters the central nervous system. Supraspinally projecting pathways containing these amines are also important in regulating nociception and in influencing the emotional state. Monoamine pathways are implicated in antidepressant antinociception because antinociception is inhibited by depletion of central NA (by α-methyl-p-tyrosine, a tyrosine hydroxylase inhibitor) and systemic administration of α-adrenergic receptor antagonists, as well as by depletion of 5-HT (by p-chlorophenylalanine, an inhibitor of 5-HT synthesis) and 5-HT receptor antagonists (Eschalier, Ardid, and Dubray, 1999; Gray, Pache, and Sewell, 1999; Otsuka et al., 2001; Yokogawa et al., 2002). Within the spinal cord, and likely at other sites affecting nociceptive transmission, there are significant interactions between NA and 5-HT systems, and this may partially contribute to the more prominent efficacy of antidepressants that interact with both NA and 5-HT systems, as noted in clinical studies.

Opioids

The key observations that support an involvement of opioid systems in antinociception by antidepressants are the ability of naloxone, an opioid receptor antagonist, to inhibit antinociception, and the ability of chronic administration of antidepressants to alter levels of met- and leu-enkephalin and opioid receptor binding in the rat central nervous system (Eschalier, Ardid, and Dubray, 1999). As antidepressants have a low affinity for opioid receptors, the opioid link may reflect an indirect mechanism involving monoamine or other systems.

Cation Channel Block

Antidepressants can block Na^+ (Pancrazio et al., 1998; Song et al., 2000) and Ca^{2+} channels (Lavoie, Beauchamp, and Elie, 1994), and, while not directly validated, such properties may contribute to antinociception following systemic administration. Local anesthetic actions are particularly prominent following local peripheral administration immediately adjacent to the nerve (Gerner et al., 2001; Khan, Gerner, and Want, 2002), and this action may contribute to peripheral antinociceptive properties of antidepressants. Antidepressants also block N-methyl-D-aspartate (NMDA) receptors (IC_{50} about 10^{-6} M), and, given the prominent role of spinal NMDA receptors in central sensitization and the contribution of this process to inflammatory and neuropathic pain, this action has been implicated in spinal antinociception by antidepressants (Eisenach and Gebhart, 1995). While sensory afferents also express ionotropic glutamate receptors on their most peripheral aspects, block of peripheral NMDA receptors does not appear to be a prominent contributor to peripheral antinociception (Sawynok, Reid, and Esser, 1999a).

Adenosine Mechanisms

Methylxanthine adenosine receptor antagonists (caffeine, theophylline) have been shown to inhibit antinociception by a number of antidepressants following both acute (Esser and Sawynok, 2000; Sierralta et al., 1995; Ulugol et al., 2002) and chronic systemic administration (Esser et al., 2001), implicating endogenous adenosine systems in such actions. The doses of caffeine that block amitriptyline actions in a neuropathic pain model are modest and comparable to daily human dietary intake levels, raising the possibility that such intake could limit the benefit that is observed with antidepressants. However, no direct data are available for humans addressing this issue. In the periphery, adenosine clearly contributes to the antinociceptive action of amitriptyline, as caffeine administered locally inhibits its actions (Esser and Sawynok, 2000; Sawynok, Reid, and Esser, 1999a; Ulugol et al., 2002).

K+ Channels

Antidepressants lead to the opening of certain K+ channels, which leads to stabilization of membranes and inhibition of neuronal activity, and this mechanism contributes to central antinociception (Galeotti, Ghelardi, and Bartolini, 2001; Galeotti et al., 1997).

Other Mechanisms

As noted above, TCAs can block receptors for various neurotransmitters, and this contributes to their side-effect profile in humans. The ability of TCAs to block histamine H1 receptors, muscarinic and nicotinic cholinergic receptors, 5-HT$_2$ receptors, and α-adrenergic receptors may potentially contribute to systemic or peripheral antinociceptive properties of antidepressants, as each of these systems is implicated in nociceptive signaling (Sawynok, Esser, and Reid, 2001). When antidepressants act to enhance the activity of a particular system, receptor, or ion channel (e.g., monoamines, opioids, adenosine, K+ channels), one can examine the role of that system by administering receptor antagonists or blocking agents selective for that system. However, when antidepressants inhibit the functioning of a receptor or ion channel (e.g., NMDA receptor, Na+ or Ca^{2+} channel, monoamine, cholinergic, or histaminergic receptor), it is much more difficult to implicate that entity; mimicry by an agent with a discrete action at this site is necessary but not sufficient to implicate its involvement, and selective deletion strategies (antisense oligonucleotides or gene deletion of the target) are required for elaboration. It is interesting to note that while the simultaneous interaction of antidepressants with multiple systems or mechanisms can lead to redundancy and confounding in terms of interpreting the involvement of a single particular mechanism from a basic science perspective, the same multiplicity of action may be a valuable asset in targeting multiple aspects of the changes in the neurobiology of nociceptive signaling that occur in chronic pain, and can contribute positively to the clinical efficacy that is observed. This positive influence may be expressed additively or even synergistically. Thus, synergistic facilitatory interactions with respect to antinociception have been reported between 5-HT/NA, opioids/NA, opioids/ adenosine, and adenosine/NA (all are individually implicated in antidepressant antinociception) following systemic or spinal administration. It is interesting to note that site-site synergy can also occur between spinal-supraspinal and peripheral-spinal compartments with respect to antinociception (this has been observed for opioids), and this multiplicity of sites of action also could potentially contribute to antidepressant efficacy.

TOPICAL ANTIDEPRESSANTS AS ANALGESICS IN CLINICAL STUDIES

The preclinical literature indicates that antidepressants can act peripherally to suppress pain, and this introduces the possibility that antidepressants can be formulated to act as topical analgesics whereby analgesic effects would occur locally near the site of drug application. This approach requires even the most peripheral aspects of sensory nerves to express changes following injury or perturbations at distal sites. Studies in primates do indicate that when the site of injury is adjacent to the spinal cord, hyperexcitability is expressed even at the most peripheral aspects of the nerve (Ali et al., 1999).

There are now clinical studies to support the notion that antidepressants produce analgesia following topical administration as a cream. Thus, in randomized controlled trials, topical doxepin cream (3-5 percent) was shown to produce analgesia in neuropathic pain of mixed etiology when administered alone (McCleane, 2000b) or in combination with capsaicin (McCleane, 2000a). There is also a case report for efficacy of topical doxepin in complex regional pain syndrome (McCleane, 2002). In open trials, a combination of amitriptyline (2 percent) and ketamine (1 percent) produced analgesia in mixed neuropathic pain (Lynch, Clark, and Sawynok, 2003). The advantage of the topical route for this class of agents is that systemic absorption would be limited (blood levels are largely not detectable following such administration), and this would minimize both adverse effects and drug interactions. Given that the elderly have multiple health problems and frequently require multiple drug regimens for management, the topical approach may be of particular benefit in this patient population.

REFERENCES

Ali Z, Ringkamp M, Hartke TC, Chien HF, Flavahan NA, Campbell JN. Uninjured C-fibre nociceptors develop spontaneous activity and α-adrenergic sensitivity following L6 spinal nerve ligation in monkey. *J Neurophysiol* 1999;81; 455-466.
Bendtsen L, Jensen R, Olesen J. A non-selective (amitriptyline), but not a selective (citalopram), serotonin reuptake inhibitor is effective in the prophylactic

treatment of chronic tension type headache. *Neurol Neurosurg Psychiatry* 1996:61; 285-290.

Bezchlibnyk-Butler KZ, Jeffries JJ. *Clinical Handbook of Psychotropic Drugs,* 13th ed. Cambridge, MA: Hogrefe and Huber, 2003; 40-45.

Cardenas DD, Warms CA, Turner JA, Marshall H, Brooke MM, Loeser JD. Efficacy of amitriptyline for relief of pain in spinal cord injury: Results of a randomized controlled trial. *Pain* 2002:96; 365-373.

Collins SL, Moore A, McQuay HJ, Wiffen P. Antidepressants and anticonvulsants for diabetic neuropathy and postherpetic neuralgia: A quantitative systematic review. *J Pain Symptom Manage* 2000:20; 449-559.

Duman RS, Malberg J, Thome J. Neural plasticity to stress and antidepressant treatment. *Biol Psychiatry* 1999:46; 1181-1191.

Dworkin RH, Backonja M, Rowbotham MC, Allen RR, Argoff CR, Bennett GJ, Bushnesll C, Tamar JP, Galer BS, Haythornthwaite JA, et al. Advances in neuropathic pain. *Arch Neurol* 2003:60; 1525-1533.

Ebrahim S, Brittis S, Wu A. The valuation of states of ill-health: The impact of age and disability. *Age Aging* 1991:20; 37-40.

Eisenach JC, Gebhart GF. Intrathecal amitriptyline acts as an N-methyl-D-aspartate receptor antagonist in the presence of inflammatory hyperalgesia in rats. *Anesthesiology* 1995:83; 1046-1053.

Eschalier A, Ardid D, Dubray C. Tricyclic and other antidepressants as analgesics. In: *Novel Aspects of Pain Management: Opioids and Beyond,* Sawynok J, Cowan A (eds.), New York: Wiley, 1999; 303-320.

Esser MJ, Chase T, Allen GV, Sawynok J. Chronic administration of amitriptyline and caffeine in a rat model of neuropathic pain: Multiple interactions. *Eur J Pharmacol* 2001:430; 211-218.

Esser MJ, Sawynok J. Caffeine blockade of the thermal anti-hyperalgesic effect of acute amitriptyline in a rat model of neuropathic pain. *Eur J Pharmacol* 2000: 399; 131-139.

Farrell MJ, Gibson SJ. Psychosocial aspects of pain in older people. In: *Psychosocial Aspects of Pain: A Handbook for Healthcare Providers, Progress in Pain Research and Management,* Vol. 27, Dworkin RH, Breitbart WS (eds.), Seattle: IASP Press, 2004; 139-178.

Galeotti N, Ghelardini C, Bartolini A. Involvement of potassium channels in amitriptyline and clomipramine analgesia. *Neuropharmacology* 2001:40; 75-84.

Galeotti N, Ghelardini C, Capaccioli S, Quattrone A, Nicolin A, Bartolini A. Blockade of clomipramine and amitriptyline analgesia by an antisense oligonucleotide to mKv1.1, a mouse *Shaker*-like K+ channel. *Eur J Pharmacol* 1997:330; 15-25.

Galer BS. Neuropathic pain of peripheral origin: Advances in pharmacologic treatment. *Neurology* 1995:45(S9); S17-S25.

Gallagher RM, Verma S. Mood and anxiety disorders in chronic pain. In: *Psychosocial Aspects of Pain: A Handbook for Healthcare Providers, Progress in Pain Research and Management,* Vol. 27, Dworkin RH, Breitbart WS (eds.), Seattle: IASP Press, 2004; 139-178.

Gerner P, Mujtaba M, Sinnott CJ, Wang GK. Amitriptyline versus bipivicaine in rat sciatic nerve blockade. *Anesthesiology* 2001; 661-667.

Gibson SJ. The measurement of pain states in older adults. *J Gerontol B Psychol Sci Soc Sci* 1997:52; 19-28.

Gray AM, Pache DM, Sewell RDE. Do a_2-adrenoceptors play an integral role in the antinociceptive mechanism of action of antidepressant compounds? *Eur J Pharmacol* 1999:378; 161-168.

Hammack JE, Michalak JC, Loprinzi CL, Sloan JA, Novpymu PJ, Soori GS, Tirona MT, Rowland KM, Stella PJ, Johnson JA. Phase III evaluation of nortriptyline for alleviation of symptoms of cisplatin-induced peripheral neuropathy. *Pain* 2002:98; 195-203.

Henderson AS, Jorm AF, Korten AE, Jacomb P, Christensen H, Rodgers B. Symptoms of depression and anxiety during adult life: Evidence for a decline in prevalence with age. *Psychol Med* 1998:28; 1321-1328.

Jorm AF. Does old age reduce the risk of anxiety and depression? A review of epidemiological studies across the adult life span. *Psychol Med* 2000:30; 11-22.

Jung AC, Staiger T, Sullivan M. The efficacy of selective serotonin reuptake inhibitors for the management of chronic pain. *J Gen Intern Med* 1997:12; 384-389.

Khan MA, Gerner P, Want GK. Amitriptyline for prolonged cutaneous analgesia in the rat. *Anesthesiology* 2002:96; 109-116.

Kieburtz K, Simpson D, Yiannoutsos C, Max MB, Hall CD, Ellis RJ, Marra CM, McKendall R, Singer E, DalPan GJ, et al. A randomized trial of amitriptyline and mexiletine for painful neuropathy in HIV infection. *Neurology* 1998:51; 1682-1688.

Lavoie PA, Beauchamp G, Elie R. Tricyclic antidepressants inhibit voltage-dependent calcium channels and Na^+-Ca^{2+} exchange in rat brain cortex synaptosomes. *Can J Physiol Pharmacol* 1994:68; 1414-1418.

Lynch ME. Antidepressants as analgesics: A review of random controlled trials examining analgesic effects of antidepressant agents. *J Psychiatry Neurosci* 2001: 26; 30-36.

Lynch ME, Clark AJ, Sawynok J. A pilot study examining topical amitriptyline, ketamine, and a combination of both in the treatment of neuropathic pain. *Clin J Pain* 2003:19; 323-328.

Lyness JM, Cox C, Curry J, Cornwell Y, King DA, Caine ED. Older age and underreporting of depressive symptoms. *J Am Geriatr Soc* 1995:43; 216-221.

Markowitz JS, Patrick KS. Venlafaxine-tramadol similarities. *Med Hypotheses* 1998:5; 167-168.

Max MB. Antidepressants as analgesics. In: *Progress in Pain Research and Management,* Fields HL, Liebeskind JC (eds.), Seattle: IASP Press, 1994; 229-246.

Max MB. Thirteen consecutive well-designed randomized trials show that anti-depressants reduce pain in diabetic neuropathy and postherpetic neuralgia. *Pain Forum* 1995:4; 248-253.

Max MB, Lynch SA, Muir J, Shoaf SE, Smoller B, Dubner R. Effects of desipramine, amitriptyline and fluoxetine on pain in diabetic neuropathy. *N Engl J Med* 1992:326; 1250-1256.

McCleane G. Topical application of doxepin hydrochloride can reduce the symptoms of complex regional pain syndrome: A case report. *Injury Int J Care Injured* 2002:33; 88-89.

McCleane GJ. Topical application of doxepin hydrochloride, capsaicin and a combination of both produces analgesia in chronic human neuropathic pain: A randomized, double-blind, placebo-controlled study. *Br J Clin Pharmacol* 2000a: 49; 574-579.

McCleane GJ. Topical doxepin hydrochloride reduces neuropathic pain: A randomized, double-blind, placebo controlled study. *Pain Clinic* 2000b:12; 47-50.

McQuay HJ, Tramer M, Nye BA, Carroll D, Wiffen PJ, Moore RA. A systematic review of antidepressants in neuropathic pain. *Pain* 1996:68; 217-227.

Mulrow CD, Williams JW, Chiguette E, Aguilar C, Hitchcock-Noel P, Lee S, Connell T, Stamm K. Efficacy of newer medications for treating depression in primary care practices. *Am J Med* 2000:108; 54-64.

Otsuka N, Kiuchi Y, Yokagawa F, Masuda Y, Oguchi K. Antinociceptive efficacy of antidepressants: Assessment of five antidepressants and four monoamine receptors in rats. *J Anesth* 2001:15; 154-158.

Pancrazio JJ, Kamatchi GL, Roscoe AK, Lynch C. Inhibition of neuronal Na^+ channels by antidepressant drugs. *J Pharmacol Exp Ther* 1998:248; 208-214.

Rapp SR, Parisi SA, Wallace CE. Comorbid psychiatric disorders in elderly medical patients: a one year prospective study. *J Am Geriatr Soc* 1991; 39:124-131.

Roose SP, Langhrissi-Thode F, Kennedy JS, Nelson JC, Bigger JT, Pollock BG, Gaffney A, Narayam M, Finkel MS, McCafferty J, Gergel I. Comparison of paroxetine and nortriptyline in depressed patients with ischemic heart disease. *JAMA* 1998:279; 287-291.

Sawynok J. Topical and peripherally acting analgesics. *Pharmacol Rev* 2003:55; 1-20.

Sawynok J, Esser MJ, Reid AR. Antidepressants as analgesics: An overview of central and peripheral mechanisms of action. *J Psychiatry Neurosci* 2001:26; 21-29.

Sawynok J, Reid AR, Esser MJ. Peripheral antinociceptive action of amitriptyline in the rat formalin test: Involvement of adenosine. *Pain* 1999a:80; 45-55.

Sawynok J, Reid AR, Esser MJ. Peripheral antinociceptive actions of desipramine and fluoxetine in an inflammatory and neuropathic pain test in the rat. *Pain* 1999b:82; 149-158.

Semenchuk MR, Sherman S, Davis B. Double blind randomized trial of bupropion SR for the treatment of neuropathic pain. *Neurology* 2001:57; 1583-1588.

Sierralta K, Pinardi G, Mendez M, Miranda HF. Interaction of opioids with antidepressant-induced antinociception. *Psychopharmacology* 1995:122; 374-378.

Sindrup SH. Antidepressants as analgesics. In: *Anesthesia: Biologic Foundations,* Yaksh TL, Maze M, Lynch C, Bieguyck JF, Zampol WM, Saidman LJ (eds.), Philadelphia: Lippincott-Raven, 1997; 987-997.

Sindrup SH, Bach FW, Madsen C, Gram LF, Jensen TS. Venlafaxine versus imipramine in painful polyneuropathy: A randomized, controlled trial. *Neurology* 2003:60; 1284-1289.

Sindrup SH, Bjerre U, Dejgaard A, Brosen K, Aaes-Jorgensen T, Gram LF. The selective serotonin reuptake inhibitor citalopram relieves symptoms of diabetic neuropathy. *Clin Pharmacol Ther* 1992:52; 547-552.

Sindrup SH, Gram LF, Brosen K, Eshoj O, Morgensen LF. The selective serotonin reuptake inhibitor paroxetine is effective in the treatment of diabetic neuropathy symptoms. *Pain* 1990:43; 135-144.

Sindrup SH, Gram LF, Skjold T, Froland A, Beck-Nielsen H. Concentration response relationship in imipramine treatment of diabetic neuropathy symptoms. *Clin Pharmacol Ther* 1990:47; 509-515.

Sindrup SH, Jensen TS. Pharmacologic treatment of pain in polyneuropathy. *Neurology* 2000:55; 915-920.

Skolnick P. Antidepressants for the new millennium. *Eur J Pharmacol* 1999:375; 31-40.

Song JH, Ham SS, Shin YK, Lee CS. Amitriptyline modulation of Na^+ channels in rat dorsal root ganglion neurons. *Eur J Pharmacol* 2000:401; 297-305.

Songer DA, Schule H. Venlafaxine for the treatment of chronic pain. *Am J Psychiatry* 1996:153; 737.

Sumptom JE, Moulin DE. Treatment of neuropathic pain with venlafaxine. *Ann Pharmacother* 2001:35; 557-559.

Tasmuth T, Hartel B, Kalso E. Venlafaxine in neuropathic pain following treatment of breast cancer. *Eur J Pain* 2002:6; 17-24.

Taylor K, Rowbotham MC. Venlafaxine hydrochloride and chronic pain. *Western J Med* 1996:165; 147-148.

Thase ME. Evaluating antidepressant therapies: remission as the optimum outcome. *J Clin Psychiatry* 2003; 64(Suppl 13):18-25.

Ulugol A, Karadag HC, Tamer M, Firat Z, Aslantas A, Dokmeci I. Involvement of adenosine in the anti-allodynic effect of amitriptyline in streptozotocin-induced diabetic rats. *Neurosci Lett* 2002:328; 129-132.

Yokogawa F, Kiuchi Y, Ishikawa Y, Otsuka N, Masuda Y, Oguchi K, Hosoyamada A. An investigation of monoamine receptors involved in antinociceptive effect of antidepressants. *Anesth Analg* 2002:95; 163-168.

Chapter 12

Antiepileptics

Gary McCleane

Historically, many of the drugs used to treat pain, and in particular neuropathic pain, were originally developed for other uses. The consequence of this has been that the classification originally used for these drugs has persisted, so that we now utilize antiepileptic drugs (AEDs) and tricyclic antidepressants as analgesics. Although this is of little consequence to those who specialize in pain management, to those who only occasionally treat neuropathic pain the use of drugs also used to treat significant conditions such as epilepsy can be off-putting.

Why then is there a need to use drugs such as the AEDs? Unfortunately, the analgesia produced by the opioid analgesics in patients with neuropathic pain is inconsistent. There has therefore been a need to identify other classes of medication that can more consistently provide pain relief in those with neuropathic pain. We know that epilepsy is a central nervous system disorder in which aberrant neural function manifests itself as seizure activity. Neuropathic pain has many similarities. It may become apparent when neural injury (macroscopic or microscopic, central or peripheral) occurs and produces symptoms and signs that are generated by abnormal neural function and in that respect have similarities to epilepsy. It is of little surprise, therefore, that the majority of drugs that reduce seizure frequency in patients with epilepsy can also reduce the severity of neuropathic pain. Although AEDs have a known effect on neuropathic pain, they, like the opioids, are not universally effective. Therefore, when they are used they should be used at an appropriate dose and for a defined period of time as part of a therapeutic trial. If they are ineffective at an appropriate dose, or if their benefits are outweighed by side effects, the individual AED should be discontinued and thought given to an appropriate alternative.

Clinical Management of the Elderly Patient in Pain
© 2006 by The Haworth Press, Inc. All rights reserved.
doi:10.1300/5356_12

NEUROPATHIC PAIN

As the AED's are used predominantly for neuropathic pain, some consideration of neuropathic pain and the conditions that precipitate it is now warranted. When we talk of neuropathic pain, we are describing a condition in which neural injury gives rise to pain. Such injury may be mild or major and the abnormal activity produced may be a manifestation of either underactivity or overactivity of the neural structures involved. To complicate matters, a complex system of central inhibition and facilitation comes into play in an attempt to minimize the consequences of the neural injury. Our therapeutic interventions are aimed at the aberrant neural function or at the descending inhibitory or excitatory processes.

From a practical perspective, neuropathic pain may at least be suspected when there are features of under- or overactivity of neural structures. At one extreme is numbness while at the other is allodynia (pain created by a normally nonpainful stimulus) or hyperesthesia. This allodynia may be static, where direct pressure produces pain, or dynamic, where a stroking of skin brings on discomfort. It may also be mechanical, where touch evokes pain, or thermal, where changes in temperature provoke discomfort. The consequences of developing allodynia in an elderly patient may be severe. The mere touch of clothing against skin in an allodynic area may be enough to bring on intense discomfort to the extent that clothing is no longer worn over that area. Fear of wind blowing against the skin or passersby rubbing against an allodynic area can be enough to prevent sufferers from leaving their homes, with all the social isolation that can ensue.

Other features include burning pain and shooting or lancinating pain. The latter is an episodic pain that is often unprovoked, coming on unexpectedly with a severity that can interrupt any other activity taking place at that time. Pins and needles are also common, with tingling or a discomfort often described by patients as being like a nettle sting. Formication, a feeling analogous to insects crawling over the skin, may also be present.

It would be expected that since neuropathic pain is often the result of a peripheral nerve insult, the consequent pain would be confined to a dermatomal distribution. Although this may well initially be the case, as time progresses the margins between areas where pain is and is not felt can become blurred. Furthermore, the exact areas over which the constituent symptoms and signs of neuropathic pain (numbness, allodynia, burning, shooting/lancinating and paresthesia) are experienced may vary with time, with, for example, an area of numbness being surrounded by a rim of allodynic skin evolving with time to a central area over which paresthesia is experienced with an increased depth of surrounding allodynia.

The converse of this is, however, that not all pain felt in a dermatomal distribution is neuropathic in its purest sense. A prolapsed intervertebral disk impinging on a spinal nerve root can cause neuropathic pain in a dermatomal distribution. However, inflammation of a facet joint at the same level will produce discomfort in the same dermatomal distribution that does have features of neuropathic pain but is described more in terms of a deep aching discomfort, and this is indicative of a referred rather than a radiated pain. Fortunately, drugs such as the AEDs can be as effective for such referred pain as they are for radiated neuropathic pain.

Although the majority of clinical studies investigating the effect of AEDs on neuropathic pain are carried out in patients with well-defined neuropathic pain conditions such as trigeminal neuralgia, postherpetic neuralgia, and painful diabetic neuropathy, they can be effective in any condition where the cardinal features of neuropathic pain are present. Therefore, patients with a broad range of conditions such as sciatica, cervical radiculopathy, meralgia paresthetica, and radiated pain from a vertebral collapse fracture may all benefit from treatment with an AED.

SELECTING AN AED

An increasing number of AEDs are now available, and choosing an appropriate AED can be difficult. Historically, phenytoin was the first such drug to have an analgesic effect attributed to it, although gabapentin and carbamazepine are now the most widely used. When selecting an AED, some thought needs to be given to their individual modes of action (see Table 12.1).

It should be remembered, of course, that just because investigation demonstrates an effect of a particular AED on a receptor or ion channel, that does not necessarily prove that the action is responsible for its analgesic or antiepileptic effect. Therefore, what relevance has a knowledge of these proposed sites of action? It indicates that the AEDs are a collection of drugs unified by clinical effects, that is, reduction in seizure frequency and an analgesic effect in neuropathic pain, but not always by mode of action. Even those with known sodium channel effects may not have identical clinical effects, as there are a number of different sodium channels and it is quite possible that individual AEDs target different channels. The critical issue is that a trial of one AED does not indicate the likelihood of response to any other member of the class. Therefore, in the face of therapeutic failure with one (that is, lack of analgesic effect at an appropriate dose or unacceptable side effects), it is entirely logical to try another member of this class. There is no such thing as the best AED. Each has its own merits and problems.

TABLE 12.1. Proposed sites of action of antiepileptic drugs.

AED	Site of action
Phenytoin	Sodium channel
Fosphenytoin	Sodium channel
Carbamazepine	Sodium channel
	Calcium channel
	Adenosine receptors
	Serotonin reuptake
	GABA
Oxcarbazepine	Sodium channel
	Calcium channels
	Adenosine receptors
Gabapentin	Alpha delta 2 subunit of calcium channel
Lamotrigine	Voltage-gated cation channels
	Glutamate release
	GABA release
Valproic acid	Central nervous system GABA
	Voltage-sensitive sodium channels
Harkoseride	Strychnine-sensitive glycine channels
Topiramate	Voltage-gated sodium channels
	GABA
	Voltage-gated calcium channels
	Glutamate receptors

SPECIFIC AEDs

Phenytoin and Fosphenytoin

As previously mentioned, phenytoin was the first AED to have an analgesic effect attributed to it. When used orally, tachyphylaxis can complicate use. That property, and its propensity to interfere with the protein binding and metabolism of other drugs make it not the AED of first choice. That said, it may have a place in the acute management of neuropathic pain. A parenteral formulation is available that allows it to be given either intravenously or intramuscularly in a patient with an acute flare-up of neuropathic pain or in whom the oral route is not available.

Unfortunately, the parenteral formulation of phenytoin contains sodium hydroxide and ethylene glycol among its diluents, giving it a highly alkaline pH. Numerous reports of skin necrosis caused by inadvertent extravascular, subcutaneous administration remind us that extreme care needs to be practiced when it is used by the intravenous route.

In an attempt to mitigate this problem, a water-soluble, ester prodrug of phenytoin has been produced. This fosphenytoin has a near-normal pH and is not associated with the danger of skin necrosis if it escapes from a vein. Its major immediate complication is a burning discomfort that is most marked in areas of the body, such as the perineum, where the concentration of phosphatases, which are responsible for its metabolism and activation, are highest. Fosphenytoin is labeled both in milligrams and phenytoin equivalent units (PE units). The reason for this is that phenytoin and fosphenytoin are not milligram-for-milligram equivalent, and 1 mg of phenytoin is equal to 1 PE unit of fosphenytoin. For acute management of a flare-up of neuropathic pain, a single 500 PE unit intramuscular injection of fosphenytoin can be effective.

Carbamazepine

Until recently the most widely used AED in the management of neuropathic pain, carbamazepine has the advantage of enormous clinical experience with its use. Structurally a tricyclic with close similarities to tricyclic antidepressants such as amitriptyline, carbamazepine achieves at least some of its effect by blocking sodium channels. Although undoubtedly effective in many neuropathic conditions, because of its side-effect profile patients may be willing to use it in effective doses during an acute flare-up, but not so willing to use it at effective doses as a prophylactic against subsequent flare-ups during more quiescent periods. Side effects that seem more prevalent in the elderly patient include water retention, decreased osmolality, and hyponatremia.

Carbamazepine is extensively metabolized in the liver, with only about 1 percent of the administered dose being excreted in an unchanged form. Although one would intuitively expect the clearance of any drug to be reduced in the elderly patient, carbamazepine is one of the few analgesic drugs for which clinical studies have verified this. Battino and colleagues (2003) concluded that the oral clearance of carbamazepine is decreased in an age-dependent manner in elderly patients when compared to younger subjects. They postulate that this may be due to a reduction in CYP3A4-mediated drug metabolism. Even with this reduction in drug metabolism, elderly patients retain their sensitivity to dose-dependent autoinduction of other liver enzymes, and their metabolic rates remain considerably below those observed in younger patients.

Oxcarbazepine

Oxcarbazepine is a keto derivative of carbamazepine that is rapidly metabolized to its active form. It appears to be at least as effective as carbamazepine and yet would appear to have fewer side effects. Approximately one in five elderly patients may expect to suffer nausea with its use, with occasional patients developing hyponatremia (a side effect also associated with the use of carbamazepine). The incidence of such hyponatremia seems to be greater if the patient is also taking a natriuretic drug.

Gabapentin

Extensive evidence testifies to a potential analgesic effect of gabapentin in patients with neuropathic pain. Rapid dose escalation is said to decrease the duration of the most prominent side effects of this drug, sedation and light-headedness. Initial rapid titration to 1800 mg daily with further increases up to 3600 mg daily can be tried. This drug has few known drug-drug interactions and is safe even in overdose. However, caution with its side effects of cognitive impairment and sedation are particularly important in elderly patients.

Lamotrigine

Perhaps the most prominent side effect seen when lamotrigine is used is skin rash. This may be minor and not interfere with continued use or may be more severe and dictate discontinuation of the drug. The incidence of skin rash seems to be related to the rate of increase in drug dose. Immediate use of a potentially therapeutic dose is complicated by skin rash in approximately one in five patients, whereas more gradual increase may reduce this rate to one in twenty. It is likely that a response to lamotrigine is dependent on reaching a certain dose level. Therefore the relationship between effect and dose is not linear. Few will get relief at a small dose; approximately one in three when a dose of 300 mg per day is reached. Other side effects individual to lamotrigine include glandular enlargement and insomnia. This insomnia is in marked contrast to many other AEDs, which tend to cause sedation.

From a practical perspective, lamotrigine can be commenced at a dose of 50 mg daily, increasing by 50 mg on a weekly basis to an initial daily total of 300 mg. If no relief is apparent within two weeks on 300 mg per day, then it is unlikely that sustained use will offer any relief, and it should be discontinued. Because of its long half-life, once-daily dosing is acceptable.

Valproic Acid

The evidence that valproic acid is effective in patients with neuropathic pain is mixed, with some studies showing no benefit while others are more positive. Perhaps its major advantage is that it is generally well tolerated and rapid dose escalation is possible. Because of this, only a short treatment period is required to decide whether it is helpful or not.

Clonazepam

Available in both oral and parenteral formulations, clonazepam tends to cause sedation. As well as potential analgesic properties it may have muscle relaxant effects and cause anterograde amnesia. It may therefore have a role in promoting sleep by virtue of its hypnotic effect, with the added advantage of providing analgesia. Its long half-life may lead to a hangover effect on the morning after administration.

Topiramate

One of the newer AEDs, topiramate has mechanisms of action which would suggest that it may be useful, although the results from human studies have been mixed. Psychosis is a recognized side effect that may discourage use.

SIDE EFFECTS OF AEDs

Side effects specific to individual AEDs have already been mentioned. However, some side effects are potentially common to all AEDs. One of these is cognitive impairment. This issue has been extensively investigated in patients with epilepsy, and the lessons learned from these investigations give some guidance when it comes to patients with neuropathic pain. That said, epilepsy and neuropathic pain, while having some similarities, are different conditions, and the issue of cognitive impairment in patients with epilepsy is complicated by effects of the epilepsy itself, frequent seizures, and psychological issues. However, it does appear that in general the newer AEDs have less effect on cognitive function than the older AEDs. Therefore, oxcarbazepine may be preferable to carbamazepine, while gabapentin and lamotrigine may have less effect on cognitive function than phenytoin.

Interestingly, the effect of AEDs on cognitive function is not necessarily dose related, and some caution is therefore needed during the titration phase of treatment. Table 12.2 lists suggested dosing regimens for the antiepileptic drugs discussed in this chapter.

Another side effect often attributed to AEDs is weight gain. Review of this feature has concluded that valproic acid and carbamazepine can increase weight, and lamotrigine and phenytoin are weight neutral, while topiramate is associated with weight loss.

EXAMPLES OF CONDITIONS THAT MAY RESPOND TO USE OF AN AED

In general, any condition that has the features of neuropathic pain may respond to the use of an AED. Unfortunately, our depth of knowledge does not, as yet, inform us which drug is most likely to be effective for particular features of neuropathic pain. For example, we do not yet have a particular drug that is known to be most effective for pins and needles, burning pain, and so on. AEDs may also be effective for referred pain, such as that arising from ligamentous trauma in the back or from an osteoporotic fracture of the spine.

TABLE 12.2. Suggested dosing regimens for antiepileptic drugs.

AED	Route of administration	Unit dose	Rate of dose increase	Total daily dose
Phenytoin	IV/IM	200 mg		Stat dose
Fosphenytoin	IV/IM	500 PE units		Stat dose
Carbamazepine	Oral	100 mg	From 100 mg twice daily increasing every second day by 200 mg	800 mg
Oxcarbazepine	Oral	150 mg	Increasing by 150 mg every third day	600 mg
Gabapentin	Oral	300 mg	Every third day	1800-2400 mg
Lamotrigine	Oral	50 mg	Every week	300 mg
Valproic acid	Oral	200 mg	Every second day	800 mg
Clonazepam	Oral	0.5 mg	Every second day	1.5 mg

Postherpetic Neuralgia

A proportion of patients who suffer from shingles go on to suffer from postherpetic neuralgia. The proportion who will develop this neuralgia increases with advancing age. There is a greater evidence base for the use of AEDs in postherpetic neuralgia than almost any other neuropathic condition.

Painful Diabetic Neuropathy

Again, substantial evidence points to a reasonable chance of success when AEDs are used for painful diabetic neuropathy. Of course, good glycemic control is desirable. The neuropathic pain seen in diabetic patients may be caused directly by the diabetes but may also be related to the vascular disease that complicates diabetes. Such ischemic neuritis often has a strong allodynic and burning component, and attempts to improve limb perfusion are important. That said, because the neural damage that occurs with this ischemia may not be reversible, an improvement in circulation is not always accompanied by a reduction in neuropathic pain.

Trigeminal Neuralgia

The intensity of the facial pain of trigeminal neuralgia may be of a severity to stop patients from eating, washing, or leaving their homes. Allodynia and shooting or lancinating pain are particularly associated with the condition.

Cervical Radiculopathy

With osteoarthritis being prevalent in elderly patients, impingement of a nerve traversing through a lateral recess or the spinal canal by an osteophyte is not that unusual. Consequent neuropathic pain in an upper limb is then common. AEDs may palliate this pain, but of course no analgesic treatment is going to lessen the nerve pressure caused by the osteophyte.

Lumbar Radiculopathy

We are used to seeing lumbar radiculopathy as a consequence of prolapsed intervertebral disk in younger patients. The same event can occur in older subjects but more often the actual origin of the neuropathic pain is harder to define. Degenerative disease increases in incidence as age advances. Ligamentous thickening, facet joint arthritis, spinal stenosis, and pathology at multiple spinal levels are all more common. If there is radiated or referred pain, a trial of an AED is still warranted.

Spinal Stenosis

Radicular pain exacerbated by lying down and associated with limb weakness on exercise all suggest spinal stenosis. This stenosis may be due to congenital narrowness of the spinal canal but may also be due to prolapsed intervertebral disk, ligamentous thickening, or osteophyte intrusion into the spinal canal. Of particular note in elderly patients is the association between the symptoms of spinal stenosis and the presence of an epidural metastatic deposit. As the epidural veins form a portal circulation between the pelvic viscera and the brain, deposits are not particularly unusual. A heightened awareness should be present when the radicular symptoms are gradually worsening and when there are concomitant symptoms and signs suggestive of cancer elsewhere.

Vertebral Collapse Fracture

Vertebral collapse fracture, whether secondary to tumor infiltration or osteoporosis, may give rise to a number of different causes of pain. The bony pain that initially accompanies fracture usually settles after a few weeks. Persistent pain may arise from ligamentous strains, usually from the interspinous ligament or facet joint irritation. With fracture, a change in vertebral architecture occurs that can throw abnormal stresses on the vertebral column and those structures such as ligaments and joints that are integral in vertebral function.

In addition, nipping of intercostal nerves can occur, giving rise to neuropathic pain in a dermatomal distribution. Facet joint irritation can give rise to referred pain in a similar distribution. These referred and radiated pains can respond to AEDs. However, difficulty often arises because of the distribution of the referred or radiated pain. If the 12th thoracic vertebra collapses, for example, the consequent pain along the 12th thoracic dermatome can be confused with renal or ureteric colic, appendicitis, ovarian pain, or pain from an inguinal or femoral hernia. Therefore, a level of awareness needs to be maintained that such pain may be radiated or referred from the spine or may be due to pathology of viscera at a similar level.

Although many other conditions could be mentioned, the overall principle is that any condition exhibiting features of neuropathic pain warrants a trial on an AED.

CONCLUSION

Antiepileptic drugs are a fairly diverse group of drugs unified by an ability to lessen epileptic seizures, and to varying degrees lessen neuropathic pain, regardless of its exact etiology.

Since these drugs have varying modes of action, no one is universally superior to the others. Personal preference is perhaps the major influence in deciding which AED to try first. Each AED is associated with differing side effects and therefore if one fails to produce analgesia at a reasonable dose, or produces unacceptable side effects, then a trial with a different agent is warranted. Lack of response to any dictates that it should be discontinued. There is no place for sustained treatment in the face of therapeutic failure.

BIBLIOGRAPHY

Aldenkamp AP. Effects of antiepileptic drugs on cognition. *Epilepsia* 2001; 42S: 46-49.

Aldenkamp AP, De Krom M, Reijs R. Newer antiepileptic drugs and cognitive issues. *Epilepsia* 2003; 44S: 21-29.

Ambrosio AF, Soaras-de-Silva P, Carvalho CM, Carvalho AP. Mechanisms of action of carbamazepine and its derivatives, oxcarbazepine, BIA 2-093, and BIA 2-024. *Neurochem Res* 2002; 27: 121-130.

Backonja M, Beydoun A, Edwards KR, Schwartz SL, Fonseca V, Hes M, LaMoreaux L, Garofalo E. Gabapentin for the treatment of painful neuropathy in patients with diabetes mellitus. *JAMA* 1998; 280: 1831-1836.

Backonja M-M. Anticonvulsants (antineuropathics) for neuropathic pain syndromes. *Clin J Pain* 2000; S16: 67-72.

Bartusch SL, Sanders BJ, D'Alessio JG, Jernigan JR. Clonazepam for the treatment of lancinating limb pain. *Clin J Pain* 1996; 12: 59-62.

Battino D, Coroci D, Rossinin A, Messina S, Mamoli D, Perucca E. Serum carbamazepine concentrations in elderly patients: A case matched pharmacokinetic evaluation based on therapeutic drug monitoring data. *Epilepsia* 2003; 44: 923-929.

Biton V. Effect of antiepileptic drugs on bodyweight: overview and clinical implications for the treatment of epilepsy. *CNS Drugs* 2003; 17: 781-791.

Brown JP, Boden P, Singh L, Gee NS. Mechanisms of action of gabapentin. *Rev Contemp Pharmacother* 1996; 7: 203-214.

Campbell FG, Graham JG, Zilkha KJ. Clinical trial of carbazepine (Tegretol) in trigeminal neuralgia. *J Neurol Neurosurg Psychiat* 1966; 29: 265-267.

Canavero S, Bonicalzi V. Lamotrigine control of central pain. *Pain* 1996; 68: 179-181.

Canavero S, Bonicalzi V. Lamotrigine control of trigeminal neuralgia: An expanded study. *J Neurol* 1997; 244: 527-532.

Canavero S, Bonicalzi V, Ferroli P, Zeme S, Montalenti E, Benna P. Lamotrigine control of idiopathic trigeminal neuralgia. *J Neurol Neurosurg Psychiat* 1995; 59: 646.

Carlton SM, Zhou S. Attenuation of formalin-induced nociceptive behaviors following local peripheral injection of gabapentin. *Pain* 1998; 76: 201-207.

Chang VT. Intravenous phenytoin in the management of crescendo pelvic cancer related pain. *J Pain Symptom Manage* 1997; 13: 238-240.

Chapman V, Wildman MA, Dickenson AH. Distinct electrophysiological effects of two spinally administered membrane stabilizing drugs, bupivicaine and lamotrigine. *Pain* 1997; 71: 285-295.

Cheshire WP. Fosphenytoin: An intravenous option for the management of acute trigeminal neuralgia crisis. *J Pain Symptom Manage* 2001; 21: 506-510.

Cunningham MO, Jones RSG. The anticonvulsant, lamotrigine decreases spontaneous glutamate release but increases spontaneous GABA release in the rat entorhinal cortex in vivo. *Neuropharmacology* 2000; 39: 2139-2146.

De Toledo JC, Lowe MR, Rabinstein A, Villaviza N. Cardiac arrest after fast intravenous infusion of phenytoin mistaken for fosphenytoin. *Epilepsia* 2001; 42: 288.

Devulder J, De Latt M. Lamotrigine in the treatment of chronic refractory neuropathic pain. *J Pain Symptom Manage* 2000; 19: 398-403.

Devulder J, Lambert J, Naeyaert JM. Gabapentin for control in cancer patients wound dressing care. *J Pain Symptom Manage* 2001; 22: 622-626.

Dickenson AH, Mathews EA, Suzuki R. Neurobiology of neuropathic pain: mode of action of anticonvulsants. *Eur J Pain* 2002; 6S: 51-60.

Drewes AM, Andreasen A, Poulsen LH. Valproate for treatment of chronic central pain after spinal cord injury: A double-blind cross-over study. *Paraplegia* 1994; 32: 565-569.

Eisenberg E, Lurie Y, Braker C, Daoud D, Ishay A. Lamotrigine reduces painful diabetic neuropathy: A randomized, controlled study. *Neurology* 2001; 57: 505-509.

Field MJ, Oles RJ, Lewis ASD, McCleary S, Hughes J, Singh L. Gabapentin (neurontin) and S-(+)-3-isobutylgaba represent a novel class of selective antihyperalgesic agents. *Br J Pharmacol* 1997; 121: 1513-1522.

Finnerup NB, Sindrup SH, Bach FW, Johannesen IL, Jensen TS. Lamotrigine in spinal cord injury pain: A randomized controlled trial. *Pain* 2002; 96: 375-383.

Fischer JH, Barr AN, Rogers SL, Fischer PA, Trudeau VL. Lack of serious toxicity following gabapentin overdose. *Neurology* 1994; 44: 982-983.

Gee NS, Brown JP, Dissanayake VU, Offord J, Thurlow R, Woodruff GN. The novel anticonvulsant drug, gabapentin (Neurontin), binds to the alpha delta 2 sub unit of a calcium channel. *J Biol Chem* 1996; 271: 5768-5776.

Goldberg JF, Burdick KE. Cognitive side effects of anticonvulsants. *J Clin Psychiatry* 2001; 62S: 27-33.

Grunze H, Wegener J, Greene RW, Walden J. Modulation of calcium and potassium currents by lamotrigine. *Neuropsychobiology* 1998; 38: 131-138.

Hill DR, Suman-Chauhan N, Woodruff GN. Localization of [3H] gabapentin to a novel site in rat brain: Autoradiographic studies. *Eur J Pharmacol* 1993; 244: 303-309.

Hirsch E, Schmitz B, Carreno M. Epilepsy, antiepileptic drugs (AEDs) and cognition. *Acta Neurol Scand* 2003; 108S: 23-32.

Houtchens MK, Richert JR, Sami A, Rose JW. Open label gabapentin treatment for pain in multiple sclerosis. *Multiple Sclerosis* 1997; 3: 250-253.

Hunter JC, Gogas KR, Hedley LR, Jacobson LO, Kassotakis L, Thompson J, Fontana DJ. The effect of novel anti epileptic drugs in rat experimental models of acute and chronic pain. *Eur J Pharmacol* 1997; 324: 153-160.

Jensen T. Anticonvulsants in neuropathic pain: rationale and clinical evidence. *Eur J Pain* 2002; 6S: 61-68.

Jun JH, Yaksh TL. The effect of intrathecal gabapentin and 3-isobutyl gamma amino butyric acid on the hyperalgesia observed after thermal injury in the rat. *Anesth Analg* 1998; 86: 348-354.

Khan OA. Gabapentin relieves trigeminal neuralgia in multiple sclerosis patients. *Neurology* 1998; 51: 611-614.

Kutluay E, McCague K, D'Souza J, Beydoun A. Safety and tolerability of oxcarbazepine in elderly patients with epilepsy. *Epilepsy Behav* 2003; 4: 175-180.

Lang DG, Wang CM, Cooper BR. Lamotrigine, phenytoin and carbamazepine interactions on the sodium current present in N4TG1 mouse neuroblastoma cells. *J Pharmacol Exp Ther* 1993; 266: 829-835.

Leandri M, Lunardi G, Inglese M, Messmer-Uccelli M, Mancardi GL, Gottlieb A, Solar C. Lamotrigine in trigeminal neuralgia secondary to multiple sclerosis. *J Neurol* 2000; 247: 556-558.

Lees G, Leach MJ. Studies on the mechanisms of action of the novel anticonvulsant lamotrigine (Lamictal) using primary neuroglial cultures from rat cortex. *Brain Res* 1993; 612: 190-199.

Lunardi G, Leandri M, Albano C, Cultera S, Fracassi M, Rubino V, Favale E. Clinical effectiveness of lamotrigine and plasma levels in essential and symptomatic trigeminal neuralgia. *Neurology* 1997; 48: 1714-1717.

Luo ZD, Calcutt NA, Higuera ES, Valder CR, Song YH, Svensson CI, Myers RR. Injury type specific calcium channel alpha delta 2 subunit up regulation in rat neuropathic pain models correlates with antiallodynic effects of gabapentin. *J Pharmacol Exp Ther* 2002; 303: 1199-1205.

Macdonald RL, Kelly KM. Antiepileptic drug mechanisms of action. *Epilepsia* 1995; 36S: 2-12.

Maneuf YP, Hughes J, McKnight AT. Gabapentin inhibits the substance P facilitated K^+ evoked release of [^{3}H] glutamate from rat caudal trigeminal nucleus slices. *Pain* 2001; 93: 191-196.

Martin R, Meador K, Turrentine L, Faught E, Sinclair K, Kuzniecky R, Gilliam F. Comparative cognitive effects of carbamazepine and gabapentin in healthy senior adults. *Epilepsia* 2001; 42: 764-771.

McCleane GJ. Gabapentin reduces chronic benign nociceptive pain: A double blind, placebo controlled crossover study. *Pain Clinic* 2000; 12: 81-85.

McCleane GJ. Intramuscular fosphenytoin reduces neuropathic pain: A randomized, double-blind, placebo-controlled, crossover study. *Analgesia* 1999; 4: 479-482.

McCleane GJ. Intravenous fosphenytoin relieves chronic neuropathic pain: A double-blind, placebo-controlled, crossover trial. *Analgesia* 2000; 5: 45-48.

McCleane GJ. Intravenous infusion of fosphenytoin produces prolonged pain relief: A case report. *J Pain* 2002; 3: 156-158.

McCleane GJ. Intravenous infusion of phenytoin relieves neuropathic pain: A randomized, double-blind, placebo-controlled crossover study. *Anesth Analg* 1999; 89: 985-988.

McCleane GJ. Lamotrigine can remove the pain associated with painful diabetic neuropathy. *Pain Clinic* 1999; 11: 69-70.

McCleane GJ. The symptoms of complex regional pain syndrome type 1 alleviated with lamotrigine: A report of 8 cases. *J Pain* 2000; 1: 171-173.

McGraw T, Kosek P. Erythromyalgia pain managed with gabapentin. *Anesthesiology* 1997; 86: 988-990.

McGraw T, Stacey BR. Gabapentin for treatment of neuropathic pain in a 12-year-old girl. *Clin J Pain* 1998; 14: 354-356.

McLean MJ. Clinical pharmacokinetics of gabapentin. *Neurology* 1994; 44: S17-S22.

McQuay H, Carroll D, Jadad ER, Wiffen P, Moore A. Anticonvulsant drugs for management of pain: A systematic review. *BMJ* 1995; 311: 1047-1052.

Mellick GA, Mellick LB. Reflex sympathetic dystrophy treated with gabapentin. *Arch Phys Rehabil* 1997; 78: 98-105.

Mellick GA, Seng ML. The use of gabapentin in the treatment of reflex sympathetic dystrophy and a phobic disorder. *Am J Pain Manage* 1995; 5: 7-9.

Mercadante S. Gabapentin in spinal cord injury pain. *Pain Clinic* 1998; 10: 203-206.

Morello CM, Leckband SG, Stoner CP, Moorhouse DF, Sahagian GA. Randomized double blind study comparing the efficacy of gabapentin with amitriptyline on diabetic peripheral neuropathy pain. *Arch Intern Med* 1999; 159: 1931-1937.

Nakamura-Craig M, Follenfant RL. Effect of lamotrigine in the acute and chronic hyperalgesia induced by PGE2 and in the chronic hyperalgesia in rats with streptozotocin induced diabetes. *Pain* 1995; 63: 33-37.

Norton JW. Gabapentin withdrawal syndrome. *Clin Neuropharmacol* 2001; 24: 245-246.

Novelli GP, Trovati F. Gabapentin and neuropathic pain. *Pain Clinic* 1998; 11: 5-32.

Pan H-L, Eisenach JC, Chen S-R. Gabapentin suppresses ectopic nerve discharges and reverses allodynia in neuropathic rats. *J Pharmacol Exp Ther* 1999; 288: 1026-1030.

Pandey CK, Bose N, Garg G, Singh N, Baronia A, Agarwal A, Singh PK, Singh U. Gabapentin for the treatment of pain in Guillain-Barre syndrome: A double-blind, placebo-controlled, crossover study. *Anesth Analg* 2002; 95: 1719-1723.

Partridge BJ, Chaplan SR, Sakamoto E, Yaksh TL. Characterization of the effects of gabapentin and 3-isobutyl gamma amino butyric acid on substance P induced thermal hyperalgesia. *Anesthesiology* 1998; 88: 196-205.

Patel J, Naritoku DK. Gabapentin for the treatment of hemifacial spasm. *Clin Neuropharmacol* 1996; 19: 185-188.

Rosner H, Rubin L, Kestenbaum A. Gabapentin adjunctive therapy in neuropathic pain states. *Clin J Pain* 1996; 12: 56-58.

Rowbotham M, Harden N, Stacey B, Bernstein P, Magnus-Miller L. Gabapentin for the treatment of postherpetic neuralgia: A randomized controlled trial. *JAMA* 1998; 280: 1837-1842.

Samkoff LM, Daras M, Tuchman AJ, Koppell BS. Amelioration of refractory dysesthetic limb pain in multiple sclerosis by gabapentin. *Neurology* 1997; 49: 304-305.

Schachter SC, Carrazana EJ. Treatment of facial pain with gabapentin. *J Epilepsy* 1997; 10: 148-149.

Schachter SC, Sauter MK. Treatment of central pain with gabapentin. *J Epilepsy* 1996; 9: 223-226.

Segal AZ, Rordorf G. Gabapentin as a novel treatment for postherpetic neuralgia. *Neurology* 1996; 46: 1175-1176.

Serpell MG, Neuropathic Pain Study Group. Gabapentin in neuropathic pain syndromes: A randomized, double-blind, placebo-controlled trial. *Pain* 2002; 99: 557-566.

Shimoyama N, Shimoyama M, Davis AM, Inturrisi CE, Elliott KJ. Spinal gabapentin is antinociceptive in the rat formalin test. *Neurosci Lett* 1997; 222: 65-67.

Shuaib A, Mahmood RH, Wishart T, Kanthan R, Murabit MA, Ijaz S, Miyashita H, Howlett W. Neuroprotective effects of lamotrigine in global ischemia in gerbils: A histological, in vivo microdialysis and behavioral study. *Brain Res* 1995; 702: 199-206.

Simpson DM, Olney R, McArthur JC, Khan A, Godbold J, Ebel-Frommer K. A placebo-controlled trial of lamotrigine for painful HIV associated neuropathy. *Neurology* 2000; 54: 2115-2119.

Singh L, Field MJ, Ferris P, Hunter JC, Oles RJ, Williams RG, Woodruff GN. The antiepileptic agent gabapentin (Neurontin) possess anxiolytic-like and antinociceptive actions that are reversed by D serine. *Psychopharmacology* 1996; 127: 1-9.

Sist T, Filadora V, Miner M, Lema M. Gabapentin for idiopathic trigeminal neuralgia: report of two cases. *Neurology* 1997; 48: 1467-1471.

Sist TC, Filadora VA, Miner M, Lema M. Experience with gabapentin for neuropathic pain in the head and neck: Report of 10 cases. *Reg Anesth* 1997; 22: 473-478.

Soderpalm B. Anticonvulsants: Aspects of their mechanisms of action. *Eur J Pain* 2002; 6S: 3-9.

Sotelo JC, Isanta MR, Felip M, Gimeno EB. Use of lamotrigine in a first line treatment for dysesthetic neuropathic pain. *Analgesia* 2000; 5: 61-62.

Stanfa LC, Singh L, Williams RG, Dickenson AH. Gabapentin, ineffective in normal rats, markedly reduces C fiber evoked responses after inflammation. *NeuroReport* 1997; 8: 587-590.

Taylor CP, Vartanian MG, Yuen PW, Bigge C, Suman-Chauhan N, Hill DR. Potent and stereospecific anticonvulsant activity of 3-isobutyl GABA relates to in vitro binding at a novel site labeled by tritiated gabapentin. *Epilepsy Res* 1993; 14: 11-15.

Taylor JC, Brauer S, Espir ML. Long term treatment of trigeminal neuralgia with carbamazepine. *Postgrad Med J* 1981; 57: 16-18.

Teoh H, Fowler LJ, Bowery NG. Effect of lamotrigine on the electrically evoked release of endogenous amino acids from slices of dorsal horn of the rat spinal cord. *Neuropharmacology* 1995; 34: 1273-1278.

Vestergaard K, Andersen G, Gottrup H, Kristensen BT, Jensen TS. Lamotrigine for central poststroke pain: A randomized controlled trial. *Neurology* 2001; 56: 184-190.

Werner MU, Perkins FM, Holte K, Pedersen JL, Kehlet H. Effects of gabapentin in acute inflammatory pain in humans. *Reg Anesth Pain Med* 2001; 26: 322-328.

Wiard RP, Dickerson MC, Beek O, Norton R, Cooper BR. Neuroprotective properties of the novel antiepileptic lamotrigine in a gerbil model of global cerebral ischaemia. *Stroke* 1995; 26: 466-472.

Xiao WH, Bennett G. Gabapentin has an antinociceptive effect mediated via a spinal site of action in a rat model of painful peripheral neuropathy. *Analgesia* 1996; 2: 267-273.

Zakrzewska JM, Chaudhry Z, Nurmikko TJ, Patton DW, Mullens EL. Lamotrigine (Lamictal) in refractory trigeminal neuralgia: Results from a double-blind placebo-controlled crossover trial. *Pain* 1997; 73: 223-230.

Zapp JJ. Poliomyeltitis pain treated with gabapentin. *Am Fam Physician* 1996; 53: 2442-2443.

Chapter 13

Spinal Analgesia in the Elderly

Thomas M. Larkin
Steven P. Cohen

DEFINITIONS

A major difficulty in reviewing spinal analgesia in the elderly lies in the fact that most clinical studies have not focused on the elderly per se. Instead, most studies cover a broad range of ages and do not separately analyze the neuraxial effects of drugs in this population. In addition, most of the pharmacology literature in the elderly is limited to the pharmacodynamic and pharmacokinetic effects of oral and parenteral medications. Thus, the effect of spinal analgesia in the elderly is for the most part an unexplored clinical area.

Epidemiology

The percentage of elderly people in the United States continues to grow. In 1900, those over 65 years of age comprised 4.1 percent of the population. Today, nearly 12.5 percent of the population is over the age of 65 (U.S. Census Bureau, 2000). This tremendous growth makes the elderly the fastest-growing segment of the U.S. population. This trend is mirrored in other industrialized countries and reflects steadily increasing life expectancies in developed nations. In 2000, the average life expectancy in the United States was 77.1 years (Kinsella and Velkoff, 2002). Since this trend shows no signs of abating, it is imperative that physicians understand the unique challenges posed by this rapidly growing group of patients.

Chronic Pain in the Elderly

As people age, they are more likely to suffer from chronic pain. The prevalence of chronic pain is estimated to be between 25 percent and

Clinical Management of the Elderly Patient in Pain
© 2006 by The Haworth Press, Inc. All rights reserved.
doi:10.1300/5356_13

50 percent in community-dwelling older persons. Among nursing home residents, the prevalence is even higher, ranging from 45 percent to 80 percent (Helm and Gibson, 1997; Fox, Raina, and Jadad, 1999). The two most common causes of pain in the elderly are rheumatological diseases and malignant pain. It is in the latter group that intrathecal medications were first used as long-term analgesics (Onofrio, Yaksh, and Arnold, 1981). It is estimated that 70 percent of all cancer patients will experience significant pain in the terminal stages of their illness (Foley, 1985). Other common causes of chronic pain in the elderly include herpes zoster, postherpetic neuralgia, peripheral vascular disease, and diabetic neuropathy.

PHYSIOLOGICAL CONSIDERATIONS

In managing elderly patients, one must take into account the inevitable changes that occur in aging organ systems. Compared with systemic delivery systems, the senescent changes in organ function have less impact on the pharmacodynamics and pharmacokinetics of neuraxial delivery due to the lower doses of drugs administered. However, this aphorism may be less applicable to age-associated central nervous system (CNS) changes.

Central nervous system changes are common in the elderly, especially those requiring assisted living. In the brain, there is a generalized loss of nervous tissue with a concomitant increase in water content. The degree of neuronal loss is controversial, but is estimated to be 10 percent (Pakkenberg and Gundersen, 1997). Over the age range of 30 to 90 years, the volume losses are about 14 percent in the cortex, 35 percent in the hippocampus, and 26 percent in cerebral white matter (Esiri et al., 1997). Accompanying these changes are reductions in CNS cholinergic, serotonergic, and catecholamine neurotransmitter levels (Baxter et al., 1999; Terry and Buccafusco, 2003; Haycock et al., 2003). These widespread changes may have myriad effects on the elderly patient's behavioral, cognitive, sensory, and motor function.

Although intrathecal delivery is less affected by the age-related diminution in organ function than parenteral or oral routes of administration, this does not mean it is devoid of potential age-related adverse effects. This is particularly true with regard to the CNS effects of neuraxially injected hydrophilic medications. These medications are more slowly redistributed to the plasma compartment and are therefore more apt to diffuse rostrally to the brain (Nordberg et al., 1983). Consequently, centrally delivered hydrophilic drugs tend to have side effect profiles similar to much larger doses of systemic medications. Systemic effects should also be taken into account for epidurally injected lipophilic drugs, as the plasma concentrations may approach those following parenteral administration (Bernards, 2002). Considering these factors, the starting dose of neuraxial medications in the elderly should be lower than in similar patients of lesser age (Krames, 2002).

ANATOMICAL CONSIDERATIONS

Anatomical alterations in the aged spine can present unique challenges for neuraxial anesthesia. As the spine ages, intervertebral disks lose height and elastic capacity and begin to bulge into the spinal canal. This results in a redistribution of weight to the vertebral end plate and facet joints. This in turn leads to hypertrophy of the facet joints which, when combined with ligamentum flavum hypertrophy, can further exacerbate spinal stenosis. If severe, the reduced size of the epidural space can lead to compression of the dural sac, impeding the flow of cerebrospinal fluid (CSF). Aging is also associated with decreased flexibility of the spine, increased lumbar lordosis, and calcification of spinal ligaments (Okada et al., 1993). These changes can all serve to make the technical performance of spinal injections very challenging. When the stenosis is above the injection site, it can also impede rostral spread of anesthetics. The obstruction of CSF flow is considered by some but not all practitioners to be a relative contraindication to implanted drug delivery systems (Levy, 1999).

NEURAXIAL ANALGESICS IN PERIOPERATIVE AND CHRONIC PAIN CONDITIONS

It is imperative to distinguish between the two main situations where neuraxial analgesics are utilized: perioperatively and in chronic pain states. The perioperative use of intrathecal analgesics is widespread. Consequently, most studies addressing the effects of spinal analgesics, and virtually all those with elderly cohorts, have been conducted in this setting.

Intrathecal therapy for chronic pain is a more recent phenomenon. Over the past 10 years the use in this setting has grown tremendously, especially in nonmalignant pain. Although the following sections describe the use of multiple agents (often in combination) for intrathecal therapy, only morphine is approved for long-term spinal delivery. No studies have specifically addressd the long-term effects of neuraxial medications in elderly patients.

LOCAL ANESTHETICS

The most widely utilized spinal analgesics are local anesthetics, which are used for both surgical anesthesia and pain relief. The mechanism of action by which local anesthetics provide analgesia is the blockade of sodium channels, the sentinel event in the depolarization of neurons. Thus, local anesthetics are capable of blocking the transmission of all nerve fibers, not just the A-delta and C fibers responsible for pain. With aging, neuronal population declines in the spinal cord and conduction velocities decrease (Dorfman and Bosley, 1979). This should make the elderly more sensitive to the effects of local anesthetics. This observation has been borne out in studies comparing the effects of local anesthetics in elderly and younger cohorts with epidural anesthesia. Older patients have a tendency to develop higher, denser blocks as well as a greater propensity for hypotension and bradycardia (Simon et al., 2002; Veering et al., 1992). This has led to the recommendation that local anesthetic doses be reduced in older patients.

Several studies demonstrate good long-term outcomes using off-label mixtures of opioids and bupivacaine (Deer et al., 2002; Hildebrand, Elsberry, and Deer, 2001; van Dongen, Crul, and van Egmond, 1999). The benefits associated with these combinations include lower intrathecal and oral opioid requirements, better relief of neuropathic pain, and slower development of tolerance. The neurological deficits observed with long-term bupivacaine infusions have been minimal. In one study involving 106 subjects, the only neurological finding was nondermatomal numbness that resolved after removal of bupivacaine (Deer et al., 2002). Typical daily dosages of bupivacaine range from 0.5 to 2.5 mg per day (Bennett, Serafini, et al., 2000; Bennett, Burchiel, et al., 2000).

Although there are no comparison trials for neuraxial opioid–local anesthetic combinations between elderly and younger cohorts, no age-related differences have been noted in the existing studies. We therefore conclude that it is safe to proceed with these combinations using lower starting dosages.

OPIOIDS

Opioid analgesics exert their actions through inhibition of target cell activity. Mediating these effects are three endogenous opioid receptors, mu (μ), delta (δ), and kappa (κ). Although peripherally located opioid receptors have been identified, the predominant analgesic sites are believed to be in the CNS. In the brain, these receptor sites include the brainstem, thalamus, forebrain, and mesencephalon. In the substantia gelatinosa, they include postsynaptic receptors located on cells originating in the dorsal horn of the spinal cord, as well as presynaptic receptors found on the spinal terminals of primary afferent fibers.

The effects of opioids are determined not only by their affinity for endogenous receptors but by their ability to reach those receptors. The onset of analgesia is similar for intrathecal and epidural narcotics, suggesting that the penetration of neural tissue (and not dura) is the rate-limiting step. Intrathecal opioids exert their analgesic properties by presynaptically inhibiting the release of substance P and calcitonin gene-related peptide, neuropeptides believed to be responsible for transmitting nociceptive signals across synapses. They also work by hyperpolarizing postsynaptic neurons. Epidurally administered narcotics may work by an additional mechanism. The systemic absorption of an epidural bolus of lipophilic opioids is similar to that which follows an intramuscular injection and thus may play a role in the analgesic effects (Nordberg, 1984; Glass et al., 1992; Guinard et al., 1992). In contrast, hydrophilic opioids such as morphine are more likely to diffuse across dural membranes where their primary analgesic effect is through receptors in the dorsal column (Bernards et al., 2003).

Lipid solubility determines in part several other important characteristics of intraspinal opioids, including the spread of analgesia and side effects. Highly water-soluble opioids such as morphine exhibit a greater degree of rostral spread when injected into the subarachnoid or epidural space than lipid-soluble compounds so that in pain conditions requiring higher spinal levels or more extensive coverage, the degree of analgesia they confer may be better. Conversely, since many adverse effects of spinal opioids such as pruritus, nausea and vomiting, and delayed respiratory depression are the result of interaction with opioid receptors in the brain, the more water-soluble compounds are associated with a higher incidence of these problems. Table 13.1 lists the recommended conversion ratios between different opioids.

Whereas the earliest studies on the chronic use of intraspinal opioids were conducted in patients suffering from cancer pain, more recent ones

TABLE 13.1. Equianalgesic doses of opioids (mg).

	Oral	Parenteral	Epidural	Intrathecal	Water solubility
Morphine	300	100	10	1	High
Hydromorphone	60	20	2	0.2	Intermediate
Meperidine	3000	1000	100	10	Low
Fentanyl	—	1	0.1	0.01	Low
Sufentanil	—	0.1	0.01	0.001	Low

have found intrathecal and epidural narcotics to be effective in nonmalignant pain as well (Paice, Winkelmuller, and Burchiel, 1997; Yue, St Marie, and Hendrickson, 1991). These conditions include not only nociceptive pain but also neuropathic pain, a heterogeneous group of disorders originally believed to be resistant to narcotics. Certain aspects of neuropathic pain such as tactile allodynia may be less responsive to the effects of spinal opiates. This may stem from the absence of opiate receptors on the spinal terminals of low-threshold mechanoreceptors thought to mediate the allodynic state. Many neuropathic conditions require nonopioid adjuvants to be added to spinal opioids for successful pain relief. When opioids are administered directly into the CSF, only a fraction of the systemic dose is required because there are no anatomical barriers to be crossed, and vascular reuptake is slow. In addition, when administered intrathecally, the ratio of two of morphine's main metabolites, morphine-3-glucoronide and morphine-6-glucuronide, to the parent compound is less than when morphine is given orally (Faura et al., 1998). Although not all side effects of intrathecal opioids are dose related, in many instances this drastic reduction in dosage translates into reduced side effects. In fact, one of the primary indications for a trial with intrathecal or epidural narcotics is a good analgesic response to systemic opioids coupled with intractable side effects. Among the adverse opioid effects reduced by switching from oral formulations to spinal administration are sedation and constipation. Those that may be increased include pruritus, urinary retention, and edema.

The mechanisms contributing to the various adverse effects of opioids are incompletely understood but probably multifactorial. These include those that are mediated via interaction with specific opioid receptors, and those that are not. Undesirable effects not mediated by opioid receptors such as CNS excitation and hyperalgesia cannot be reversed with naloxone. The incidence of the various opioid-induced side effects depends on a number of different factors including the opioid infused, route of administration and dosage, extent of disease, concurrent drug use to include oral narcotics, age, concomitant medical problems, and prior exposure to opioids. The most frequent side effects of intrathecal morphine are constipation, urinary retention, nausea and vomiting, and libido disturbances (Winkelmuller and Winkelmuller, 1996). With the exceptions of sweating, peripheral edema, and constipation, most of these adverse effects tend to diminish with time.

Most studies assessing neuraxial opioids in the elderly (all with cohorts over 65 years as entry criteria) have been perioperative and in combination with local anesthetics, and none offer direct comparisons with younger cohorts. Based on existing data, it appears that both dose responses and side effects in the elderly are similar to those of younger patients. The optimal dose for intrathecal morphine in large operations such as hip arthroplasty is

100 to 200 µg, and 50 µg in smaller surgeries (Murphy et al., 2003; Walsh et al., 2003; Fleron et al., 2003).

Although no studies have focused on the long-term administration of intrathecal opioids in elderly cohorts, most have had participants over the age of 65 (Angel, Gould, and Casey, 1998; Paice, Penn, and Shott, 1996; Rauck et al., 2003; Becker et al., 2000; Onofrio and Yaksh, 1990). In these studies, the mean ages ranged from 54 to 63 years of age with the median ages tending to be slightly higher. Not surprisingly, all trials demonstrated long-term efficacy with intrathecal morphine treatment, with more rapid dose escalations being required in patients with malignant pain. No study mentioned any unique treatment finding in the elderly or age-related adverse effects. We therefore conclude that spinal opioids are a safe and effective treatment option in patients over 65.

ALPHA-2 ADRENERGIC AGONISTS

The intraspinal administration of alpha-2 agonists to provide analgesia has been utilized since 1985. Although several different subtypes of alpha-2 receptors have been identified that may play a role in antinociception, recent studies have suggested that the alpha-2$_A$ receptor is primarily responsible for analgesia (Lakhlani et al., 1997). The mechanism of action of spinally administered alpha-2 agonists is similar to that of opioids (Lakhlani et al., 1997). Presynaptically, they bind to alpha-2 adrenergic receptors on small primary afferent neurons, thus decreasing the release of neurotransmitters involved in relaying pain signals. On postsynaptic neurons, alpha-2 agonists hyperpolarize the cell by increasing potassium conductance through Gi-coupled K^+ channels (North et al., 1987). Alpha-adrenergic agonists have also been shown to activate spinal cholinergic neurons, which may contribute to their analgesic effects. In addition to their antinociceptive properties, alpha-2 agonists produce dose-dependent sedation, presumably by inhibitory mechanisms involving the locus coeruleus in the brainstem.

The most studied alpha-2 agonist is the antihypertensive medication clonidine. Although it is currently FDA approved for epidural use only in cancer pain, clinical reports have shown it to be effective intrathecally and epidurally for nonmalignant pain as well (Ackerman, Follett, and Rosenquist, 2003; Raphael et al., 2002; Rainov, Heidecke, and Burkert, 2001). These studies had cohorts with mean ages in the fifties. No age-related analgesic or side effects were noted in these investigations. Several studies show clonidine may prolong and enhance the effects of spinal and epidural anesthesia with local anesthetics and that adding it to opioids for labor analgesia may extend the duration of pain relief (Dobrydnjov and Samarutel, 1999;

Milligan et al., 2000). It has also been reported to be effective in treating spasticity and central pain following spinal cord injury (Middleton et al., 1996). As with opiates, clonidine is effective in animal models of thermal hyperalgesia. Unlike opiates, it displays considerable potency in models of nerve injury-evoked tactile allodynia (Yaksh et al., 1995). Clonidine may be most effective in patients with neuropathic or sympathetically maintained pain (Rauck et al., 1993).

The most common side effects of neuraxial clonidine are sedation, hypotension, and bradycardia (Eisenach et al., 1995). These are more frequent following the larger doses needed to provide epidural analgesia than with intrathecal administration, and may be due in part to systemic absorption of the drug. In low doses by either route, these effects are usually well tolerated.

With regard to the specific effects of alpha-2 adrenergic agonists in the elderly, there is little data to draw upon. All of the studies involving elderly patients assessed clonidine in the operative setting. None compared the effects of the drug between younger and older cohorts (Gehling et al., 2003; Sites et al., 2003; Fournier et al., 2002; Santiveri et al., 2002). A review of these studies did not reveal significant response differences in elderly patients. Most show that whereas clonidine prolongs and enhances local anesthetic blockade and improves postoperative analgesia, hypotension is a common side effect, especially with higher doses. Therefore, reasonable caution is advised when using neuraxial clonidine in geriatric patients.

There are no clinical trials on the long-term intrathecal use of alpha-2 adrenergic agonists in the elderly. The evidence is further complicated by the fact that most trials on the subject have used clonidine in combination with opioids or local anesthetics (Ackerman, Follett, and Rosenquist, 2003; Rainov, Heidecke, and Burkert, 2001; Uhle et al., 2000). Even though these studies included elderly patients in the cohort, age-related issues were not addressed. Two studies found reduced opioid requirements and better analgesia with clonidine, but one showed only limited and short-lived benefits. In a randomized, placebo-controlled trial evaluating epidural clonidine in 85 patients with severe cancer pain, Eisenach et al. (1995) found that while pain relief was better in the epidural-clonidine group than the placebo group, there was no difference in rescue epidural morphine requirements. Although this study did not specifically target geriatric patients, the average age of the subjects was 57 years. Because of the limited data on the long-term use of neuraxial alpha-2 adrenergic agonists in elderly patients, no conclusions can be drawn at this time.

N-METHYL-D-ASPARTATE
RECEPTOR ANTAGONISTS

The most studied *N*-methyl-D-aspartate (NMDA) receptor antagonist for neuraxial use is ketamine, a noncompetitive NMDA antagonist that has been administered both epidurally and intrathecally in humans for acute and chronic pain relief. Following tissue injury, the activation of spinal NMDA receptors induces a state of facilitated processing from repetitive small afferent fiber stimulation, leading to an increased response to high- and low-threshold stimulation and enhanced receptor field size. This process, known as windup, is responsible for such phenomena such as allodynia and hyperalgesia. When delivered spinally, NMDA receptor antagonists have little effect on acute activation, but may block windup induced by small afferent input.

In a randomized, double-blind study (Choe et al. 1997) ketamine (mean age 53) was found to prolong the duration of analgesia and decrease the number of patients requiring supplemental injections when combined with epidural morphine for upper abdominal surgery. In combination with intrathecal morphine alone or with other agents in patients suffering from cancer pain, the addition of intraspinal ketamine has been shown to enhance the analgesic effects of opioids and the other drugs, while reducing the development of tolerance (Muller and Lemos, 1996). However, in several other studies examining the effects of adding ketamine spinally or epidurally to the local anesthetic bupivacaine for surgical anesthesia, investigators were not able to demonstrate additional benefit (Weir and Fee, 1998; Kathirvel et al., 2000). The Weir study had a mean age of 71, with the only epidural ketamine-related side effect being sedation (Weir and Fee, 1998).

Although intrathecal ketamine was reported to provide adequate short-term anesthesia by Bion (1984) in a young group of patients, a more recent study by Hawksworth and Serpell (1998) conducted in elderly patients undergoing prostate surgery found that the high frequency of psychomimetic disturbances, the short duration of action, and the high incidence of incomplete anesthesia precluded its use as a sole anesthetic agent. The average age of the 10 male patients in this pilot study was 73 years. In a case report by Kristensen, Svensson, and Gordh (1992), the spinal administration of CPP [3-(2-carboxypoperazin-4-yl) propyl-1-phosphonic acid], a competitive NMDA antagonist, was noted to suppress windup but not spontaneous pain or allodynia in a patient with a peripheral nerve injury. Four hours after the last injection of CPP, psychomimetic side effects developed that were attributed to the rostral spread of medication.

Epidural ketamine alone or in combination with opioids has been shown to produce enhanced analgesia without significant side effects for major abdominal surgery (Subramaniam et al., 2001). In a study involving older patients (mean age 60 years) with cirrhosis having hepatic resection, the combination of epidural ketamine and morphine was found to provide superior pain relief to morphine alone. In elderly patients, the epidural ketamine dose was reduced by 33 percent (20 vs. 30 mg; Taura et al., 2003). There were no reports of psychomimetic effects, neurological findings, or any other complications in this study. In a study by Himmelseher and colleagues (2001) assessing the impact of adding S (+) ketamine to epidural anesthesia with ropivacaine in elderly patients undergoing knee arthroplasty, the combination group experienced significantly longer pain relief than patients receiving local anesthetic alone. The average age in this study was 65 years. The existing literature demonstrates that epidural ketamine in doses ranging from 0.5 to 1 mg/kg is well tolerated in patients of all age groups and is most effective when combined with opioids or local anesthetics. The potential neurotoxicity of intraspinal ketamine remains a subject of controversy. Karpinski and colleagues (1997) reported a terminal cancer patient who received a three-week intrathecal infusion of ketamine and was found to have subpial vacuolar myelopathy on autopsy. Stotz, Oehen, and Gerber (1999) reported a similar finding. On postmortem examination of a terminal cancer patient who received a seven-day trial of intrathecal ketamine, focal lymphocytic vasculitis close to the catheter injection site was found. Ketamine is not currently FDA approved for neuraxial use in the United States.

There are no published studies evaluating neuraxial NMDA antagonists in the perioperative setting or with long-term infusions that specifically compare older and younger cohorts. For this reason, neuraxial NMDA antagonists should be used with caution and at lower starting doses in the elderly. Low-dose (0.5 mg/kg) epidural ketamine in the operative setting appears to be well tolerated in older patients. In the only study evaluating intrathecal ketamine as the main anesthetic, the failure rate and incidence of side effects was too high to be practical (Hawksworth and Serpell, 1998). Because of the reports of possible neurotoxicty with ketamine, the drug is considered a fourth-line drug for long-term chronic pain therapy and should be used only in end-of-life situations where all other options have been exhausted (Bennett, Serafini, et al., 2000).

CALCIUM CHANNEL BLOCKERS

Voltage-sensitive calcium channel conduction is essential for the transmission of pain. In clinical and laboratory studies, both N- and L-type calcium channel antagonists have been shown to contain analgesic properties in the settings of somatic and neuropathic pain. N-type calcium channels are found in high concentrations in the substantia gelatinosa and dorsal root ganglia, where they play a role in the release of transmitters involved in nociceptive pathways such as substance P. In animals, tolerance to the antinociceptive effects of calcium channel blockers develops very slowly (Bowersox et al., 1996; Wang et al., 2000).

In a double-blind study examining the effects of a continuous intrathecal infusion of the N-type calcium channel blocker ziconotide started prior to surgical incision and continued for 48 to 72 hours postoperatively in patients who received spinal anesthesia, patients in the two treatment groups had lower pain scores and decreased postoperative PCA (patient-controlled analgesia) morphine requirements compared to those receiving a placebo infusion (Atanassoff et al., 2000). In four of six patients receiving high-dose ziconotide (7 µg per hour vs. 0.7 µg per hour), adverse effects such as blurred vision, nystagmus, dizziness, and sedation necessitated discontinuing the infusion. These effects, which disappeared after discontinuing the medication, were likely due to delayed clearance of ziconotide from neural tissues. There was no difference in postoperative pain scores between those who had received the high-dose ziconotide infusion and those receiving the low dose. Even with prolonged delivery, there does not appear to be significant tolerance with intrathecal ziconotide use (Jain, 2000).

In a multicenter, double-blind, placebo-controlled study evaluating intrathecal ziconotide for the treatment of refractory pain in 111 patients with cancer and AIDS, Staats et al. (2004) found the treatment group fared markedly better than the control group (53 percent vs. 18 percent improvement). The observation that there was no loss of efficacy for ziconotide in the maintenance phase is consistent with animal studies showing the absence of tolerance with this class of medications. Several adverse side effects were noted in the titration phase, with the most notable being confusion, somnolence, and urinary retention. In patients over 60, confusion was more common. All side effects were reversible, with their incidence decreasing after the initial dosing period. The average age in this clinical trial was 55.3 years.

In a double-blind study conducted in a younger population (mean age 44 years), adding a low dose of the L-type calcium channel blocker verapamil (5 mg) to epidural bupivacaine both before and after surgical incision was found to reduce postoperative analgesic requirements in patients undergoing abdominal surgery (Choe et al., 1998). The authors reported no increased incidence of sedation, mood disturbances, or hypotension as defined by a blood pressure drop greater than 25 percent below baseline in the treatment group. Animal studies have failed to show independent antinociceptive effects for the intrathecal administration of various L-type calcium channel blockers, although in combination with morphine, their interactions appear to be synergistic (Omote et al., 1993). In a study done in rats, coadministration of verapamil or the N-type calcium channel blocker omega-conotoxin MVIIA with morphine resulted in dose-dependent and sustained decreases in blood pressure. Administered independently in high doses, both drugs caused significant hypotension. When given with clonidine, verapamil but not omega-conotoxin MVIIA potentiated the hypotension caused by alpha-2 agonist (Horvath, Brodacz, and Holzer-Petsche, 2002).

No studies have been published assessing calcium channel blockers in the perioperative setting or long-term intrathecal infusions that specifically deal with elderly patients. Although the preliminary data are auspicious, these drugs should be used with caution in older patients, who appear to be at increased risk to develop sedation, confusion, and adverse hemodynamic changes (Staats et al., 2004).

ADENOSINE

Adenosine A1 receptors are found in high concentrations in the substantia gelatinosa, most notably on nonprimary afferent terminals. In both animal and human experiments, neuraxial adenosine has been found to have antinociceptive activity. This effect appears to be mediated by A1 receptors. Proposed mechanisms include a reduction in glutamate release from spinal afferents and a decrease in substance P concentrations in the CSF. The analgesic effects of both systemic and intrathecal adenosine may be abolished by adenosine receptor antagonists such as methylxanthines.

In a phase I clinical safety study published in 1998 by Rane et al. in twelve healthy volunteers (age range 18-52 years), the intrathecal injection of adenosine reduced areas of secondary allodynia after skin inflammation and decreased forearm ischemic tourniquet pain. Ice water-induced cold pain was unchanged by adenosine. No adverse side effects were noted, although one patient who received a 2000 μg injection (ranges tested were from 500 to 2000 μg) experienced transient low back pain. In a case report on a patient with neuropathic leg pain and tactile allodynia, a single intrathecal injection of the A1 agonist R-phenylisopropyl adenosine (R-PIA) provided long-term relief (10 days) of the patient's stimulus-dependent pain (Karlsten and Gordh, 1995). Pain relief has also been reported follow-ing intrathecal administration in a patient suffering from secondary erythro-melalgia (Lindblom et al., 1997). However, in a randomized, double-blind study by Rane et al. (1998) evaluating the effects of intrathecal adenosine on anesthetic and postoperative analgesic requirements in 40 women under-going hysterectomies (mean age 50 years, range 37-66), no difference was found between the adenosine and placebo groups. With the 500 µg dose range, no adverse side effects were reported (Helm and Gibson, 1997). In an assessment using a different formulation of adenosine marketed in the United States, Eisenach, Hood, and Curry (2002) found that intrathecal adenosine reduced hyperalgesia and allodynia associated with intradermal capsaicin injection, but had no effect on acute noxious chemical or thermal stimulation in young volunteers. A follow-up study by the same group of in-vestigators showed that intrathecal adenosine reduced areas of allodynia by 25 percent in volunteers given subdermal capsaicin. These findings are con-sistent with those of Rane (Rane et al., 1998; Rane, Sollevi, and Segerdahl, 2000) and indicate that adenosine may be more effective for neuropathic pain than it is for nociceptive pain. The only side effects noted in the initial safety studies, all done on younger patients, were headache and back pain (Eisenach, Hood, and Curry, 2002; Belfrage et al., 1999; Eisenach, Rauck, and Curry, 2003).

There are no published studies investigating the long-term infusion of intrathecal adenosine in patients with chronic pain. To date, all human stud-ies assessing neuraxial adenosine have been in either the perioperative set-ting or experimental pain models. Although adenosine shows promise as a treatment for chronic pain, it is premature to comment on its safety or effi-cacy in elderly patients.

CHOLINERGIC AGONISTS

In animal models, the spinal administration of cholinergic agonists and acetylcholinesterase inhibitors results in antinociception. When adminis-tered neuraxially, nicotinic agonists can initially produce paradoxical noci-ceptive behavior, followed by a subsequent increase in nociceptive thresh-olds. The spinal delivery of cholinesterase inhibitors has been similarly demonstrated to increase pain thresholds. The analgesic effects of neuraxial cholinergic drugs may in part be mediated by muscarinic M1 and M3 recep-tors, found in dorsal root ganglia and superficial laminae of the dorsal horn. Furthermore, studies have shown that the stimulation of muscarinic recep-tors in the spinal cord can enhance the release of gamma-aminobutyric acid

(GABA) and nitric oxide. In animal models, tolerance to the analgesic effects of cholinergic agents develops rapidly.

In a phase I safety assessment conducted in young volunteers by Hood, Eisenach, and Tuttle (1995), the administration of intrathecal neostigmine reduced visual analog pain scores to painful cold stimulation. In a study examining the drug's postoperative analgesic effects in middle-aged women undergoing abdominal hysterectomies with and without opioids, the administration of intrathecal neostigmine reduced postoperative pain scores and opioid requirements comparable to the fentanyl group, with the greatest effect seen in patients receiving both fentanyl and high-dose (25 µg) intrathecal neostigmine (Lauretti, Mattos, et al., 1998). These results support those of another study demonstrating synergistic effects between intrathecal neostigmine and opioids (Chung et al., 1998). Some studies have suggested that intrathecal neostigmine is more effective for somatic than visceral pain (Lauretti and Lima, 1996). In a clinical trial performed in healthy volunteers, combining spinal neostigmine with epidural clonidine provided additive but not synergistic analgesic effects, with the authors attributing part of neostigmine's antinociceptive properties to alpha-2 adrenergic enhancement (Hood et al., 1996). The addition of intrathecal neostigmine in this study diminished clonidine-induced reductions in blood pressure and norepinephrine levels. In an experiment comparing different combinations of neuraxial analgesics for labor analgesia in healthy parturients, patients receiving bupivacaine, fentanyl, clonidine, and neostigmine had significantly longer analgesia than those receiving bupivacaine and fentanyl, or bupivacaine, fentanyl, and clonidine (Owen et al., 2000).

Tan et al. (2001) compared intrathecal neostigmine, morphine, and normal saline in combination with bupivacaine for postoperative analgesia in 60 patients undergoing total knee replacement under spinal analgesia. The morphine group had a later onset of postsurgical pain and longer time to first rescue analgesics than the neostigmine group, which in turn had a longer duration of analgesia than the saline group. Motor blockade lasted significantly longer in the neostigmine group than the morphine and saline groups. The morphine group experienced a higher incidence of pruritus than the other two groups (14 of 20 vs. 0 in the saline and neostigmine groups). The overall satisfaction rate was considerably higher in the neostigmine (11/20) than the morphine (4/20) and saline (1/20) groups. The mean age in the 20 patients who received neostigmine with bupivacaine was 63 years (Tan et al., 2001). This study represents the only trial of intrathecal neostigmine conducted in an elderly patient population.

The most common side effects of intrathecal neostigmine are nausea, vomiting, and, at doses exceeding 150 µg, sedation and leg weakness. At low doses, neostigmine is not associated with significant hemodynamic effects. However, at higher doses (750 μg), increases in blood pressure, heart rate, respiratory rate, and anxiety may occur (Hood, Eisenach, and Tuttle, 1995). When combined with other spinal analgesics, the drug-sparing effects of neostigmine may actually decrease side effects.

Clinical trials assessing epidural neostigmine have shown similar promise. In a comparative study done in patients undergoing knee surgery, epidural neostigmine was found to provide superior analgesia compared to intra-articular administration of the drug (Lauretti et al., 2000). A placebo-controlled study evaluating three different epidural doses of neostigmine (1, 2, or 4 μg/kg) mixed with lidocaine resulted in sustained, dose-independent analgesic effects (lasting approximately 8 hours) and reduced postoperative analgesic requirements with no increase in side effects (Lauretti et al., 1999). Low-dose (60 μg) epidural neostigmine has also been used in combination with morphine to prolong analgesia and reduce opioid-related side effects in patients having orthopedic surgery (Omais, Lauretti, and Paccola, 2002).

There are no studies to date on the long-term intrathecal use of neostigmine for chronic pain, which is partly due to the fact that no preservative-free formulation is available in the United States. Despite its proven efficacy, neostigmine is currently considered a fourth-line drug for long-term intrathecal use in chronic pain patients (Bennett et al., 2000).

GAMMA-AMINOBUTYRIC ACID AGONISTS

In clinical studies, both GABA-A and GABA-B agonists have been shown to contain analgesic effects when injected neuraxially. The GABA-A receptor is part of a chloride channel ionophore complex modulated by barbiturates, benzodiazepines, alcohol, propofol, and etomidate. Stimulation of this receptor increases chloride conductance, thereby hyperpolarizing and inhibiting the postsynaptic neuron. This alteration in neuronal function changes the spinal cord processing of nociceptive input in such a way that animals receiving intrathecal midazolam exhibit a dermatomal level of decreased pinprick sensation. Since the antinociceptive effect of intrathecal midazolam can be reversed in rats by the administration of naloxone, an additional mechanism of action may involve a spinal cord-opioid pathway that does not involve mu receptors.

The GABA-B receptor is a G-protein-linked complex whose activation results in augmentation of potassium channel currents. This results in the hyperpolarization of the neuronal cell membrane, leading to a decrease in opening of voltage-sensitive calcium channels and a reduction in transmitter release. Although GABA-B receptors are found throughout the spinal cord, they are present in the highest concentrations in the substantia gelatinosa, being located both pre- and postsynaptically. The GABA-B agonist most studied in humans is baclofen.

Clinical studies are not consistent in demonstrating antinociceptive effects of neuraxially administered GABA-A and B agonists. The addition of both intrathecal and epidural midazolam to local anesthetics with and without opioids was found in several studies to enhance postoperative analgesia and reduce the need for narcotics (Batra et al., 1999; Nishiyama, Matsukawa, and Hanaoka, 1999; Valentine, Lyons, and Bellamy, 1996). In a double-blind study evaluating the effects of adding intrathecal midazolam to bupivacaine in patients undergoing hemorrhoidectomy, the addition of midazolam was found to expedite the onset of spinal analgesia in a dose-dependent manner (Kim and Lee, 2001). Other studies have found intrathecal midazolam to be effective in treating chronic mechanical low back pain, musculoskeletal pain, and neurogenic pain (Serrao et al., 1992; Borg and Krijnen, 1996). However, the administration of subarachnoid midazolam was not shown to be effective in treating pain associated with peripheral vascular disease and malignancy (Borg and Krijnen, 1996).

Interestingly, two well-designed animal studies published after the pilot studies in humans showed evidence of neurotoxicity with intrathecal midazolam. Svensson et al. (1995) found histological evidence of neuronal death in the spinal cords of rats after 20 consecutive days of 100 μg intrathecal injections of midazolam. In a similar experiment by Erdine et al. (1999), the investigators found that rabbits infused with both preservative-containing and preservative-free intrathecal midazolam (300 μg daily) over 5 days displayed vascular and other histological spinal cord lesions on microscopic examination. In addition to possible neurotoxicity, potential side effects of spinal midazolam include dose-dependent sedation and amnesia. Although the relative doses in the animal studies were much higher than in clinical studies, it is still considered ill-advised to use long-term neuraxial midazolam infusions in patients of any age until more safety studies are conducted.

A plethora of literature attests to the safety of intrathecal baclofen in humans, with most of the research done on patients with spinal spasticity. Numerous studies have shown the effectiveness of intrathecal baclofen to treat central pain states, including those following stroke, spinal cord injury, cerebral palsy, and multiple sclerosis (Taira et al., 1995; Van Schaeybroeck et al., 2000; Dario et al., 2001; Becker et al., 2000). Intrathecal baclofen has also been found to be an effective treatment for noncentral neuropathic pain conditions including complex regional pain syndrome and phantom limb pain (Zuniga, Perera, and Abram, 2002; Zuniga, Schlicht, and Abram, 2000). Since the most common use of baclofen is as a muscle relaxant, it is not surprising that several authors report intrathecal baclofen to be beneficial for spasm-related pain (Thompson and Hicks, 1998; Meythaler et al., 2001). Not all studies assessing the effects of intrathecal baclofen for pain have been positive. Loubser and Akman (1996) found intrathecal baclofen reduced musculoskeletal but not neurogenic pain in 12 patients with chronic pain secondary to spinal cord injury. In view of the results of this study and the temporal disparity regarding its analgesic effects on central pain and muscle spasm, it is likely that different pain-relieving mechanisms exist for these two conditions. Potential side effects of neuraxial baclofen include weakness and sedation.

No studies have specifically addressed intrathecal baclofen in the elderly. However, most clinical studies have contained geriatric patients, and in these trials no age-specific side effects were reported. As with other neuraxial medications, caution should be used when dosing intrathecal baclofen in older patients (Middel et al., 1997; Meythaler et al., 2001, 2003).

SOMATOSTATIN

There is extensive literature on the use of spinal somatostatin for pain relief. To date, at least six somatostatin receptors have been identified, which are dispersed throughout the periacqueductal gray, ventral horn, primary afferent neurons, and substantia gelatinosa. The antinociceptive effects of somatostatin result from presynaptic inhibition. Stimulation of somatostatin receptors results in hyperpolarization of the cell via a G-protein-coupled inwardly rectifying potassium current. This serves to block coupled calcium channels, reduce transmitter release, and decrease the synthesis of cAMP.

Epidural somatostatin has been demonstrated in several studies to provide postoperative pain relief for patients undergoing major surgical procedures (Taura et al., 1994; Bagarani et al., 1989; Chrubasik et al., 1985). In an open-label study assessing the effect of 250 μg of epidural somatostatin on postoperative pain after abdominal surgery, complete pain relief (no other analgesics required) was obtained in all eight patients. In two patients, an epidural somatostatin infusion also provided adequate intraoperative analgesia. There were no side reported side effects in this pilot study. The mean age of the patients was 56 years.

There are also reports of intrathecal and epidural somatostatin being used in cancer pain (Meynadier et al., 1985; Mollenholt et al., 1994). In a study performed by Mollenholt et al. (1994) examining the efficacy of continuous intrathecal and epidural infusions of somatostatin in eight patients with intractable cancer pain unresponsive to opioids, the authors described demyelination of spinal nerve roots and dorsal columns in two of their eight patients at autopsy. None demonstrated any clinical signs of neurological deficits during their treatment. As the patients were receiving other treatments for cancer including chemotherapy and radiation treatment, the pathological changes could not definitively be attributed to somatostatin. All patients in this investigation required a rapid escalation of dose over a relatively short period, perhaps indicating the development of tolerance. Analgesia was rated as either good or excellent in six of the eight patients. One patient experienced nausea, headache, and vertigo during the last five days of somatostatin treatment, and another became agitated and tremulous during the first night of therapy. The average age in this study was 55 years.

In another report, intrathecal octreotide, a synthetic analogue of somatostatin with a longer half-life, was noted to provide long-term pain relief in two patients, one of whom was a 62-year-old man suffering from refractory central pain secondary to multiple sclerosis (Paice, Penn, and Kroin, 1996). In this patient, a double-blinded "*N* of 1" trial with saline resulted in a sharp increase in pain during the two-week placebo period, necessitating an increase in supplemental opioids. The patient continued on the intrathecal somatostatin therapy for five years with no adverse side effects. The increase in somatostatin required during this period was modest, from 20 to 29 µg per hour.

Not all studies examining spinal somatostatin for pain relief have found the drug to be of benefit (Desborough et al., 1989). In a randomized, controlled trial assessing epidural diamorphine and somatostatin in 24 patients undergoing cholecystectomy, only the patients who received intraoperative diamorphine required less postoperative analgesics. Aside from the possibility of neurotoxicity, the neuraxial use of somatostatin is associated with minimal side effects.

Because of the reports of possible neurotoxicity, there have been no recent clinical trials assessing neuraxial somatostatin as an analgesic. At the present time, it is inadvisable to consider using this drug or its analogues in the elderly or any other patient population.

NEUROLEPTICS

The mechanism by which neuraxial droperidol exerts its antinociceptive effects has not been fully delineated, but may involve D1 and D2 receptors in descending dopaminergic tracts in the spinal medulla (Gao, Zhang, and Wu, 2001). When administered parenterally, neuroleptic drugs have been demonstrated to have analgesic as well as sedative and antiemetic effects in humans. In several clinical studies including two randomized, controlled trials, the butyrophenone droperidol has been shown to potentiate epidural analgesia with opioids (Wilder-Smith et al., 1994; Naji et al., 1990; Bach et al., 1986). In a double-blind study, Wilder-Smith et al. (1994) demonstrated that the combination of epidural droperidol and sufentanil significantly reduced both the duration of analgesia and adverse effects compared to sufentanil alone. Less nausea, vomiting, and pruritus were reported in the group receiving combination epidural therapy. The average age in this study was 52 years. A more recent randomized, controlled study by Gurses et al. (2003) showed that epidural droperidol in combination with epidural tramadol increased the quality and duration of analgesia over tramadol alone. The average age in the tramadol-droperidol group was 51 years. Last, Bach et al. (1986) conducted a retrospective study assessing the effect of adding epidural droperidol to epidural opioids in 20 patients with chronic pain, 17 of whom suffered from malignancy. The authors found that the addition of droperidol to epidural morphine resulted in significantly reduced opioid requirements and improved pain relief (80 percent of patients reported decreased pain), with 7 patients reporting reversible side effects. The mean age of the patients in this study was 64.5 years (range 32-87 years).

The potential benefits of combining epidural droperidol with opioids include a reduction in opioid-related side effects including nausea, vomiting, pruritus, urinary retention, and hypotension (Gurses et al., 2003; Aldrete, 1995; Hayashi et al., 2002). Side effects of epidural droperidol include sedation, respiratory depression, and Parkinsonian effects. One case report described the development of akathisia in a 75-year-old cancer patient after long-term use of epidural droperidol to treat intractable vomiting (Athanassiadis and Karamanis, 1992). A more recent article revealed two cases of extrapyramidal reactions after epidural droperidol was given to prevent postoperative nausea and vomiting. In one case, extrapyramidal symptoms developed after intravenous droperidol was administered to a patient who had previously received the medication epidurally (Yotsui et al., 2000).

There are no studies to date on the long-term intrathecal use of neuroleptics. The literature that does exist on neuraxial neuroleptics primarily deals with either the intrathecal effects of droperidol in animals, or epidural droperidol in the perioperative setting. None of these studies have specifically addressed the use of the drug in elderly patients, although several clinical trials enrolled significant numbers of older patients. In geriatric patients, low-dose epidural droperidol in combination with opioids appears to be a useful adjuvant to combat opioid-related side effects.

ASPIRIN AND NSAIDs

As with oral administration, the mechanism of action for spinally administered nonsteroidal anti-inflammatory drugs (NSAIDs) is inhibition of prostaglandin synthesis, most likely at the spinal level. There is a growing body of research that implicates the COX-1 and COX-2 isoenzymes in the maintenance of spinal neuropathic pain (Lashbrook et al., 1999). In an animal experiment using a peripheral nerve injury model, the COX-1-selective NSAID ketorolac provided significantly longer antinociception than the COX-2 selective NSAID NS-398 (six days vs. two hours). Interestingly, no effect was noted for the nonspecific COX inhibitor piroxicam (Ma, Du, and Eisenach, 2002).

In humans, several studies have examined the analgesic effects of intrathecal aspirin in patients with chronic, refractory pain (Pellerin et al., 1987; Devoghel, 1983). In a large study conducted in 60 cancer patients with intractable pain, a single dose of isobaric lysine acetylsalicylate (doses ranged from 120 to 720 mg) resulted in excellent relief in 78 percent of cases, with the duration of analgesia lasting from three weeks to one month on average (Pellerin et al., 1987). The only significant side effect was fatigability. The mean age in this series was 60 years (range 30 to 88).

An open-label, dose-escalating, phase I safety study assessing preservative-free intrathecal ketorolac in young, healthy volunteers demonstrated no adverse side effects aside from a dose-dependent decrease in heart rate lasting one hour after injection. Of note, the threshold to heat in these volunteers was unaffected by any dose of neuraxial ketorolac (Eisenach et al., 2002). This finding is in contrast to recent experiments showing potent antinociceptive effects in rats without evidence of neurotoxicity following intrathecal ketorolac tromethamine administration (Korkmaz et al., 2004). In a study by Parris et al. (1996) investigating intrathecal ketorolac and morphine in an animal model of neuropathic pain, the authors demonstrated that both drugs possessed antinociceptive properties, with morphine being more potent than ketorolac for most outcome measures (Parris et al., 1996). For cold allodynia, the analgesic effects of the two drugs were found to be similar. In an interesting report by Lauretti, Reis, et al. (1998), inadvertent epidural diclofenac injection by family members in two terminal cancer patients was reported to provide pain relief ranging from several hours to two days after several previous failed epidural trials.

Whereas the intrathecal use of COX-1 inhibitors appears to hold promise in the treatment of neuropathic pain, long-term efficacy and safety studies are lacking. It is therefore impossible to make any recommendations for the neuraxial use of these drugs in elderly patients.

CONCLUSION

The use of spinal analgesics to modulate pain is a rapidly expanding field, with broad implications in the management of acute and chronic pain. Although numerous compounds that are currently available have been shown to contain antinociceptive properties in preclinical studies, only those that have been examined in humans are discussed in this chapter. Other substances that have shown promise for future study in humans include nitric oxide inhibitors, dynorphins, calcitonin, neurotensin, tricyclic antidepressants, beta-blockers, and cannabinoids.

It is difficult to determine age-related effects for the acute and chronic administration of spinal analgesics in the elderly. This is not surprising, given the lack of clinical trials with these drugs in any age cohort. Even for the more widely used neuraxial analgesics such as opioids and clonidine, one can only cautiously extrapolate the data in older patients due to the absence of age-specific research studies. Clearly, there is a need for further study in this area of medicine.

REFERENCES

Ackerman LL, Follett KA, Rosenquist RW. Long-term outcomes during treatment of chronic pain with intrathecal clonidine or clonidine/opioid combinations. *J Pain Symptom Manage* 2003; 26: 668-677.

Aldrete JA. Reduction of nausea and vomiting from epidural opioids by adding droperidol to the infusate in home-bound patients. *J Pain Symptom Manage* 1995; 10: 544-547.

Angel IF, Gould HJ Jr., Carey ME. Intrathecal morphine pump as a treatment option in chronic pain of nonmalignant origin. *Surg Neurol* 1998; 49: 92-98.

Atanassoff PG, Hartmannsgruber MWB, Thrasher J, et al. Ziconotide, a new N-type calcium channel blocker, administered intrathecally for acute postoperative pain. *Reg Anesth Pain Med* 2000; 25: 274-278.

Athanassiadis C, Karamanis A. Akathisia after long-term epidural use of droperidol: A case report. *Pain* 1992; 50: 203-204.

Bach V, Carl P, Ravlo O, et al. Potentiation of epidural opioids with epidural droperidol. A one-year retrospective study. *Anaesthesia* 1986; 41: 1116-1119.

Bagarani M, Amodei C, Beltramme P, et al. Effects of somatostatin peridurally administered in the treatment of postoperative pain. *Minerva Anestesiol* 1989; 55: 513-516.

Batra YK, Jain K, Chari P, et al. Addition of intrathecal midazolam to bupivacaine produces better post-operative analgesia without prolonging recovery. *Int J Clin Pharmacol Ther* 1999; 37: 519-523.

Baxter MG, Frick KM, Price DL, Breckler SJ, Markowska AL, Gorman LK. Presynaptic markers of cholinergic function in the rat brain: Relationship with age and cognitive status. *Neuroscience* 1999; 89: 771-779.

Becker R, Jakob D, Uhle EI, Riegel T, Bertalanffy H. The significance of intrathecal opioid therapy for the treatment of neuropathic cancer pain conditions. *Stereotact Funct Neurosurg* 2000; 75: 16-26.

Becker R, Uhle EI, Alberti O, Bertalanffy H. Continuous intrathecal baclofen infusion in the management of central deafferentation pain. *J Pain Symptom Manage* 2000; 20: 313-315.

Belfrage M, Segerdahl M, Arner S, Sollevi A. The safety and efficacy of intrathecal adenosine in patients with chronic neuropathic pain. *Anesth Analg* 1999; 89: 136-142.

Bennett G, Burchiel K, Buchser E, et al. Clinical guidelines for intraspinal infusion: report of an expert panel. PolyAnalgesic Consensus Conference 2000. *J Pain Symptom Manage* 2000; 20: S37-S43.

Bennett G, Serafini M, Burchiel K, et al. Evidence-based review of the literature on intrathecal delivery of pain medication. *J Pain Symptom Manage* 2000; 20: S12-S36.

Bernards CM. Understanding the physiology and pharmacology of epidural and intrathecal opioids. *Best Pract Res Clin Anesth* 2002; 16: 489-505.

Bernards CM, Shen DD, Sterling ES, et al. Epidural, cerebrospinal fluid, and plasma pharmacokinetics of epidural opioids (part 1): differences among opioids. *Anesthesiology* 2003; 99: 455-465.

Bion JF. Intrathecal ketamine for war surgery: A preliminary study under field conditions. *Anaesthesia* 1984; 39: 1023-8.

Borg PA, Krijnen HJ. Long-term intrathecal administration of midazolam and clonidine. *Clin J Pain* 1996; 12: 63-68.

Bowersox SS, Gadbois T, Singh T, Pettus M, Wang YX, Luther RR. Selective N-type neuronal voltage-sensitive calcium channel blocker, SNX-111, produces spinal antinociception in rat models of acute, persistent and neuropathic pain. *J Pharmacol Exp Ther* 1996; 279: 1243-1249.

Choe H, Choi YS, Kim YH, et al. Epidural morphine plus ketamine for upper abdominal surgery: Improved analgesia from preincisional versus postincisional administration. *Anesth Analg* 1997; 84: 560-563.

Choe H, Kim JS, Ko SH, et al. Epidural verapamil reduces analgesic consumption after lower abdominal surgery. *Anesth Analg* 1998; 86: 786-790.

Chrubasik J, Meynadier J, Scherpereel P, Wunsch E. The effect of epidural somatostatin on postoperative pain. *Anesth Analg* 1985; 64: 1085-1088.

Chung CJ, Kim JS, Park HS, Chin YJ. The efficacy of intrathecal neostigmine, intrathecal morphine, and their combination for post-cesarean section analgesia. *Anesth Analg* 1998; 87: 341-346.

Dario A, Scamoni C, Bono G, et al. Functional improvement in patients with severe spinal spasticity treated with chronic intrathecal baclofen infusion. *Funct Neurol* 2001; 16: 311-315.

Deer TR, Caraway DL, Kim CK, Dempsey CD, Stewart CD, McNeil KF. Clinical experience with intrathecal bupivacaine in combination with opioid for the treatment of chronic pain related to failed back surgery syndrome and metastatic cancer pain of the spine. *Spine J* 2002; 2: 274-278.

Desborough JP, Edlin SA, Burrin JM, et al. Hormonal and metabolic responses to cholecystectomy: Comparison of extradural somatostatin and diamorphine. *Br J Anaesth* 1989; 63: 508-515.

Devoghel J-C. Small intrathecal doses of lysine-acetylsalicylate relieve intractable pain in man. *J Int Med Res* 1983; 11: 90-91.

Dobrydnjov I, Samarutel J. Enhancement of intrathecal lidocaine by addition of local and systemic clonidine. *Acta Anaesthesiol Scand* 1999; 43: 556-562.

Dorfman LJ, Bosley TM. Age-related changes in peripheral and central nerve conduction in man. *Neurology* 1979; 29: 38-44.

Eisenach JC, Curry R, Hood DD, Yaksh TL. Phase I safety assessment of intrathecal ketorolac. *Pain* 2002; 99: 599-604.

Eisenach JC, DuPen S, Dubois M, et al. Epidural clonidine analgesia for intractable cancer pain: The epidural clonidine study group. *Pain* 1995; 61: 391-399.

Eisenach JC, Hood DD, Curry R. Preliminary efficacy assessment of intrathecal injection of an American formulation of adenosine in humans. *Anesthesiology* 2002; 96: 29-34.

Eisenach JC, Rauck RL, Curry R. Intrathecal, but not intravenous adenosine reduces allodynia in patients with neuropathic pain. *Pain* 2003; 105: 65-70.

Erdine S, Yucel A, Ozyalcin S, et al. Neurotoxicity of midazolam in the rabbit. *Pain* 1999; 80: 419-423.

Esiri MM, Hyman BT, Beyreuther K, Masters CL. Ageing and dementia. In: Graham D, Lantos PL, eds. *Greenfield's Neuropathology*, London: Arnold, 1997, pp. 153–233.

Faura CC, Collins SL, Moore RA, McQuay HJ. Systematic review of factors affecting the ratios of morphine and its major metabolites. *Pain* 1998; 74: 43-53.

Ferrell BA. Pain management in elderly people. *J Am Geriatr Soc* 1991; 39: 64-73.

Fleron MH, Weiskopf RB, Bertrand M, et al. A comparison of intrathecal opioid and intravenous analgesia for the incidence of cardiovascular, respiratory, and renal complications after abdominal aortic surgery. *Anesth Analg* 2003; 97: 2-12.

Foley KM. The treatment of cancer pain. *N Engl J Med* 1985; 313: 84-95.

Fournier R, Van Gessel E, Weber A, Gamulin Z. Epinephrine and clonidine do not improve intrathecal sufentanil analgesia after total hip replacement. *Br J Anaesth* 2002; 89: 562-566.

Fox PL, Raina P, Jadad A. Prevalence and treatment of pain in older adults in nursing homes and other long-term care institutions: A systematic review. *CMAJ* 1999; 160: 329-333.

Gao X, Zhang Y, Wu G. Effects of dopaminergic agents on carrageenan hyperalgesia after intrathecal administration to rats. *Eur J Pharmacol* 2001; 418: 73-77.

Gehling M, Tryba M, Lusebrink T, Zorn A. [Can the addition of clonidine improve the analgesic efficacy of low dose intrathecal morphine? A randomized double-blind trial]. *Anaesthetist* 2003; 52: 204-209. German.

Glass PS, Estok P, Ginsberg B, Goldberg JS, Sladen RN. Use of patient-controlled analgesia to compare the efficacy of epidural to intravenous fentanyl administration. *Anesth Analg* 1992; 74: 45-51.

Guinard JP, Mavrocordatos P, Chiolero R, Carpenter RL. A randomized comparison of intravenous versus lumbar and thoracic epidural fentanyl for analgesia after thoracotomy. *Anesthesiology* 1992; 77: 1108-1115.

Gurses E, Sungurtekin H, Tomatir E, Balci C, Gonullu M. The addition of droperidol or clonidine to epidural tramadol shortens onset time and increases duration of postoperative analgesia. *Can J Anaesth* 2003; 50: 147-152.

Hawksworth C, Serpell M. Intrathecal anaesthesia with ketamine. *Reg Anesth Pain Med* 1998; 23: 283-288.

Hayashi K, Higuchi J, Sakio H, Tanaka Y, Onoda N. Continuous epidural administration of droperidol to prevent postoperative nausea and vomiting. *Masui* 2002; 51: 124-127.

Haycock JW, Becker L, Ang L, Furukawa Y, Hornykiewicz O, Kish SJ. Marked disparity between age-related changes in dopamine and other presynaptic dopaminergic markers in human striatum. *J Neurochem* 2003; 87: 574-585.

Helm RD, Gibson SJ. Pain in the elderly. In: Jensen J'S, Turner JA, Wiesenfeld-Hallin Z, eds., *Proceedings of the 8th World Congress on Pain, Progress in Pain Research and Management,* vol. 8. Seattle: IASP Press, 1997, pp. 919-944.

Hildebrand KR, Elsberry DD, Deer TR. Stability, compatibility, and safety of intrathecal bupivacaine administered chronically via an implantable delivery system. *Clin J Pain* 2001; 17: 239-244.

Himmelseher S, Ziegler-Pithamitsis D, Argiriadou H, Martin J, Jelen-Esselborn S, Kochs E. Small-dose S(+)-ketamine reduces postoperative pain when applied with ropivacaine in epidural anesthesia for total knee arthroplasty. *Anesth Analg* 2001; 92: 1290-1295.

Hood DD, Eisenach JC, Tuttle R. Phase I safety assessment of intrathecal neostigmine methylsulfate in humans. *Anesthesiology* 1995; 82: 331-343.

Hood DD, Mallak KA, Eisenach JC, Tong C. Interaction between intrathecal neostigmine and epidural clonidine in human volunteers. *Anesthesiology* 1996; 85: 315-325.

Horvath G, Brodacz B, Holzer-Petsche U. Blood pressure changes after intrathecal co-administration of calcium channel blockers with morphine or clonidine at the spinal level. *Naunyn Schmiedebergs Arch Pharmacol* 2002; 366: 270-275.

Jain KK. An evaluation of intrathecal ziconotide for the treatment of chronic pain. *Expert Opin Investig Drugs* 2000; 9: 2403-2410.

Karlsten R, Gordh T Jr. An A_1-selective adenosine agonist abolishes allodynia elicited by vibration and touch after intrathecal injection. *Anesth Analg* 1995; 80: 844-847.

Karpinski N, Dunn J, Hansen L, Masliah E. Subpial vacuolar myelopathy after intrathecal ketamine: Report of a case. *Pain* 1997; 73: 103-105.

Kathirvel S, Sadhasivam S, Saxena A, et al. Effects of intrathecal ketamine added to bupivacaine for spinal anaesthesia. *Anaesthesia* 2000; 55: 899-904.

Kim MH, Lee YM. Intrathecal midazolam increases the analgesic effects of spinal blockade with bupivacaine in patients undergoing haemorrhoidectomy. *Br J Anaesth* 2001; 86: 77-79.

Kinsella K, Velkoff VA. Life expectancy and changing mortality. *Aging Clin Exp Res* 2002; 14: 322-332.

Korkmaz HA, Maltepe F, Erbayraktar S, et al. Antinociceptive and neurotoxicologic screening of chronic intrathecal administration of ketorolac tromethamine in the rat. *Anesth Analg* 2004; 98: 148-152.

Krames E. Implantable devices for pain control: Spinal cord stimulation and intrathecal therapies. *Best Pract Res Clin Anesth* 2002; 16: 619-649.

Kristensen JD, Svensson B, Gordh T Jr. The NMDA-receptor antagonist CPP abolishes neurogenic "wind-up pain" after intrathecal administration in humans. *Pain* 1992; 51: 249-253.

Lakhlani PP, MacMillan LB, Guo TZ, et al. Substitution of a mutant alpha 2a-adrenergic receptor via "hit and run" gene targeting reveals the role of this subtype in sedative, analgesic, and anesthetic-sparing responses in vivo. *Proc Natl Acad Sci USA* 1997; 94: 9950-9955.

Lashbrook JM, Ossipova MH, Hunter JC, Raffa RB, Tallarida RJ, Porreca F. Synergistic antiallodynic effects of spinal morphine with ketorolac and selective COX1- and COX2-inhibitors in nerve-injured rats. *Pain* 1999; 82: 65-72.

Lauretti GR, de Oliveira R, Perez MV, Paccola CA. Postoperative analgesia by intraarticular and epidural neostigmine following knee surgery. *J Clin Anesth* 2000; 12: 444-448.

Lauretti GR, de Oliveira R, Reis MP, Juliao MC, Pereira NL. Study of three different doses of epidural neostigmine coadministered with lidocaine for postoperative analgesia. *Anesthesiology* 1999; 90: 1534-1538.

Lauretti GR, Lima ICPR. The effects of intrathecal neostigmine on somatic and visceral pain: Improvement by association with a peripheral anticholinergic. *Anesth Analg* 1996; 82: 617-620.

Lauretti GR, Mattos AL, Reis MP, Pereira NL. Combined intrathecal fentanyl and neostigmine: Therapy for postoperative abdominal hysterectomy pain relief. *J Clin Anesth* 1998; 10: 291-296.

Lauretti GR, Reis MP, Mattos AL, Gomes JM, Oliveira AP, Pereira NL. Epidural nonsteroidal antiinflammatory drugs for cancer pain. *Anesth Analg* 1998; 86: 117-118.

Levy RM. Implanted drug delivery systems for control of chronic pain. In Benzon HT, Raja SN, Molloy RE, Strichartz G, eds., *Essentials of Pain Medicine and Regional Anesthesia,* Philadelphia: Churchill Livingstone, 1999; 96-103.

Lindblom U, Nordfors L-O, Sollevi A, Sydow O. Adenosine for pain relief in a patient with intractable secondary erythromelalgia. *Eur J Pain* 1997; 1: 299-302.

Loubser PG, Akman NM. Effects of intrathecal baclofen on chronic spinal cord injury pain. *J Pain Symptom Manage* 1996; 12: 241-247.

Ma W, Du W, Eisenach JC. Role for both spinal cord COX-1 and COX-2 in maintenance of mechanical hypersensitivity following peripheral nerve injury. *Brain Res* 2002; 937: 94-99.

Meynadier J, Chrubasik J, Dubar M, Wunsch E. Intrathecal somatostatin in terminally ill patients: A report of two cases. *Pain* 1985; 23: 9-12.

Meythaler JM, Guin-Renfroe S, Brunner RC, Hadley MN. Intrathecal baclofen for spastic hypertonia from stroke. *Stroke* 2001; 32: 2099-2109.

Meythaler JM, Guin-Renfroe S, Hadley MN. Improvement in walking speed in poststroke spastic hemiplegia after intrathecal baclofen therapy: A preliminary study. *Arch Phys Med Rehabil* 2003; 84: 1194-1199.

Middel B, Kuipers-Upmeijer H, Bouma J, et al. Effect of intrathecal baclofen delivered by an implanted programmable pump on health related quality of life in patients with severe spasticity. *J Neurol Neurosurg Psychiatry* 1997; 63: 204-209.

Middleton JW, Siddall PJ, Walker S, et al. Intrathecal clonidine and baclofen in the management of spasticity and neuropathic pain following spinal cord injury: A case study. *Arch Phys Med Rehabil* 1996; 77: 824-826.

Milligan KR, Convery PN, Weir P, et al. The efficacy and safety of epidural infusions of levobupivicaine with and without clonidine for postoperative pain relief in patients undergoing total hip replacement. *Anesth Analg* 2000; 91: 393-397.

Mollenholt P, Rawal N, Gordh T Jr, Olsson Y. Intrathecal and epidural somatostatin for patients with cancer. *Anesthesiology* 1994; 81: 534-542.

Muller A, Lemos D. Cancer pain: beneficial effect of ketamine addition to spinal administration of morphine-clonidine-lidocaine mixture. *Ann Fr Anesth Reanim* 1996; 15: 271-276.

Murphy PM, Stack D, Kinirons B, Laffey JG. Optimizing the dose of intrathecal morphine in older patients undergoing hip arthroplasty. *Anesth Analg* 2003 Dec; 97: 1709-1715.

Naji P, Farschtschain M, Wilder-Smith OH, Wilder-Smith CH. Epidural droperidol and morphine for postoperative pain. *Anesth Analg* 1990; 70: 583-588.

Nishiyama T, Matsukawa T, Hanaoka K. Continuous epidural administration of midazolam and bupivacaine for postoperative analgesia. *Acta Anaesthesiol Scand* 1999; 43: 568-572.

Nordberg G. Pharmacokinetic aspects of spinal morphine analgesia. *Acta Anaesthesiol Scand* 1984; 28: 1-38.

Nordberg G, Hedner T, Mellstrand T, Dahlstrom B. Pharmacokinetic aspects of epidural morphine analgesia. *Anesthesiology* 1983; 58: 545-551.

North RA, Williams JT, Surprenant A, Christie MJ. Mu and delta receptors belong to a family of receptors that are coupled to potassium channels. *Proc Natl Acad Sci USA* 1987; 84: 5487-5491.

Okada A, Harida S, Takeda Y, Nakamura T, Takagaki K, Endo M. Age-related changes in proteoglycans of human ligamentum flavum. *Spine* 1993; 18: 2261-2266.

Omais M, Lauretti GR, Paccola CA. Epidural morphine and neostigmine for postoperative analgesia after orthopedic surgery. *Anesth Analg* 2002; 95: 1698-1700.

Omote K, Sonoda H, Kawamata M, et al. Potentiation of antinociceptive effects of morphine by calcium-channel blockers at the level of the spinal cord. *Anesthesiology* 1993; 79: 746-752.

Onofrio BM, Yaksh TL. Long-term pain relief produced by intrathecal morphine infusion in 53 patients. *J Neurosurg* 1990; 72: 200-209.

Onofrio BM, Yaksh TL, Arnold PG. Continuous low-dose intrathecal morphine administration in the treatment of chronic pain of malignant origin. *Mayo Clin Proc* 1981; 56: 516-520.

Owen MD, Ozsarac O, Sahin S, et al. Low-dose clonidine and neostigmine prolong the duration of intrathecal bupivicaine-fentanyl for labor analgesia. *Anesthesiology* 2000; 92: 361-366.

Paice JA, Penn RD, Kroin JS. Intrathecal octreotide for relief of intractable nonmalignant pain: 5-year experience with two cases. *Neurosurgery* 1996; 38: 203-207.

Paice JA, Penn RD, Shott S. Intraspinal morphine for chronic pain: a retrospective, multicenter study. *J Pain Symptom Manage* 1996; 11: 71-80.

Paice JA, Winkelmuller W, Burchiel K. Clinical realities and economic considerations: Efficacy of intrathecal pain therapy. *J Pain Symptom Manage* 1997; 14: S14-S26.

Pakkenberg B, Gundersen HJ. Neocortical neuron number in humans: effect of sex and age. *J Comp Neurol* 1997; 384: 312-320.

Parris WC, Janicki PK, Johnson B Jr, Horn JL. Intrathecal ketorolac tromethamine produces analgesia after chronic constriction injury of sciatic nerve in rat. *Can J Anaesth* 1996; 43: 867-870.

Pellerin M, Hardy F, Abergel A, et al. Chronic refractory pain in cancer patients: Usefulness of intrathecal lysine acetylsalicylate in 60 cases. *Presse Med* 1987; 16: 1465-1468.

Rainov NG, Heidecke V, Burkert W. Long-term intrathecal infusion of drug combinations for chronic back and leg pain. *J Pain Symptom Manage* 2001; 22: 862-871.

Rane K, Segerdahl M, Goiny M, Sollevi A. Intrathecal adenosine administration. *Anesthesiology* 1998; 89: 1108-1115.

Rane K, Sollevi A, Segerdahl M. Intrathecal adenosine administration in abdominal hysterectomy lacks analgesic effect. *Acta Anaesthesiol Scand* 2000; 44: 868-872.

Raphael JH, Southall JL, Gnanadurai TV, Treharne GJ, Kitas GD. Long-term experience with implanted intrathecal drug administration systems for failed back syndrome and chronic mechanical low back pain. *BMC Musculoskelet Disord* 2002; 20(3): 17.

Rauck RL, Cherry D, Boyer MF, Kosek P, Dunn J, Alo K. Long-term intrathecal opioid therapy with a patient-activated, implanted delivery system for the treatment of refractory cancer pain. *J Pain* 2003; 4: 441-447.

Rauck RL, Eisenach JC, Jackson K, et al. Epidural clonidine treatment for refractory reflex sympathetic dystrophy. *Anesthesiology* 1993; 79: 1163-1169.

Santiveri X, Arxer A, Plaja I, et al. Anaesthetic and postoperative analgesic effects of spinal clonidine as an additive to prilocaine in the transurethral resection of urinary bladder tumors. *Eur J Anaesthesiol* 2002; 19: 589-593.

Serrao JM, Marks RL, Morley SJ, Goodchild CS. Intrathecal midazolam for the treatment of chronic mechanical low back pain: A controlled comparison with epidural steroid in a pilot study. *Pain* 1992; 48: 5-12.

Simon MJ, Veering BT, Stienstra R, van Kleef JW, Burm AG. The effects of age on neural blockade and hemodynamic changes after epidural anesthesia with ropivacaine. *Anesth Analg* 2002; 94: 1325-1330.

Sites BD, Beach M, Biggs R, et al. Intrathecal clonidine added to a bupivacaine-morphine spinal anesthetic improves postoperative analgesia for total knee arthroplasty. *Anesth Analg* 2003; 96: 1083-1088.

Staats PS, Yearwood T, Charapata SG, et al. Intrathecal ziconotide in the treatment of refractory pain in patients with cancer or AIDS: A randomized controlled trial. *JAMA* 2004; 291: 63-70.

Stotz M, Oehen HP, Gerber H. Histological findings after long-term infusion of intrathecal ketamine for chronic pain: a case report. *J Pain Symptom Manage* 1999; 18: 223-228.

Subramaniam K, Subramaniam B, Pawar DK, Kumar L. Evaluation of the safety and efficacy of epidural ketamine combined with morphine for postoperative analgesia after major upper abdominal surgery. *J Clin Anesth* 2001; 13: 339-344.

Svensson BA, Welin M, Gordh T Jr, Westman J. Chronic subarachnoid midazolam (Dormicum) in the rat: Morphologic evidence of spinal cord neurotoxicity. *Reg Anesth* 1995; 20: 426-434.

Taira T, Kawamura H, Tanikawa T, et al. A new approach to control central deafferentation pain: Spinal intrathecal baclofen. *Stereotact Funct Neurosurg* 1995; 65: 101-105.

Tan PH, Chia YY, Lo Y, Liu K, Yang LC, Lee TH. Intrathecal bupivacaine with morphine or neostigmine for postoperative analgesia after total knee replacement surgery. *Can J Anaesth* 2001; 48: 551-556.

Taura P, Fuster J, Blasi A, et al. Postoperative pain relief after hepatic resection in cirrhotic patients: The efficacy of a single small dose of ketamine plus morphine epidurally. *Anesth Analg* 2003; 96: 475-480.

Taura P, Planella V, Balust J, et al. Epidural somatostatin as an analgesic in upper abdominal surgery: A double-blind study. *Pain* 1994; 59:135-140.

Terry AV Jr, Buccafusco JJ. The cholinergic hypothesis of age and Alzheimer's disease-related cognitive deficits: Recent challenges and their implications for novel drug development. *J Pharmacol Exp Ther* 2003; 306: 821-827.

Thompson E, Hicks F. Intrathecal baclofen and homeopathy for the treatment of painful muscle spasms associated with malignant spinal cord compression. *Palliat Med* 1998; 12: 119-121.

Uhle EI, Becker R, Gatscher S, Bertalanffy H. Continuous intrathecal clonidine administration for the treatment of neuropathic pain. *Stereotact Funct Neurosurg* 2000; 75: 167-175.

U.S. Census Bureau, Population Division. Annual Estimates of the Civilian Population by Selected Age Groups for the United States and States: April 1, 2000. Washington, DC: U.S. Census Bureau.

Valentine JM, Lyons G, Bellamy MC. The effect of intrathecal midazolam on postoperative pain. *Eur J Anaesthesiol* 1996; 13: 589-593.

van Dongen RT, Crul BJ, van Egmond J. Intrathecal coadministration of bupivacaine diminishes morphine dose progression during long-term intrathecal infusion in cancer patients. *Clin J Pain* 1999; 15: 166-172.

Van Schaeybroeck P, Nuttin B, Lagae L, et al. Intrathecal baclofen for intractable cerebral spasticity: A prospective, placebo-controlled, double-blind study. *Neurosurgery* 2000; 46: 603-609.

Veering BT, Burm AG, Vletter AA, van den Heuvel RP, Onkenhout W, Spierdijk J. The effect of age on the systemic absorption, disposition and pharmacodynamics of bupivacaine after epidural administration. *Clin Pharmacokinet* 1992; 22: 75-84.

Walsh KH, Murphy C, Iohom G, Cooney C, McAdoo J. Comparison of the effects of two intrathecal anesthetic techniques for transurethral prostatectomy on haemodynamic and pulmonary function. *Eur J Anaesthesiol* 2003; 20: 560-564.

Wang YX, Gao D, Pettus M, Phillips C, Bowersox SS. Interactions of intrathecally administered ziconotide, a selective blocker of neuronal N-type voltage-sensitive calcium channels, with morphine on nociception in rats. *Pain* 2000; 84: 271-281.

Weir PS, Fee JP. Double-blind comparison of extradural block with three bupivacaine-ketamine mixtures in knee arthroplasty. *Br J Anaesth* 1998; 80: 299-301.

Wilder-Smith CH, Wilder-Smith OH, Farschtschian M, Naji P. Epidural droperidol reduces the side effects and duration of analgesia of epidural sufentanil. *Anesth Analg* 1994; 79: 98-104.

Winkelmuller M, Winkelmuller W. Long-term effects of continuous intrathecal opioid treatment in chronic pain of nonmalignant etiology. *J Neurosurg* 1996; 85: 459-467.

Yaksh TL, Pogrel JW, Lee YW, Chaplan SR. Reversal of nerve ligation-induced allodynia by spinal alpha-2 adrenoceptor agonists. *J Pharmacol Exp Ther* 1995; 272: 207-214.

Yotsui H, Matsunaga M, Katori K, Kohno S, Higa K. Extrapyramidal reactions after epidural droperidol. *Masui* 2000; 49: 1152-1154.

Yue SK, St Marie B, Henrickson K. Initial clinical experience with the SKY epidural catheter. *J Pain Symptom Manage* 1991; 6: 107-114.

Zuniga RE, Perera S, Abram SE. Intrathecal baclofen: A useful agent in the treatment of well-established complex regional pain syndrome. *Reg Anesth Pain Med* 2002; 27: 90-93.

Zuniga RE, Schlicht CR, Abram SE. Intrathecal baclofen is analgesic in patients with chronic pain. *Anesthesiology* 2000; 92: 876-880.

Chapter 14

Oral and Intravenous Local Anesthetics

Gary McCleane

When we talk of local anesthetics, we are conventionally considering agents known to produce local anesthesia when injected into tissue and to cause distal anesthesia when administered perineurally. As a group, these agents are unified by a sodium channel-blocking effect, and it is this action that reduces neural function to the extent of producing anesthesia. That said, a number of other widely used analgesic agents also possess sodium channel-blocking effects and yet are not classified as local anesthetics. For example, carbamazepine, oxcarbazepine, phenytoin, fosphenytoin, and many of the tricyclic antidepressants have significant sodium channel-blocking actions. The fact that these drugs possess sodium channel effects that are directly implicated in their analgesic actions and yet do not cause tissue anesthesia emphasizes that their effect is systemic as well as local and that the systemic administration of a sodium channel blocker, or local anesthetic, can produce analgesia by modes other than "freezing" the painful area.

It has been mentioned that local anesthetics exert at least some of their effect by blocking sodium channels. It is now clear that a sodium channel is not a single entity but rather a collection of channels with differing characteristics. We know that voltage-activated sodium channels consist of a pore-forming alpha subunit, of which nine have been cloned, as well as three associated beta subunits. Consequently, not all drugs with sodium channel-blocking effects necessarily produce identical therapeutic effects, as each has a propensity to interact at differing types of sodium channels.

We have seen in previous chapters that local anesthetics can be used topically and perineurally. The emphasis of this chapter is the systemic use of these agents when administered either orally or intravenously.

Clinical Management of the Elderly Patient in Pain
© 2006 by The Haworth Press, Inc. All rights reserved.
doi:10.1300/5356_14

ORAL LOCAL ANESTHETICS

Mexiletine

Clinically, the most widely used oral local anesthetic is mexiletine. Electrophysiological studies in rats suggest that spinally administered mexiletine has a predominant effect on spinal A-delta and C fibers, with little effect on A-beta fibers.

Whereas we instinctively associate the use of drugs such as mexiletine with neuropathic pain, animal studies suggest that it may also have an effect on other types of pain. For example, one model of chronic inflammatory pain is the formalin test. In this type of study, formalin is applied to the paw of a rat and the behavioral reaction to the irritation is measured by counting the times the animal flinches. Mexiletine has been shown to reduce the flinching behavior in such a formalin test.

Erichsen and colleagues (2003) have shown that in a rat model of neuropathic pain, mexiletine significantly reduced mechanical allodynia, while lidocaine had no such effect. Therefore, despite the fact that both lidocaine and mexiletine are both active on sodium channels, in this experimental paradigm, their effect was different. In a similar vein, Xu and colleagues (1992) examined the effect of mexiletine and carbamazepine (also known to be active at sodium channels) along with morphine, baclofen, and muscimol, in a rat model of ischemic spinal cord injury. The allodynia produced by this injury was resistant to treatment with carbamazepine (and morphine, baclofen, and muscimol) but did respond to mexiletine. The logic, therefore, of using a small dose of intravenous lidocaine to test the likely responsiveness to oral mexiletine is not necessarily based on scientific evidence.

It has been suggested by some that mexiletine exerts its effect by blocking nociception in capsaicin-sensitive primary afferent fibers, perhaps by causing a reduction in substance P release from the afferent terminals. As usual with many of the drugs used in pain management, the actual actions are diverse and rarely attributable to one single action.

Clinical Use of Mexiletine

When the pharmacokinetics of mexiletine in elderly patients are considered, it has been shown that the elimination half-life, oral clearance, and urinary elimination of mexiletine are similar in young and elderly patients. However, the rate of absorption of the drug from the gastrointestinal tract is significantly slower in elderly patients.

A number of human studies have been performed examining the effect of mexiletine in a variety of pain conditions. Dejgard and colleagues (1988) examined subjects with chronic painful diabetic neuropathy and showed that mexiletine reduced pain significantly when compared with placebo. They also showed that there were no changes in tendon reflexes, vibration threshold levels, beta-to-beat variation in heart rate during deep breathing, or postural blood pressure during mexiletine treatment. These workers used a dose of mexiletine of 10 mg/kg. Other studies have examined the effect of mexiletine in spinal cord injury dysesthetic pain (using a dose of only 450 mg per day) and allodynia of mixed etiology (using a dose of 900 mg per day) and found no significant reduction in measured pain parameters. It does appear that mexiletine has a narrow therapeutic window and it may be hard to find an effective dose without inducing unacceptable side effects.

Flecainide

The antiarrhythmic drug flecainide has sodium channel-blocking effects like mexiletine and lidocaine. Little clinical evidence exists for its effect on neuropathic pain, and many practitioners may be put off from using it because of lack of experience in its use and because of reports of withdrawal arrhythmias when it is suddenly stopped in patients who have been using it for its antiarrhythmic properties. That said, from an anecdotal clinical perspective it is both more effective and better tolerated than mexiletine.

In an isolated study, Ichimata and colleagues (2001) showed that flecainide significantly reduced the pain of postherpetic neuralgia when it was used over a one-month period.

INTRAVENOUS LOCAL ANESTHETICS

Few therapeutic acts go against the grain as much as the prospect of injecting a local anesthetic agent deliberately into a vein. We have all been brought up to carefully aspirate before injection of any local anesthetic to avoid the inadvertent systemic administration of the substance. Yet the concept to be outlined involves the deliberate injection of what will seem like enormous amounts of specific local anesthetics by the intravenous (IV) route. To many, it will be difficult to ignore years of ingrained practice and yet the potential benefit of systemic administration of certain local anesthetics is enormous. Reference to the IV use of local anesthetics dates back over 60 years with many subsequent reports of pain relief in a wide variety of clinical scenarios appearing, often as case reports, in the literature since then.

Mode of Action of Systemically Administered
Local Anesthetics

At a cellular level, ionic disequilibrium across semipermeable membranes provides the potential energy for impulse conduction. For nerve cells, the most important ionic disequilibria are created and maintained by the electrogenic, energy-requiring, membrane-bound enzyme Na^+-K^+ ATPase, which pumps Na^+ ions out of the cell and K^+ ions in. The steady-state resting potential is due to the combined effects of Na^+-K^+ ATPase (three Na^+ ions are extruded for every two K^+ ions that are absorbed), which results in a hyperpolarizing, outward current, plus an inward "leak" current. Changes in either of these current components as well as minimum activation of voltage-gated conductances will alter the resting potential.

During an action potential, voltage-gated Na^+ channels open briefly, allowing a small quantity of extracellular Na^+ ions to flow into the cell, thus depolarizing the plasma membrane. Sodium channels close spontaneously (inactivate), and thus the duration of the depolarizing inward Na^+ current is limited. A more slowly developing outward current, often of K^+ ions flowing through voltage-gated K^+ channels, helps to repolarize the membrane rapidly and restore electrical neutrality. A local ionic current flowing through cytoplasm helps propagate the regenerative wave of depolarization throughout the cell's excitable membrane. Local anesthetics block impulses by inhibiting individual Na^+ channels and thereby reducing the aggregate inward sodium current of the nerve fiber.

When administered systemically, lidocaine has specific spinal cord effects. Devor and colleagues (1992) have shown that systemic lidocaine suppresses ectopic impulse discharge generated both at sites of experimental nerve injury and in axotomized dorsal root ganglia cells. The doses effective for blocking ectopic discharge failed to block the initiation or propagation of impulses by electrical stimulation and only minimally affected normal sensory receptors. It therefore seems that systemic administration of lidocaine has the potential for reducing the injury-induced discharge of peripheral nerves, in particular A-delta and C fibers, as well as having an effect on dorsal root ganglia cells.

Animal Models

A strong body of evidence from animal studies supports the contention that systemic lidocaine reduces neuropathic pain. The reduction in pain observed appears to be dose dependent. Indeed, the antinociceptive effect may not be confined to neuropathic pain. Ness (2000) reports that intravenous lidocaine inhibits visceromotor and cardiovascular reflexes and the evoked and spontaneous activity of neurons excited by colorectal distension in a rat model, with the implication that systemic lidocaine may be useful in the treatment of visceral pain conditions.

Significant insight into the potential clinical use of IV lidocaine is gained by examination of the work of Chapman and colleagues (1995). They examined the effect of intravenous lidocaine in a rat spinal nerve ligation model of neuropathic pain and confirmed the findings of others who had observed a reduction in tactile allodynia when lidocaine is administered in this fashion (see Figure 14.1). Two further highly significant results were obtained. First, when lidocaine was given by the intravenous route over a short infusion period, the reduction of tactile allodynia observed persisted for significantly longer than the half-life of the drug. Indeed, in this experiment, 21 days after the lidocaine infusion, 30 to 40 percent of the maximum possible reduction in tactile allodynia persisted. When the authors applied lidocaine intrathecally and regionally, no such reduction in allodynia was observed.

The second highly relevant finding was that the effect was related to the speed of lidocaine administration rather than the total dose (see Figure 14.2). When a dose was given slowly, little reduction in baseline, preinfusion

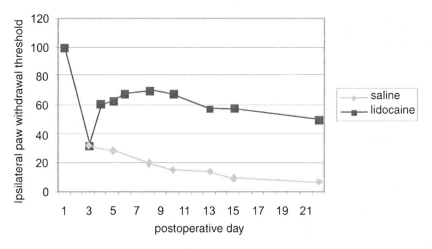

FIGURE 14.1. Ipsilateral paw withdrawal threshold, normalized to the preoperative level (=100 percent) in rats with SNL (spinal nerve ligation) on day 0 and then infused for 30 min by lidocaine orsaline. *Source:* Chapman, S.R., Bach, F.W., Shafer, S.L., and Yaksh, T.L. Prolonged alleviation of tactile allodynia by intravenous lidocaine in neuropathic rats. *Anesthesiology,* 1995; 83(4): 780. Reprinted by permission.

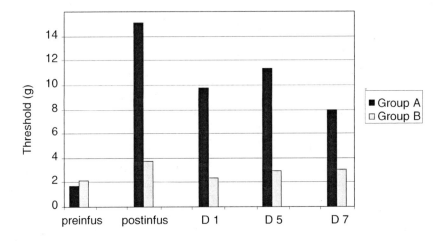

FIGURE 14.2. Two groups of neuropathic rats receiving identical dose of IV lidocaine, group A receiving infusion at faster rate than group B. Paw withdrawal thresholds. *Source:* Reprinted from *Pain* 103(1), Araujo et al., Multiple phases of relief from experimental mechanical allodynia by systemic lidocaine: Responses to early and late infusions, pp. 21-29. © 2003 with permission from the International Association for the Study of Pain®.

allodynia was observed. However, when exactly the same dose was given more rapidly, a pronounced and prolonged antiallodynic effect was recorded.

Further fascinating insight into the effect of systemic lidocaine is given by the work of Araujo and colleagues (2003). They examined rats that underwent spinal nerve ligation and who suffered from consequent allodynia. Lidocaine infusions were compared with saline infusions and the effect of allodynia measured. They also examined the timing of infusions, with some being given on the second day after ligation while others were given seven days after this procedure (see Figure 14.3). They were able to show that there were three phases of response to lidocaine. First there was an acute reduction of allodynia during lidocaine infusion that disappeared within 30 to 60 minutes after the end of the infusion. Second, there was a transient reduction in allodynia several hours after infusion and third, a sustained reduction that developed slowly over 24 hours after infusion and was maintained over the following 21-day study period.

Their second major finding was that infusion given two days after spinal nerve ligation was more effective than infusion of an equal dose on postoperative day seven in reducing allodynia.

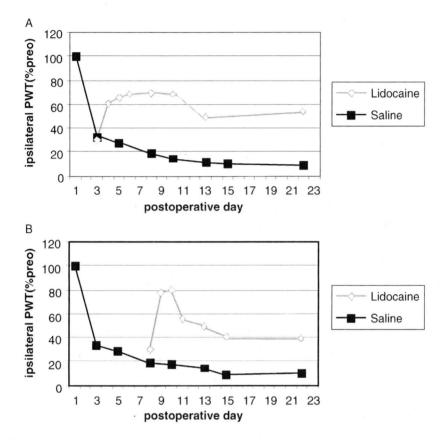

FIGURE 14.3. Effect of IV lidocaine versus saline on ipsilateral paw withdrawal threshold (PWT) normalized to preoperative level (=100 percent). A. Lidocaine at postop day 2. B. Lidocaine at postop day 7. *Source:* Reprinted from *Pain* 103(1), Araujo et al., Multiple phases of relief from experimental mechanical allodynia by systemic lidocaine: Responses to early and late infusions, pp. 21-29. © 2003 with permission from International Association for the Study of Pain®.

Three major conclusions can be gleaned from the animal studies. First, IV lidocaine reduces the animal signs of neuropathic pain in a dose-dependent fashion. Second, the rate of infusion has a significant effect on consequent antinociception, and third, the antinociception can persist for a period far in excess of the plasma half-life of the lidocaine.

Safety of Intravenous Lidocaine

If we accept that the animal evidence strongly supports the contention that the IV administration of lidocaine can reduce pain, then the issue of the safety of such administration becomes crucial. Most practitioners would have an instinctive reluctance to consider the IV use of any local anesthetic. Many would associate the use of IV local anesthetics with a significant potential for cardiovascular suppression or even collapse. Perhaps one of the reasons for this fear is the historical use of intravenous lidocaine in the treatment of arrhythmias associated with acute myocardial infarction. In this scenario, infarcted and hypoxic myocardium produces an impairment of ventricular performance and lessening of cardiac output along with a propensity for dysrhythmia. The issue is, therefore, whether lidocaine used in this type of patient worsens the cardiac dysfunction or is merely tarnished by association. Reference to the literature, which itself is based largely on animal experimentation, gives a mixed picture, with some articles suggesting a negative inotropic effect of lidocaine while others suggest an improvement in coronary blood flow, increase in myocardial oxygenation, and reduction in arrhythmia potential.

Clinical use of lidocaine in pain management also gives an indication of its safety. Extensive clinical use by some points to a high degree of safety. Anecdotal reports of use in over 6,000 cases without untoward cardiovascular events should increase confidence in its use. In one small case series, McCleane (2001) reports on the effect of lidocaine infusions of over 1000 mg given over six hours in patients with significant concomitant illnesses, including those of a cardiac nature. No significant effect on heart rate, arterial blood pressure, or cardiac rhythm was observed.

In the anecdotal reports of experience of lidocaine infusions in over 6,000 patients, over two thirds were given as domiciliary infusions—in other words, the patient went home with a disposable infusion device and received the lidocaine infusion outside a hospital environment. Still no major cardiovascular or other complications have been observed.

That said, as usual with many aspects of medical practice, common sense in the use of such techniques is important. Adjustment of dose because of size, general health, and age are all sensible, and an admission to hospital for administration where major health issues exist would be wise.

The major side effect of IV lidocaine is in fact inflammation of the vein through which the lidocaine is administered. This can be of the extent to require premature withdrawal of the administration cannula. This propensity to cause venous irritation is related to the concentration of the lidocaine infused and, strangely, to the proprietary brand of lidocaine used. It does not appear to be related to the pH or the presence of preservatives. One method of reducing this infusion-related pain and inflammation is to place a glyceryl trinitrate patch above the infusion site. This nitrate possesses local anti-inflammatory properties that can be sufficient to negate the chances of this particular complication.

Human Experimental Pain

Several published studies have examined the effect of systemic lidocaine on human experimental pain. In one, Koppert and colleagues (2000) compared the effect of lidocaine administered systemically and by a regional technique on the pain and secondary hyperalgesia produced by intradermal injection of capsaicin. Lidocaine administered in both fashions reduced slightly the pain produced by capsaicin injection. However, only systemically administered lidocaine had a significant effect on the secondary hyperalgesia, as measured by pinpricks. This suggests a central mode of action for lidocaine when used in this fashion.

Mattsson and colleagues (2000) examined the effect of systemic lidocaine on the tissue response to partial-thickness skin burns. When compared to placebo infusion, lidocaine had no effect in the first four hours after the burn was inflicted. However, by 12 hours after the burn, the lidocaine-treated subjects had a significantly quicker resolution of residual erythema compared to control sites.

CONDITIONS BENEFITING FROM INTRAVENOUS LIDOCAINE

The balance of animal and human experimental data would suggest a potential role for IV lidocaine in pain management. Unfortunately, much of the clinical evidence is based on case reports, although there are a few randomized controlled trials.

Burn Pain

Historically, the first report of the successful use of a local IV anesthetic dates from 1943, reporting analgesia in burn patients when IV novocaine was used. We have seen already that human experimental investigation supports the contention that local IV anesthetics may be analgesic when used in burn patients with the added advantage of quickening the resolution of the erythematous flare that surrounds the burn site. Jonsson and colleagues (1991) report successful use of IV lidocaine in patients immediately after hospital admission with a burn and confirm that the use of IV lidocaine can significantly reduce the need to give rescue opioid analgesia.

Neuropathic Pain

The evidence confirming a potential analgesic effect when IV lidocaine is used is perhaps strongest in the case of neuropathic pain. Even then, certain contraindications arise. Attal and colleagues (2000) report a significant reduction in central pain when IV lidocaine is compared to placebo infusion, while Galer and colleagues (1993) have found that IV lidocaine had significantly less analgesic effect in patients with central pain when compared to those with peripheral nervous system injury. The results they obtained are nevertheless impressive: 58 percent of those with peripheral nervous system injury pain gained relief, 83 percent in patients with trigeminal neuralgia, 78 percent in those with lumbosacral arachnoiditis, and 70 percent with polyneuropathy.

Baranowski and colleagues (1999) examined the effect of IV infusions of lidocaine (1 and 5 mg/kg) given over two hours and compared them with saline (placebo) infusions in patients with postherpetic neuralgia. They found that both pain and allodynia were reduced in the active treatment group and that in this scenario, the higher-dose infusion inferred no additional benefit.

It also seems that the pain of diabetic neuropathy can respond to IV lidocaine and that the duration of relief can extend to 21 days after infusion.

Postamputation Pain

Wu and colleagues (2002) have compared the effect of IV lidocaine to IV morphine infusion in patients with phantom limb and stump pain. Lidocaine 1 mg/kg bolus and 4 mg/kg infusions repeated on three consecutive days were used. They found that IV lidocaine reduced stump but not phantom pain.

Fibromyalgia

Several studies have looked at fibromyalgia. Infusions up to 500 mg of lidocaine were used and response rates as high as 48 percent were reported. Indeed, in the study by Raphael and colleagues (2002), the duration of relief after infusion was prolonged; 21 out of 50 responders had relief that extended between 13 and 18 weeks.

Pain Associated with Malignancy

Although it could be argued that when treating pain associated with cancer an attempt should be made to define which tissue is giving rise to the pain (nerve, viscera, muscle, etc.) and to choose the most appropriate pharmacological method of treatment used for that type of pain, there are circumstances where this is not possible. Intravenous lidocaine has distinct advantages in pain associated with malignancy. It can work for pain arising from any tissue. A short treatment may give prolonged relief, and it does not have the potential cognitive and sedative side effects of opiate analgesics.

Postoperative Pain

As long ago as 1961, Bartlett and Hutaserani reported significant alleviation of postoperative pain with IV lidocaine when doses up to 800 mg were used. In their sample, 85 percent reported either no or mild pain after IV lidocaine, compared to only 31 percent in the control group.

Groudine and colleagues (1998) report that IV lidocaine was associated with a significantly reduced time to first flatulence, more rapid return of normal bowel function, and shorter stay in hospital of 1.1 days in patients undergoing radical retropubic prostatectomy.

Chronic Daily Headache

Hand and Stark (2000) report the use of IV lidocaine in 19 patients with severe chronic daily headache. There was resolution in 82 percent of patients. Four subjects derived lasting relief.

Sciatica

Medrik-Goldberg and colleagues (1999) report the effect of a two-hour infusion of 5 mg/kg in patients with sciatica. Use of lidocaine was associated with a significant reduction in sciatic pain and increase in straight leg raising.

Fractured Ribs

Although the gold standard of treatment for multiple fractured ribs may be a thoracic epidural injection, this form of treatment is not available to the elderly patient at home or in community hospital settings. Furthermore, it can sometimes be difficult to decide when the threshold has been crossed to merit a thoracic epidural. Yet one hopes to avoid respiratory impairment produced by the pain from the fractured ribs, secretion retention, and the analgesic drugs used in an attempt to alleviate the pain. Anecdotal evidence suggests that IV lidocaine can be highly effective in reducing the pain of fractured ribs. Because the pain relief provided by infusion is not associated with sedation or cough suppression, the chances of further respiratory complications can be lessened.

Pain of Mixed Etiology

Although it is usually unsatisfactory to examine the effect of any pain treatment on pain of mixed etiology, the report of Edwards and colleagues (1985) does provide interesting data. They looked at 211 patients who were treated with IV lidocaine at a dose of 1 and 5 mg/kg given over 5-35 minutes, and 46 percent reported complete pain relief.

Proctalgia Fugax

Proctalgia fugax is characterized by sudden internal anal sphincter and anorectic ring attacks of pain of short duration. A case report of a single patient reports a resolution of pain after a single intravenous dose of lidocaine.

SUGGESTED CLINICAL USE

Although the animal and human experimental and clinical data suggest an analgesic effect, the exact place of IV, systemic use of lidocaine needs to be defined.

On the negative side, lidocaine clearly does not alleviate all types of pain and may or may not be effective in individuals with conditions known to be amenable to the use of lidocaine. But then no pain treatment, no matter how good it is, is effective in all patients. Lidocaine may have cardiovascular side effects, but in practice these do not seem to present a major problem with the doses used. The major practical problem with its use is venous irritation when concentrated solutions are used.

On the positive side, lidocaine has no major effects on cognition and does not induce somnolence. The concept of providing a treatment with a drug of relatively short half-life that is given over a short period of time and yet may give substantial relief for days, weeks, or even months after infusion must have appeal. With most other treatments, it would be necessary to continually administer the treatment to obtain relief. Not so with lidocaine.

In the elderly patient, the ability to reduce oral analgesics, avoid drugs with definite and marked side-effect profiles, and yet have a realistic chance of getting relief must offer some advantage. With few other treatments do we have as much chance of relieving neuropathic as well as nonneuropathic pain. Furthermore, incident pain such as that caused by changes in dressings, rib fracture pain, and pain arising from long bone fractures is often reduced along with the background pain that more conventional analgesics seem to preferentially target.

It may be perceived that the use of IV lidocaine is a hospital-based treatment. Although it can be usefully applied for a wide range of conditions seen in hospital practice, it may also have domiciliary application. We have extensive clinical experience with around 5000 uses of disposable elastomeric infusion devices for the administration of lidocaine infusion for domiciliary infusions (see Figure 14.4). Patients come to a practice for cannula insertion and attachment of the prefilled infusor and then go home. At a defined time, the cannula is removed. Because 2 percent lidocaine is used, the risk of venous irritation is relatively high, and so a glyceryl trinitrate patch is applied above the infusion site to lessen the risk of venous pain and swelling.

Dose

The most thorny issue is that of dose used. In some studies, a single bolus is given. In others, infusion over several hours is used. This may be repeated

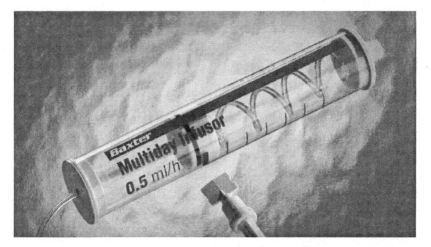

FIGURE 14.4. Baxter elastomeric infusion device. Image copyright Baxter Healthcare Ltd. Reprinted by permission.

over subsequent days. In our practice, a single infusion is used. When a disposable infusor is used, the infusion is given over 30 hours. When used as a hospital inpatient treatment, the infusion may be over 6 to 8 or 24 hours.

We have seen that the total dose given has some influence on the resultant analgesia. Speed of infusion seems to be more important. Quicker infusion of a given dose is more likely to produce analgesia than a slower infusion of an equal dose. Furthermore, quicker infusion is associated with either better quality pain relief, pain relief of greater duration, or both.

Total dose and speed of administration are influenced by the age, size, and general health of the patient. It is therefore hard to give exact guidance. Perhaps the best approach is to think of maximum doses and for one to modify them for the older, smaller, or sicker patient.

We use a maximum of 1200 mg lidocaine in the disposable infusion device (60 ml 2 percent lidocaine). Because the particular infusor we use has a 2 ml per hour flow restrictor, this infusion is completed in 30 hours.

For inpatient treatments, a commercially prepared 0.2 percent lidocaine in 500 ml 5 percent dextrose solution is used (total lidocaine content 1000 mg). This can be given over 24 hours (in younger patients, 1500 mg may be given in a similar period). Alternatively, where pain is more resistant, or a longer period of relief is hoped for, this 1000 mg lidocaine infusion can be given over 6 to 8 hours. Although dizziness and light-headedness are not uncommon with such rapid infusion, cardiovascular changes are infrequent. Clearly, dose modification is appropriate to tailor the dose to an individual patient.

CONCLUSION

Clinical experience and investigation support the contention that oral membrane stabilizers, such as mexiletine, can have an analgesic effect in various pain states. The use of mexiletine may be limited by its narrow therapeutic window.

The use of IV local anesthetics, such as lidocaine, is clearly more contentious. However, the potential advantages of IV lidocaine, which include effectiveness in a broad range of pain conditions, a short half-life yet long duration of pain relief, and lack of sedative and cognitive side effects, make it a potentially useful tool in the management of pain in elderly patients. Arguably, it is much better to give infusions of lidocaine over a few hours than to continually dose these vulnerable patients with opioids, TCAs, or the like.

It does seem that there is, to some extent, a dose-response relationship, but also that speed of infusion is crucial in both the quality and duration of relief.

BIBLIOGRAPHY

Abdi S, Lee DH, Chung JM. The anti-allodynic effects of amitriptyline, gabapentin, and lidocaine in a rat model of neuropathic pain. *Anesth Analg* 1998; 87: 1360-1366.

Ackerman WE, Colclough GW, Juneja MM, Bellinger K. The management of oral mexiletine and intravenous lidocaine to treat chronic painful symmetrical distal diabetic neuropathy. *KMA J* 1991; 89: 500-501.

Araujo MC, Sinnott CJ, Strichartz GR. Multiple phases of relief from experimental mechanical allodynia by systemic lidocaine: Responses to early and late infusions. *Pain* 2003; 103: 21-29.

Attal N, Gaude L, Brasseur L, Dupuy M, Guirimand F, Bouhassira D. Intravenous lidocaine in central pain: A double-blind, placebo-controlled, psychophysical study. *Neurology* 2000; 54: 564-574.

Baranowski AP, De Courcey J, Bonello E. A trial of intravenous lidocaine on the pain and allodynia of postherpetic neuralgia. *J Pain Symptom Manage* 1999; 17: 429-433.

Bartlett EE, Hutaserani O. Xylocaine for the relief of postoperative pain. *Anesth Analg* 1961: 40: 296-304.

Bennett MI, Tai TM. Intravenous lignocaine in the management of primary fibromyalgia syndrome. *Int J Clin Pharm Res* 1995; 15: 115-119.

Blackburn-Munro G, Ibsen N, Erichsen HK. A comparison of the anti-nociceptive effects of voltage-activated Na^+ channel blockers in the formalin test. *Eur J Pharmacol* 2002; 445: 231-238.

Boas RA, Covino BG, Shahnarian A. Analgesic responses to IV lignocaine. *Br J Anaesth* 1982; 54: 501-505.

Butterworth JF, Strichartz GR. Molecular mechanisms of local anesthesia: A review. *Anesthesiology* 1990; 72: 711-734.

Catterall WA. Common modes of drug action on Na^+ channels: Local anesthetics, antiarrhythmics and anticonvulsants. *Tips* 1987; 8: 57-65.

Chabal C, Russell LC, Burchill KJ. The effect of intravenous lidocaine, tocainide, and mexiletine on spontaneously active fibers originating in rat sciatic neuromas. *Pain* 1989; 38: 333-338.

Chapman SR, Bach FW, Shafer SL, Yaksh TL. Prolonged alleviation of tactile allodynia by intravenous lidocaine in neuropathic rats. *Anesthesiology* 1995; 83: 775-785.

Chapman V, Ng J, Dickenson AH. A novel spinal action of mexiletine in spinal somatosensory transmission of nerve injured rats. *Pain* 1998; 77: 289-296.

Chiou-Tan FY, Tuel SM, Johnson JC, Priebe MM, Hirsh DD, Strayer JR. Effect of mexiletine on spinal cord injury dysesthetic pain. *Am J Phys Med Rehabil* 1996; 75: 84-87.

De Jong RH, Nace RA. Nerve impulse conduction during intravenous lidocaine injection. *Anesthesiology* 1968; 29: 22-28.

Dejgard A, Petersen P, Kastrup J. Mexiletine for treatment of chronic painful diabetic neuropathy. *Lancet* 1988; 8575: 9-11.

Devor M, Wall PD, Catalan N. Systemic lidocaine silences ectopic neuromas and DRG discharge without blocking nerve conduction. *Pain* 1992; 48: 261-268.

Dirks J, Fabricius P, Petersen KL, Rowbotham MC, Dahl JB. The effect of systemic lidocaine on pain and secondary hyperalgesia associated with the heat/capsaicin sensitization model in healthy volunteers. *Anesth Analg* 2000; 91: 967-972.

Edwards WT, Habib F, Burney RG, Begin GB. Intravenous lidocaine in the management of various chronic pain states. *Reg Anesthesia* 1985; 10: 1-6.

Erichsen HK, Hao J-X, Xu X-J, Blackburn-Munro G. A comparison of the antinociceptive effects of voltage-activated Na^+ channel blockers in two rat models of neuropathic pain. *Eur J Pharmacol* 2003; 458: 275-282.

Fassoulaki A, Patris K, Sarantopoulos C, Hogan Q. The analgesic effect of gabapentin and mexiletine after breast surgery for cancer. *Anesth Analg* 2002; 95: 985-991.

Fujita Y, Endoh S, Yasukawa T, Sari A. Lidocaine increases the ventricular fibrillation threshold during bupivicaine-induced cardiotoxicity in pigs. *Br J Anaesth* 1998; 80: 218-222.

Galer BS, Miller KV, Rowbotham MC. Response to intravenous lidocaine infusion based on clinical diagnosis and site of nervous system injury. *Neurology* 1993; 43: 1233-1235.

Gee D, Wilson R, Angello D. Acute effect of lidocaine on coronary blood flow and myocardial function. *Angiology* 1990; 41: 30-35.

Glazer S, Portenoy RK. Systemic local anesthetics in pain control. *J Pain Symptom Manage* 1991; 6: 30-39.

Gordon RA. Intravenous novocaine for analgesia in burns. *Can MAJ* 1943; 49: 478-481.

Grech-Belanger O, Barbeau G, Kishka P, Fiset C, LeBoeuf E, Blouin M. Pharmacokinetics of mexiletine in the elderly. *J Clin Pharmacol* 1989; 29: 311-315.

Groudine SB, Fisher HA, Kaufman RP, Patel MK, Wilkins LJ, Mehta SA, Lumb PD. Intravenous lidocaine speeds the return of bowel function, decreases postoperative pain, and shortens hospital stay in patients undergoing radical retropubic prostatectomy. *Anesth Analg* 1998; 86: 235-239.

Hand PJ, Stark RJ. Intravenous lignocaine infusions for severe chronic daily headache. *Med J Aust* 2000; 172: 157-159.

Ichimata M, Ikebe H, Yoshitake S, Hattori S, Iwasaka H, Noguchi T. Analgesic effects of flecainide on postherpetic neuralgia. *Int J Clin Pharmacol Res* 2001; 21: 15-19.

Jonsson A, Cassuto J, Hanson B, Inhibition of burn pain by intravenous lignocaine infusion. *Lancet* 1991; 338: 151-152.

Kamei J, Hitosugi H, Kawashima N, Aoki T, Ohhashi Y, Kasuya Y. Antinociceptive effect of mexiletine in diabetic mice. *Res Comm Chem Path Pharmacol* 1992; 77: 245-248.

Kamei J, Zushida K. Effect of mexiletine on thermal allodynia and hyperalgesia in diabetic mice. *Jpn J Pharmacol* 2000; 84: 89-92.

Kaslo E, Tramer MR, McQuay HJ, Moore RA. Systemic local anesthetic type drugs in chronic pain: A systematic review. *Eur J Pain* 1998; 2: 3-14.

Kastrup J, Bach FW, Petersen P, Dejgard A, Ekman R, Jensen S, Angelo H. Lidocaine treatment of painful diabetic neuropathy and endogenous opioid peptides in plasma. *Clin J Pain* 1989; 5: 239-244.

Kastrup J, Petersen P, Dejgard A, Angelo HR, Hilsted J. Intravenous lidocaine infusion—A new treatment of chronic painful diabetic neuropathy? *Pain* 1987; 28: 69-75.

Koppert W, Ostermeier N, Sittl R, Weidner C, Schmelz M. Low dose lidocaine reduces secondary hyperalgesia by a central mode of action. *Pain* 2000; 85: 217-224.

Mao J, Chen LL. Systemic lidocaine for neuropathic pain relief. *Pain* 2000; 87: 7-17.

Massey GV, Pedigo S, Dunn NL, Grossman NJ, Russell EC. Continuous lidocaine infusion for the relief of refractory malignant pain in a terminally ill pediatric cancer patient. *J Pediatr Hematol Oncol* 2002; 24: 566-568.

Matos L, Hankoczy J, Torok E. Effects of lidocaine on myocardial function and on isoprenaline-induced circulatory changes in man. *Int J Clin Pharmacol* 1976; 14: 119-125.

Mattsson U, Cassuto J, Tarnow P, Jonsson A, Jontell M. Intravenous lidocaine infusion in the treatment of experimental human skin burns—Digital color image analysis of erythema development. *Burns* 2000; 26: 710-715.

McCleane GJ. Does intravenous lidocaine reduce fibromyalgia pain? A randomized, double-blind, placebo-controlled crossover study. *Pain Clinic* 2000; 12: 181-185.

McCleane GJ. Intravenous infusion of lidocaine is not associated with changes in cardiovascular parameters: A study of 15 patients. *Pain Clinic* 2001; 13: 83-96.

Medrik-Goldberg T, Lifschitz D, Pud D, Adur R, Eisenberg F. Intravenous lidocaine, amantadine, and placebo in the treatment of sciatica: A double-blind, randomized, controlled trial. *Reg Anesth Pain Med* 1999; 24: 534-540.

Ness TJ. Intravenous lidocaine inhibits visceral nociceptive reflexes and spinal neurons in the rat. *Anesthesiology* 2000; 92: 1685-1691.

Peleg R, Shvartzman P. Low dose intravenous lidocaine as treatment for proctalgia fugax. *Reg Anesth Pain Med* 2002; 27: 97-99.

Raphael JH, Southall JL, Treharne GJ, Kitas GD. Efficacy and adverse effects of intravenous lignocaine therapy in fibromyalgia syndrome. *BMC Musculoskeletal Disord* 2002; 3: 21-29.

Smith LJ, Shih A, Miletic G, Miletic V. Continual systemic infusion of lidocaine provides analgesia in an animal model of neuropathic pain. *Pain* 2002; 97: 267-273.

Strichartz G. Protracted relief of experimental neuropathic pain by systemic local anesthetics. *Anesthesiology* 1995; 83: 654-655.

Strichartz GR, Zhou Z, Sinnott C, Khodorova A. Therapeutic concentrations of local anesthetics unveil the potential sodium of channels in neuropathic pain. *Novartis Found Symp* 2002; 241: 189-201.

Tanelian DL, Brose WG. Neuropathic pain can be relieved by drugs that are use-dependent sodium channel blockers: Lidocaine, carbamazepine, and mexiletine. *Anesthesiology* 1991; 74: 949-951.

Tanelian DL, MacIver MB. Analgesic concentrations of lidocaine suppress tonic A delta and C fiber discharges produced by acute injury. *Anesthesiology* 1991; 74: 934-936.

Tanelian DL, Victory RA. Sodium channel blocking agents: Their use in neuropathic pain conditions. *Pain Forum* 1995; 4: 75-80.

Wallace MS, Magnuson S, Ridgeway B. Efficacy of oral mexiletine for neuropathic pain with allodynia: A double-blind, placebo-controlled, crossover study. *Reg Anesth Pain Med* 2000; 25: 459-467.

Woolf CJ, Wiesenfeld-Hallin Z. The systemic administration of local anesthetics produces a selective depression of C afferent fiber evoked activity in the spinal cord. *Pain* 1985; 23: 361-374.

Wu CL, Tella P, Staats PS, Vaslav R, Kazim DA, Wesselmann U, Raja SN. Analgesic effects of intravenous lidocaine and morphine on postamputation pain: A randomized double-blind, active placebo-controlled, crossover trial. *Anesthesiology* 2002; 96: 841-848.

Xu XJ, Hao JX, Seiger A, Arner S, Lindblom U, Wiesenfeld-Hallin Z. Systemic mexiletine relieves chronic allodynia-like symptoms in rats with ischemic spinal cord injury. *Anesth Analg* 1992; 74: 649-652.

Chapter 15

Muscle Relaxants

Howard Smith

Muscle relaxants are an extremely heterogenous group of agents that are used primarily in an effort to improve spasticity, muscular conditions (e.g., muscle spasm), or pain.

Spasticity (resulting from upper motor neuron pathology) can be caused by various processes affecting the spinal cord or cortical tissues (e.g., multiple sclerosis, spinal cord injury, poststroke syndrome). Spasticity is often painful and disabling and may lead to significant deterioration of functional abilities and quality of life.

Musculoskeletal conditions associated with pain, tenderness, muscle spasms, and dysfunction may be related to mechanical insult and include myofascial pain syndrome, chronic low back pain, chronic neck pain, and tension headache. In these conditions, acute or chronic pain and spasms may respond to a variety of muscle relaxants. Muscle spasms in musculoskeletal conditions are generally related to local processes involving affected muscle groups; however, most orally administered muscle relaxants do not have specific local muscle effects.

Muscle relaxants should not be confused with nondepolarizing or depolarizing muscle relaxants, which produce neuromuscular blockade, yielding paralysis of muscles (including respiratory muscles). Most muscle relaxants do not possess significant muscle relaxant properties but rather are thought to work through general central nervous system depressant activities (see Table 15.1).

Additionally, most muscle relaxants are intended for relatively short-term use. Exceptions to this are baclofen and tizanidine, agents that can be used on a long-term or chronic basis and also stand out as seeming to possess specific antinociceptive qualities (both agents have been used as therapy for trigeminal neuralgia, a condition without associated musculoskeletal features). It remains to be seen whether orphenadrine may be counted among these agents as well.

Clinical Management of the Elderly Patient in Pain
© 2006 by The Haworth Press, Inc. All rights reserved.
doi:10.1300/5356_15

TABLE 15.1. Standard drugs used to treat spasticity.

Drug	Dose (for older patients)	Frequently reported side effects
Baclofen	PO: Initial dose 5 mg QD titrated to BID	Drowsiness, psychiatric disorder, urinary retention, constipation, hypersensitivity reactions
Carisoprodol	PO: 350 mg TID-QID	Drowsiness, dizziness, GI upset, ataxia, tremor
Cyclobenzaprine	PO: 10 mg TID	Drowsiness, dry mouth, diarrhea
Diazepam	PO: 2-5 mg TID-QID	Drowsiness, dizziness, diarrhea
Metaxalone	PO: 400-800 mg TID-QID Initial dose may be 200 mg in the elderly	Drowsiness, dizziness, nausea
Methocarbamol	PO: 750-1500 mg QID	Drowsiness, dizziness, GI upset
Orphenadrine	PO: 50-100 mg BID IV/IM 60 mg q12 hours	Anticholinergic effects, restlessness, agitation
Tizanidine	PO: initial dose 2 mg, may be titrated slowly up to 8 mg TID or as tolerated	Dry mouth, dizziness, fatigue, hypotension

Source: Smith and Barton, 2000. Reproduced with permission.

PHARMACOLOGICAL CONSIDERATIONS FOR THE USE OF MUSCLE RELAXANTS IN THE ELDERLY

People older than age 65 years constitute roughly 14 percent of the U.S. population (approximately 35 million people). The "oldest old" (over 85) are the most rapidly growing segment of the population. Multiple factors put elderly patients at increased risk for adverse drug events. The average elderly patient takes (on average) six different medications per day, increasing the risk of drug-drug interaction. In 1986, persons over age 60 accounted for 51 percent of all deaths caused by adverse reactions to medication. Pharmacokinetic changes with age include the following:

- Decreased first-pass metabolism
- Decreased rate of absorption
- Decreased lean mass
- Increased fat content

- Decreased serum protein concentrations and binding
- Decreased cytochrome P450 metabolic pathways (especially Phase 1 reaction, e.g., oxidation, hydroxylation, and demethylation)
- Decreased renal elimination/clearance

Pharmacodynamic changes associated with aging include these:

- Increased postsynaptic receptor effect (e.g., GABA)
- Decreased concentration of endogenous opioids and opioid receptors
- Altered receptor sensitivity
- Decreased cholinergic neurons and choline acetyltransferase (drugs with anticholinergic activity more likely to lead to delirium, e.g., diphenhydramine, clonidine)
- Decreased D1 and D2 receptors
- Decreased adenylate cyclase
- Decreased baroreceptor function

The Beers criteria, updated in 2003 (Fick et al., 2003) remain a widely used guideline for medication use in the elderly. The criteria, developed by consensus of a panel of experts, attach a severity rating (e.g., high or low) to various medications, or classes of medication, which they feel have concerns (as described) for usage in patients. Agents with a high severity are potentially inappropriate in older adults and should generally be avoided in people who are 65 years old or older, regardless of diagnosis or condition, either because the agents are deemed ineffective or because they are thought to pose unnecessarily high risks.

Fick et al. (2003) attached a high-risk rating to muscle relaxants and antispasmodics (methocarbamol, carisoprodol, chlorzoxazone, metaxalone, cyclobenzaprine, and oxybutynin), stating doctors should not consider the use of extended-release oxybutynin. Fick et al. stated that most muscle relaxants and antispasmodic drugs are poorly tolerated by older patients since they may cause anticholinergic adverse effects, sedation, and weakness. They also stated that the effectiveness of most muscle relaxants at doses tolerated by elderly patients is questionable.

I disagree with the vigorous dismissal of all musculoskeletal muscle relaxants in the elderly as being inappropriate and contraindicated and feels that particular agents in particular patients may be clinically useful and reasonably safe. Certainly, in evaluating older patients clinicians should appreciate the myriad of relevant concerns and issues. Practitioners should be aware of the individual patient's comorbid medical conditions and organ reserve (e.g., mental status, renal function, hepatic function, intravascular volume status, etc.). However, after a careful evaluation, including weighing the risks and benefits, it seems reasonable to proceed with a trial of a skeletal muscle relaxant in certain situations. The slow titration of tizanidine in an elderly patient with pain or muscle spasm refractory to other agents may be medically appropriate (in spite of the updated Beers criteria; e.g., 2 mg given once at night, when the patient is already in bed, is a reasonable starting point) in various circumstances.

Muscle relaxants are an extremely heterogenous group of medications: they are chemically unrelated, have different activities and mechanisms of action, and may exhibit significant differences in efficacy and safety in different medical conditions or populations.

The current literature is extremely limited and cannot be used as an evidence-based guide for clinicians in selecting an initial or second-line skeletal muscle relaxant, especially in the treatment of musculoskeletal conditions. There exists even less published evidence regarding the effectiveness of certain specific muscle relaxants: chlorzoxazone, methocarbamol, metaxalone, dantrolene, and baclofen, especially for the treatment of musculoskeletal conditions. In addition, many clinical trials of skeletal muscle relaxants have used unvalidated or poorly described methods to measure significant clinical outcomes such as spasticity, pain, or muscle strength. Even studies that use the same measurement instrument may report results differently (e.g., improvement from baseline versus number of patients improved). Also, even if a moderately reproducible tool for spasticity (the Ashworth scale) is used, resistance to passive movement may measure tone better than it does spasticity, and therefore the Ashworth scale may not correlate well with symptoms of functional ability.

Most studies of muscle relaxants in the literature (especially for musculoskeletal conditions) suffer from small numbers or poor design, short time period, inadequate record of adverse events or functional outcomes, and are extremely heterogenous in methods and interpretations.

In spite of the lack of high-quality evidence regarding muscle relaxants, widespread use of these agents in all ages continues. Furthermore, systematic reviews (although not confined to the elderly) have found that at least some muscle relaxants appear to be reasonably safe and effective for the treatment of spasticity and musculoskeletal conditions.

Chou et al. (2004) reviewed 101 randomized trials of muscle relaxants for spasticity and musculoskeletal conditions. They stated that no randomized trial was rated as good and that there was little evidence of rigorous adverse event assessment in included trials and observational studies. Chou and colleagues found that there is fair evidence that baclofen, tizanidine, and dantrolene are effective compared to placebo in patients with spasticity (predominantly in multiple sclerosis). They found fair evidence that baclofen and tizanidine have essentially equivalent efficacy for spasticity but insufficient evidence to determine the efficacy of dantrolene compared to baclofen or tizanidine. Also, they found fair evidence that the overall rate of adverse effects is similar between baclofen and tizanidine. However, tizanidine is associated with more dry mouth and baclofen with more weakness. Dantrolene (and chlorzoxazone, but much less so) have been associated with rare serious hepatotoxicity. In patients with musculoskeletal conditions (predominantly low back or neck pain), Chou and colleagues found fair evidence that cyclobenzaprine, carisoprodol, orphenadrine, and tizanidine are effective compared to placebo (cyclobenzaprine being involved in the most clinical trials, with consistent efficacy). In addition, Chou and colleagues found very limited or inconsistent data about the efficacy of metaxalone, methocarbamol, chlorzoxazone, baclofen, or dantrolene compared to placebo in patients with musculoskeletal conditions. They found insufficient evidence to compare the relative safety or efficacy between cyclobenzaprine, carisoprodol, orphenadrine, tizanidine, metaxalone, methocarbamol, and chlorzoxazone.

MUSCLE RELAXANT AGENTS

Baclofen

Baclofen (Lioresal) is the p-chlorophenyl derivative of gamma-aminobutyric acid (GABA). Baclofen is a GABA B agonist that has been utilized in the treatment of spasticity, musculoskeletal conditions, and neuropathic pain states. Side effects include sedation, weakness, and confusion. Abrupt cessation (especially with long-term therapy at high doses) may cause a withdrawal syndrome (e.g., hallucinations, anxiety, tachycardia, seizures).

In general, baclofen is not especially well tolerated in the elderly. Additionally, because it is excreted by the kidney, it should not be used in patients with a significant impairment in renal function (renal insufficiency is not infrequent in the elderly).

However, baclofen can be used judiciously in elderly patients where on occasion it may yield significant benefit. Peak serum concentrations generally occur within three to eight hours after oral ingestion. The half-life of baclofen is roughly four hours but may effectively be more in elderly or renal-impaired patient. A reasonable starting dose is half a tablet (5 mg) orally once or twice daily. A usual dose for young adults is 10 mg orally three times a day.

The precise mechanisms by which baclofen produces skeletal muscle relaxation or analgesia are unknown but appear to involve both pre- and postsynaptic GABA B receptor actions. At the presynaptic site, baclofen decreases calcium conduction with resultant decreased neurotransmitter/excitatory amino acid uptake. At the postsynaptic site, baclofen increases potassium conductance (with resultant neuronal hyperpolarization) and also may inhibit the release of substance P.

Baclofen is a racemic mixture, with L-baclofen being the active form. Pure L-baclofen (not currently available in the United States) was more effective than racemic baclofen (especially with regard to analgesic actions).

Baclofen has been utilized as a continuous intrathecal infusion in attempts to improve refractory spasticity (e.g., multiple sclerosis).

Benzodiazepines

Benzodiazepines are commonly used as muscle relaxant agents (especially in spasticity associated with spinal cord injury). They bind to benzodiazepine receptors located in the terminals of primary fibers leading to increased chloride flux across the terminal membrane, with a resultant increase in membrane potential. Although typically long acting, benzodiazepines are utilized to control spastic symptoms in young adults. In the elderly, lorazepam may exhibit favorable pharmacokinetics, and clonazepam (which also possesses analgesic qualities) may be used in small doses (e.g., half a 0.5 mg tablet or 0.25 mg orally) once at night. In most clinical situations, clonazepam and baclofen should not be used together as they are both GABA B agonists. Benzodiazepines should not be used as first-line agents since they may be associated with significant sedation as well as serious withdrawal syndromes.

Cyclobenzaprine

Cyclobenzaprine (Flexeril) is structurally closely related to the tricyclic antidepressants. It differs from amitriptyline by only one double bond.

Cyclobenzaprine is not always well tolerated in the elderly, who may be prone to develop hallucinations and significant anticholinergic side effects (e.g., tachycardia, sedation) as well as lethargy and agitation. Cyclobenzaprine is used for acute and intermittent musculoskeletal conditions including low back pain, muscle spasms, and fibromyalgia. The usual young adult dose is 10 mg orally three times a day. The starting dose in the elderly should be half a tablet (5 mg) orally once or twice a day.

Metaxalone

Metaxalone (Skelaxin) is an oxazolidone derivative that appears to be potentially useful for the acute management of peripheral musculoskeletal complaints but not all that effective in the treatment of spasticity secondary to neurological disorders. Although sedation is a potential side effect, it is generally well tolerated. A cautious initial dose in the elderly is half a tablet (200 mg) once or twice daily.

Methocarbamol

Methocarbamol (Robaxin) is a carbamate derivative of guaifenesin and structurally related to mephenesin. The agent is available both orally and parenterally and is indicated for short-term management of musculoskeletal conditions. It may conceivably provide perioperative analgesia in certain situations with muscular manipulation.

Carisoprodol

Carisoprodol (Soma) is an agent that should be used with great caution in the elderly, and in general, and on a short-term basis.

Carisoprodol is primarily metabolized in the liver to multiple metabolites, including meprobamate. Although only a relatively small amount is metabolized to meprobamate, there is potential for dependence, withdrawal, and abuse issues. There exist poor metabolizers of carisoprodol (usually metabolized by *N* deacetylation via CYP 2C19). These poor metabolizers are at increased risk of experiencing concentration-based side effects (e.g., drowsiness, hypotension, central nervous system depression) at usual doses. Additionally, carisoprodol may be associated with significant respiratory depression (which may be especially dangerous if carisoprodol is used simultaneously with propoxyphene).

The precise mechanisms of action of carisoprodol remain uncertain. However, it is conceivable that flumazenil may have potential as an antidote to carisoprodol toxicity.

Orphenadrine

Orphenadrine citrate (Norflex), a monomethylated derivative of diphenhydramine, has been used as a muscle relaxant and may possess analgesic qualities as well. Orphenadrine has been used alone and in combination with acetaminophen, aspirin, and nonsteroidal anti-inflammatory drugs. Orphenadrine may exhibit characteristics of an *N*-methyl-D-aspartate receptor antagonist. The major side effects experienced with orphenadrine seem to be related to its anticholinergic action (e.g., dry mouth, urinary retention, constipation, blurred vision, agitation, and restlessness). A reasonable starting dose in the elderly may be half a tablet (50 mg) orally once or twice daily or 30 mg parenterally every 12 to 24 hours.

Tizanadine

Tizanidine (Zanaflex) is an imidazoline derivative and an alpha-2 agonist that is structurally related to clonidine (however, its hypotensive effects are much less). The precise mechanisms of action are uncertain but appear to relate to a reduction of sympathetic nervous system outflow and presynaptic effects in the spinal cord, resulting in direct inhibition of excitatory release of amino acids with concomitant inhibition of facilitatory coeruleospinal pathways.

The elimination half-life of tizanidine is reported to be roughly one to three hours but may be effectively longer in elderly patients. The metabolism of tizanidine is predominantly hepatic, yielding biologically relatively inactive metabolites. Tizanidine should not be used in patients with hepatic impairment, and monitoring of liver function tests seems prudent. The excretion of tizanidine and its metabolites is primarily renal. Side effects include drowsiness, sedation, muscle weakness, and hypotension. A reasonable starting dose in the elderly is 2 mg orally, once at night (while in bed), which can be titrated up slowly.

In addition to its effects as a skeletal muscle relaxant, tizanidine appears to possess dose-dependent antinociceptive activity, which may be mediated via alpha-2 adrenoreceptors involving inhibition of glutamate, aspartate, or substance P release. Also, tizanidine may facilitate induction of sleep and play a role as a useful adjunct for the patient being weaned from high-dose opioids as well as a therapeutic option for restless leg syndrome.

OTHER AGENTS AND TREATMENTS

Anecdotally, numerous agents have been used for various conditions and complaints felt to be related to the musculoskeletal system. Although there exists little to no evidence for this, these agents include the following:

- Quinine sulfate
- Diphenhydramine hydrochloride
- Procainamide
- Phenytoin (and other antiepileptics)
- Propoxyphene (an agent generally not advised to be administered in the elderly)
- Cyproheptadine

- Chlorpromazine
- Dronabinol
- L-threonine (a precursor of glycine)

Physical

Physical and behavioral medicine techniques can be extremely useful in conjunction with pharmacological therapy in the elderly. Additionally, neuromodulation (electrical stimulation) may be helpful. Programs that attempt to improve coordination (e.g., ambidextrous skills, balance, proprioception, and kinesthetic awareness) along with increasing joint range of motion and enhancement of strength, power, and endurance may be beneficial in symptom palliation.

For extremely disabling and refractory spastic musculoskeletal conditions, clinicians have resorted to surgery, neuroablative procedures, or intrathecal agents.

Botulinum Toxin

Efforts to directly relax specific spastic muscles locally have been utilized, traditionally using intramuscular injections of local anesthetics with or without steroids. Botulinum toxins are also being utilized via local muscular injection for this purpose by affecting exocytosis of acetylcholine-containing vesicles. The duration of relief is variable but seems to last roughly three to six months or more. It also appears conceivable that botulinum toxins may possess inherent analgesic properties, although mechanisms of botulinum toxin-induced analgesia remain elusive. The two clinically available botulinum toxins in the United States are botulinum toxin type A (Botox) and type B (Myobloc; in Europe type B is marketed as Neurobloc). A different formulation of botulinum toxin type A known as Dysport has been issued in Europe and a type A version is also available in China (Lanzhou Biologic Products Institute).

SUMMARY

Spasticity and various musculoskeletal conditions can be extremely painful and disabling, leading to severe deterioration in quality of life. With the proper knowledge, appropriate attention to detail, and judicious slow dose titration, skeletal muscle relaxants can be utilized in the elderly and conceivably may provide significant improvements in quality of life.

BIBLIOGRAPHY

Chou R, Peterson K, Helfand M. Comparative efficacy and safety of skeletal muscle relaxants for spasticity and musculoskeletal conditions: A systematic review. *J Pain Symptom Manage* 2004; 28: 140-175.

Fick DM, Cooper JW, Wade WE, et al. Updating the Beers criteria for potentially inappropriate medication use in older adults: Results of a US consensus panel of experts. *Arch Intern Med* 2003; 1638: 2716-2724.

Smith HS. Miscellaneous analgesic agents. In Smith HS, ed. *Drugs for Pain.* Philadelphia: Hanley and Belfus, 2003; 271-287.

Smith HS, Barton AE. Tizanadine in the management of spasticity and musculoskeletal complaints in the palliative care population. *Am J Hosp Palliat Care* 2000; 17: 50-58.

Chapter 16

Physical Therapy and Pain Management with the Elderly

Dennis Martin

The aim of this chapter is to present the case for a rehabilitation perspective in the management of pain in older people and to discuss a central role for physical therapy. The discussion is based on a personal view that a pharmacological approach to pain management in older people is necessary but insufficient on its own, and that both approaches can work together on an equal footing—a view that is shared by some other authors (e.g., Ahmad and Goucke, 2002).

Pain in older people can have a significant negative impact on their performance of physical activities (Thomas et al., 2004; Reyes-Gibby et al., 2002; Scudds and Robertson, 2000; Mobily et al., 1994), but this does not have to be an inevitable product of aging. Addressing this impact of pain by way of physical therapy should help to maintain and improve their function and quality of life.

Physical therapists have a particularly valuable role in the management of pain. They are experts in the maintenance and restoration of function in the human body, and they work in the rehabilitation of people with all kinds of health conditions (CSP, 2002).

Broadly speaking, the role of physical therapy in the management of pain can be described as prevention and modification of the effects of primary and secondary mediators of pain (such as inflammation) and prevention and modification of the effects of factors that may negatively impact on function (Fields, 1995). The focus on function is particularly important.

FUNCTION

Function is at the forefront of 21st century health care thinking as articulated by the International Classification of Function, Disability and

Clinical Management of the Elderly Patient in Pain
© 2006 by The Haworth Press, Inc. All rights reserved.
doi:10.1300/5356_16

Health (ICF; WHO, 2001). Functioning, in terms of the ICF, is positive health, and negative health is dysfunction or disability. The ICF, endorsed by the World Health Organization in 2001, is a classification system with two parts: function and context.

The two components of function are body structure and body functions, and activity and participation. Body structures are anatomical, such as those involved in movement and the nervous system. Body functions are physiological and psychological, including sensory functions and pain, mental functions, and neuromusculoskeletal/movement-related functions. The ICF uses the terms *activity* and *participation* to distinguish between what an individual can do and what an individual actually does. The former relates to the person's capacity to carry out a task or an action. The latter is related to their performance or involvement in social situations. Using the same terms, the ICF discusses disability at three levels. *Impairments* describe problems with body structures and body functions. *Activity limitations* describe problems with capacity. Problems with performance are *participation restrictions*.

CONTEXT

The two components of context are personal factors (e.g., age, sex, coping styles, and experience) and environmental factors (e.g., social support and attitudes, policies, and technology). Performance is described in the context of an individual's standard environment.

Before the ICF, the accepted model as articulated by the International Classification of Impairments, Disabilities and Handicaps (ICIDH) facilitated thinking that was somewhat different (Ustan et al., 1995). (Advocates of the ICIDH argued that this thinking resulted from misinterpretation of the model.) Health and disability were conceptualized as two separate states and there was a heavy emphasis on a disease-based biomedical model. The perception of the role of the environment was, at best, marginal. Health problems were conceptualized as beginning with disease or disorder, which progressed serially and dependently through impairment and disability to handicap.

The ICF is different in that it replaces the serial dependence among body structures and body functions, activity, and participation with relationships that are dynamic and not necessarily dependent. It also gives importance to context in function and disability and sits comfortably alongside a biopsychosocial model of health.

The ICF has been shown to be of value in understanding the impact of pain (Soukup and Vollestad, 2001; Chwastiak and Von Korff, 2003; Steiner et al., 2002) as well as being relevant in other conditions (Fransen et al., 2002; Chopra et al., 2002; Chwastiak and Von Korff, 2003).

By linking function with disability and focusing on the positive side of health, the ICF gives a prominent place in health care to rehabilitation—the improvement of function (Stucki et al., 2002). The need to reduce pain-related activity limitation and participation restriction associated with pain in older people has been put forward as a high public health priority (Thomas et al., 2004). Therefore, physical therapists and other rehabilitation professionals have a valuable role in helping older people to manage their pain.

Estimates of the prevalence of persistent pain in populations are higher in older people than in their younger counterparts (Elliot et al., 1999; Smith, 2001; Helme and Gibson, 2001; Thomas et al., 2004). Age-related changes in neurophysiological processing of nociception have been reported (Gibson et al., 1994), but much less is known about the influences of psychosocial age-associated factors on the impact of pain on older people. These include beliefs about the cause and meaning of pain, presence of other diseases, loss of social support networks, and bereavement (Helme and Gibson, 2001).

The weight of current opinion is that older people are especially vulnerable to the disabling effects of pain that significantly and severely reduce quality of life (Helme and Gibson, 2001), and recent evidence points to a greater interference in function with age (Thomas et al., 2004). Others, however, have observed that the impact of pain on daily activities of older people is not as marked as that in younger people (Jakobsson et al., 2004). Regardless of relativity with age, pain has been shown to significantly limit function in older people (Mobily et al., 1994; Thomas et al., 2004).

CONSEQUENCES OF PAIN IN THE ELDERLY

The older person with pain is at risk of hospitalization or admission to long-term care. Persistent pain compromises independent function, leading to a cycle of disuse, inactivity, and further reduction in function. Unfortunately, although activity is what is required to break this cycle, activity is, understandably, often the last thing that someone wants to consider when in pain. Prolonged inactivity is damaging in many ways. The physiological effects of decreased aerobic fitness, strength, and flexibility, for example, make it all the more difficult to resume and then sustain activity. Psychological effects such as focusing on pain, lack of confidence, fear of damage, and worsening mood reduce the motivation to be active. A spiral of descent into further inactivity and disability is likely. In short, inactivity does nothing to make the pain more manageable and it only serves to make the person more vulnerable to the impact of pain on function.

MODELS OF PAIN MANAGEMENT

Because of its historical position as a profession close to medicine, physical therapy adopted and grew within a biomedical model of health that focused on disease and cure. In traditional physical therapy, people with pain are viewed as relatively passive recipients of treatment aimed at reducing their pain by curing the underlying condition. Within this context, physical therapists use a combination of methods that fall under the broad headings of electrotherapy, heat/cold, massage and manipulation, and exercise. Acupuncture has also become popular. Although the evidence base of the techniques used is sparse, the model has a certain validity in the management of acute pain. However, its utility falls short in the management of persistent or chronic pain (Harding and Williams, 1995; Martin and Palmer, 2004).

In response to an acknowledgment of the shortcomings of the biomedical model in dealing with people with pain, there has been a significant development of physical therapy practice within a biopsychosocial model. Within the biopsychosocial approach, physical therapy aims to address the impact of pain on function rather than just focusing on the pain itself (Harding and Williams, 1995; Jones and Martin, 2003). In this context, physical therapy aims to help people to live with pain. It sets out to help them learn skills to deal with the disabling effects of pain, and learn skills to deal with the distress caused by being in pain.

ROLE OF THE PHYSICAL THERAPIST

Physical therapists have an expert role to play in all but one of the core elements of pain management recommended by the Pain Society (2003) in the United Kingdom, as follows (the exception is medication review and advice).

- Physical reconditioning
- Posture and body mechanics training
- Applied relaxation techniques
- Information and education about pain and pain management
- Medication review and advice
- Psychological assessment and intervention
- Gradual return to activities of daily living

At the same time, the biopsychosocial approach to pain management emphasizes the benefits of interdisciplinary working (Wagner, 2000). Physical therapists, therefore, should be prepared to work in partnership with colleagues, including those from occupational therapy, psychology, medicine, nursing, and workers in support groups. As the roles of the different professions have many overlaps, there needs to be a shared vigilance to avoid unhelpful turf wars over ownership of roles while at the same time recognizing the value of different professional perspectives (Jones and Martin, 2003).

The biopsychosocial approach to pain management places great significance on cognitive-behavioral therapy. Cognitive-behavioral therapy reflects the understanding that the impact of pain on people is mediated to a large extent by their feelings and beliefs about their pain (Stroud et al., 2000). People with persistent, chronic pain often have negative thoughts such as, *Why me?* and *I can't take this pain anymore.*

These thoughts, which are perfectly normal, give rise to, and are subsequently reinforced by, negative emotions such as anger, frustration, and low mood. Cognitive-behavioral therapy recognizes that negative thoughts and feelings can lead to negative behavior such as withdrawing from social contact and inactivity—behavior that makes things worse for the person with chronic pain.

The aim of cognitive-behavioral therapy is to help people with chronic pain acknowledge negative thoughts and feelings, to understand the problems associated with them and to offer guidance on how to challenge negative thoughts and develop positive ways of behavior. People are encouraged to take control of pain rather than letting pain control them. Cognitive-behavioral therapy for people with chronic pain has support in research evidence (Morley et al., 1999; Williams et al., 1993). Various concepts have been developed linking cognitive variables and the impact of pain on function (Keefe et al., 2004). Modern physical therapy can embrace and adapt these ideas into its approach to managing pain (Moseley, 2002; Johnstone et al., 2003; Harding and Williams, 1995).

Within the biopsychosocial approach, information provision and education of people with pain are central to successful pain management. Education may be effective by way of addressing misplaced beliefs about pain, beliefs that can exacerbate its associated problems. Educational information packages have been shown to help promote self-management, and there is support for their use in reducing disability (Moseley, 2004; Burton et al., 1999). There is also room for education of family members and carers (Ferrell and Ferrell, 1991). A well-developed form of education about nociception and pain has been produced by Butler and Moseley (2003).

PHYSICAL THERAPY TREATMENTS

Exercise is one of the main physical therapies that can benefit people with chronic pain. Among the benefits are improved fitness, activity levels, mood, and physiological function in all of the main systems. In older patients in whom physical capacity may be declining, exercise can be used to maintain levels for a longer time or to slow down the rate of decline.

Although many different forms of exercise are promoted by physiotherapists, an interpretation of a systematic review of the literature to date is that any type of exercise is worth trying and that benefits can be found after nine months and more (Liddle et al., 2004). The review also concluded that physical therapists' supervision can enhance the benefits of exercise by providing feedback and increasing compliance (Liddle et al., 2004).

Progressive thinking is that exercise should promote well-being rather than aiming to address illness behavior, and so a purpose of exercise is to improve activity and participation. This is important because everyday activities such as housework, home maintenance, and even self-care can cause a lot of difficulty for many people with pain.

Pacing and goal setting are two of the most useful skills that can help improve activity and participation (Harding and Williams, 1995; Fey and Fordyce, 1983). A characteristic behavior of some people with chronic pain is to overdo it when they feel active. In simple terms, they carry on with tasks until reaching the limits of their physical capacity. The payback comes later on or the next day in the form of debilitating fatigue and flare-up of pain that leaves them inactive for a period of time. Once this period has passed and the person feels somewhat better, there is a tendency to try to compensate for lost time by overdoing things again, and the likelihood of subsequent flare-up is strong. The typical overactivity-underactivity cycle is harmful because its natural progression is toward prolonged inactivity.

Pacing is used to smooth out the excessive peaks of overactivity and the excessive troughs of underactivity. The underlying concept of pacing is to replace activity that is guided by capacity and motivation with activity guided by predetermined quota. The skills of pacing are to determine tolerances for actions, to set baselines for actions well within the tolerance limits, and to intersperse baseline activity with rest from that action. The most important actions to consider initially are usually sitting, standing, and walking. (There are, of course, many other actions with varying importance for different people.)

Tolerances and baselines are defined in quantifiable dimensions— usually time or distance. For example, in terms of time, sitting tolerance would be how long someone can sit before becoming fatigued or before the pain flares up to a higher level. A complicating factor is that often these consequences of carrying out the action for too long may not be felt immediately—there may be a delay until the next day. Thus, there is often a period of exploration and trial and error, and it is beneficial for the person to receive expert guidance. This is an important role for the physical therapist when discussing exercise and activity (though again not an exclusive one). The next step is to calculate an appropriate baseline—in this case a time for sitting that is well within the limits of the tolerance time. Opinions vary on the proportion and the calculation can be arbitrary, but some practitioners recommend setting baselines at 50 percent of tolerance while others may recommend 80 percent.

Pacing is about finding a balance between doing too much and doing too little, being too active and not being active enough. The skill helps people to learn to get into a pattern of operating in small chunks of activity interspersed with regular breaks from that activity (Nielson et al., 2001).

GOAL SETTING

Alongside pacing, goal setting can be useful in helping people with chronic pain to carry out tasks and take part in activities such as work and social events that they can find difficult. Goal setting involves defining aims and setting targets to achieve. Goal setting is a skill and again physical therapists are well placed to help. Very often people with chronic pain set goals that are too difficult to achieve in the time allotted. This causes problems, because when people cannot achieve their goal, they can become frustrated and give up trying. Another problem is that often people with chronic pain set goals that are unclear. It is then impossible to say if they have been reached or not. It is recommended that goals should be SMART:

Specific
Measurable
Activity related
Realistic
Time related

- *Specific* means that the goal is very clearly defined. Wanting to dance is not specific. Wanting to dance for ten minutes with the groom's father at your daughter's wedding is a more specific goal.
- *Measurable* means that it is clear when the goal has been achieved.
- *Activity related* means that the goal involves actually doing something.

- *Realistic* means that the goal is possible. Many things other than chronic pain can stop the achievement of a goal, such as lack of finance.
- *Time related* means that a date is set by which time the goal should be achieved.

Physical therapists can help to break the main goal into smaller minigoals so that achievement of each minigoal gives success and takes the person closer to the main goal. Goal setting is helped by feedback—receiving information back about how well things are progressing toward the goal—a role for physical therapists.

Within pacing and goal setting, the physical therapist can offer guidance on improving participation by prioritizing tasks, delegating, and planning ahead. Physical therapists can give guidance about how to reduce the frequency of flare-ups of pain, and make flare-up more manageable when it happens. A flare-up occurs when pain increases dramatically to a higher level than usual.

To reduce the frequency of flare-ups, it is necessary to try to identify what brings them on. Examples of triggers are

- staying in a certain position for too long;
- carrying out a certain activity for too long;
- carrying out a task such as lifting that is excessive; and
- emotional stress.

What is too long, excessive, or too much is different for different people and often a period of time will pass between the trigger and the flare-up.

The physical therapist can work with people in pain to develop a plan to manage flare-up. During flare-up it can be difficult for people to think clearly to work out what they should do. It is much better if they have a plan worked out beforehand so that they can start to manage flare-up once it starts. The physical therapist can help to formulate the plan and discuss the use of common strategies such as these:

Reducing stress
Pacing and goal setting
Heat, cold, TENS (transcutaneous nerve stimulation)
Relaxation
Medication
Stretching
Dealing with negative thoughts
Communication with others
Sleep
Distraction, viewing pictures, visualization, listening to music

Physical therapists' knowledge about the impact of pain and their beliefs about people with pain are important factors for appropriate and adequate pain management. There is often room for improvement (Jones and Martin, 2003). (This point applies equally to all health professionals.) Blomqvist (2003) reported a study showing that physical therapists along with other health professionals were not comfortable in working with older people with chronic pain when they did not present, or respond to treatment, in a manner consistent with a biomedical model. There is the risk that pain-related needs of older people can be obscured by physical therapists' and other health professionals' misinterpretation of what they are observing and hearing and that this is unlikely to result in the selection and accurate direction of appropriate and adequate pain management strategies. As a result, the older person with pain may be left with unnecessary suffering and disability.

Services incorporating the principles of pain management have been shown to be effective in reducing the disabling effects of chronic pain in populations that are not age specific (Morley et al., 1999): the incorporation of these principles into services for the older person has the potential to be of benefit to them as well. Much of the knowledge and opinion about physical therapy in the management of pain has been generated from a background that is not age specific. In fact, older people are often excluded from trials because of an age ceiling in inclusion criteria. The physical and psychological impact of pain is of a similar degree and pattern in older people as it is in younger people (Gibson et al., 1994; Sorkin et al., 1990). The challenge for physical therapists working with older people in pain is to understand the diverse needs and circumstances of older people and adapt these approaches to fit. Evidence suggests that there is good reason to believe that this is an achievable goal (Barry et al., 2003; Lansbury, 2000).

CONCLUSION

Pain can have a major negative impact on function in older people. Physical therapists, as rehabilitation professionals, are well placed to work with older people in pain to help counter any such impact. A biopsychosocial approach to pain management is advocated and this can be applied to older people. In many ways, the role of the physical therapist is a coaching one—understanding the specific needs of the person, involving people as active participants in their own pain management, agreeing on goals, and explaining why activity is feasible and beneficial, not just telling them what to do and when.

REFERENCES

Ahmad M, Goucke CR. Management strategies for the treatment of neuropathic pain in the elderly. *Drugs Aging* 2002; 19:929-945.

Barry LC, Guo Z, Kerns RD, Duong BD, Reid MC, Funotuinal A. Self-efficacy and pain-related disability among older veterans with chronic pain in a primary care setting. *Pain* 2003; 104:131-137.

Blomqvist K. Older people in persistent pain: Nursing and paramedical staff perceptions and pain management. *J Adv Nursing* 2003; 41:575-584.

British Pain Society. *Understanding and managing pain: Information for patients.* London: Author, 2003.

Burton A, Waddell G, Tilloston KM, Summerton N. Information and advice to patients with back pain can have a positive effect: A randomized controlled trial of a novel educational booklet in primary care. *Spine* 1999; 24:2484-2491.

Butler D, Moseley GL. *Explain pain.* Adelaide, Australia: NOI Group Publishing, 2003.

Chopra P, Couper J, Herman H. The assessment of disability in patients with psychotic disorders: An application of the ICIDH-2. *Aus New Zealand J Psychiatry* 2002; 36:127-132.

Chwastiak LA, Von Korff M. Disability in depression and back pain: Evaluation of the World Health Organization Disability Assessment Schedule (WHO DAS II) in a primary care setting. *J Clin Epidemiol* 2003; 56:507-514.

CSP. *Curriculum framework for qualifying programs in physiotherapy.* London: Chartered Society of Physiotherapy, 2002.

Elliot A, Smith BH, Penny KI, Smith WC, Chambers WA. The epidemiology of chronic pain in the community. *Lancet* 1999; 354:1248-1252.

Ferrell BA, Ferrell BR. Pain management at home. *Clin Ger Med* 1991; 7:765-76.

Fey SG, Fordyce WE. Behavioral rehabilitation of the chronic pain patient. *Ann Rev Rehabil* 1983; 3:32-63.

Fields HL. *Core curriculum for professional education in pain,* 2nd ed. Seattle: IASP Press, 1995.

Fransen J, Uebelhart D, Stucki G, Langeneggert T, Seitz M, Michel BA. The ICIDH-2 as a framework for the assessment of functioning and disability in rheumatoid arthritis. *Ann Rheum Dis* 2002; 61:225-231.

Gibson SJ, Katz B, Corran TM, Farrell MJ, Helme RD. Pain in older persons. *Disab Rehab* 1994; 16:127-139.

Harding V, Williams AC de C. Extending physiotherapy skills using a psychological approach: Cognitive-behavioral management of chronic pain. *Physiotherapy* 1995; 81:681-688.

Helme RD, Gibson SJ. The epidemiology of pain in elderly people. *Clin Ger Med* 2001; 17:417-431.

Jakobsson U, Hallberg RI, Westergren A. Pain management in elderly persons who require assistance with activities of daily living: A comparison of those living at home with those in special accommodation. *Eur J Pain* 2004; 8:335-344.

Johnstone R, Donaghy M, Martin DJ. A pilot study of a cognitive-behavioral therapy approach to physiotherapy, for acute low back pain patients, who show signs of developing chronic pain. *Adv Physiother* 2003; 2:182-188.

Jones D, Martin DJ. Chronic pain. In Everett T, Donaghy M, Feaver S, eds. *Interventions for mental health: an evidence based approach for physiotherapists and occupational therapists.* Edinburgh: Butterworth-Heinemann, 2003, 136-145.

Keefe FJ, Rumble ME, Scipio CD, Giordano LA, Perri LM. Psychological aspects of persistent pain: current state of the science. *J Pain* 2004; 5:195-211.

Lansbury G. Chronic pain management: A qualitative study of elderly people's preferred coping strategies and barriers to management. *Disabil Rehabil* 2000; 22: 2-14.

Liddle SD, Baxter GD, Gracey JH. Exercise and chronic low back pain: What works? *Pain* 2004; 107:176-190.

Martin DJ, Palmer ST Soft tissue pain and physical therapy. *Anaes Inten Care Med* 2004; 6:23-24.

Mobily PR, Kerr HA, Wallace R, Chung Y. An epidemiological analysis of pain in the elderly: The Iowa 65-plus Rural Health Study. *J Aging Health* 1994; 6:139-154.

Morley S, Eccleston C, Williams AC de C. Systematic review and meta-analysis of randomized controlled trials of cognitive behavior therapy for chronic pain in adults, excluding headache. *Pain* 1999; 80:1-13.

Moseley GL. Evidence for a direct relationship between cognitive and physical change during an education intervention in people with chronic low back pain. *Eur J Pain* 2004; 8:39-45.

Moseley GL. Physiotherapy is effective for chronic low back pain: A randomized controlled trial. *Aus J Physiotherapy* 2002; 48:297-302.

Nielson WR, Jensen MP, Hill ML. An activity pacing scale for the chronic pain coping inventory: Development in a sample of patients with fibromyalgia syndrome. *Pain* 2001; 89:111-115.

Reyes-Gibby CC, Aday L, Cleeland C. Impact of pain on self-rated health in the community-dwelling older adults. *Pain* 2002; 95:75-82.

Scudds RJ, Robertson JM. Pain factors associated with physical disability in a sample of community-dwelling senior citizens. *J Gerontol A* 2000; 55:M393-M399.

Smith B. Chronic pain: A challenge for primary care. *Br J Gen Pract* 2001; 51:524-526.

Sorkin BA, Rudy TE, Hanlon RB, Turk DC, Steig RL. Chronic pain in old and young patients: differences appear less important than similarities. *J Gerontol* 1990; 45:64-68.

Soukup MG, Vollestad NK. Classification of problems, clinical findings and treatment goals in patients with low back pain using the ICIDH-2 beta-2. *Dis Rehab* 2001; 23:462-473.

Steiner WA, Ryser L, Huber E, Uebelhart D, Aeschlimann A, Stucki G. Use of the ICF model as a clinical problem-solving tool in physical therapy and rehabilitation medicine. *Phys Ther* 2002; 82:1098-1107.

Stroud MW, Thorn BE, Jensen MP, Boothby JL. The relation between pain beliefs, negative thoughts, and psychosocial functioning in chronic pain patients. *Pain* 2000; 84:347-352.

Stucki G, Ewert T, Cieza A. Value and application of the ICF in rehabilitation medicine. *Dis Rehab* 2002; 24: 932-938.

Thomas E, Peat G, Harris H, Wilkie R, Croft PR. The prevalence of pain and pain interference in a general population of older adults: Cross-sectional findings from the North Staffordshire Osteoarthritis Project (NorStOP). *Pain* 2004; 110:361-368.

Ustan TB, Cooper JE, Van Duuren-Kristen S, Kennedy C, Hendershot G, Sartoriusn. Revision of the ICIDH. *Disabil Rehab* 1995; 17:202-209.

Wagner EH. The role of patient care teams in chronic disease management. *BMJ* 2000; 320:569-572.

WHO. *International classification of functioning, disability and health: ICF.* Geneva: WHO, 2001.

Williams AC de C, Nicholas MK, Richardson PH, Pither CE, Justins DM, Chamberlain JH, Harding VR, Ralphs JA, Jones SC, Dieudonne I, et al. Evaluation of a cognitive behavioral program for rehabilitating patients with pain. *Br J Gen Prac* 1993; 43:513-518.

Chapter 17

Psychosocial Factors in Pain Management of the Older Patient

Edmund J. Burke

Even a cursory reading of the literature on pain and its management, current or historical, leads one to the clear conclusion that pain is a multifaceted, multiply determined, and individually experienced phenomenon. It is true that everyone "knows pain." It is also true that everyone knows pain differently.

In trying to understand the experience of human physical pain, researchers have been able to identify a plethora of physiological, psychological, and sociocultural factors that reliably, though often not predictably, affect this experience. In recent years, several authors have begun to turn their attentions to an examination of the ways in which progressing age may act as a modulating variable in the experience of pain, its assessment, and treatment. It is the purpose of this chapter to review some of the most recent work in this area, with an eye toward providing the practicing clinician with some useful advice regarding the assessment and treatment of pain in older adults.

Attention to the issues of pain experience and response to pain treatment in the elderly patient comes naturally as a result of the dramatic increases in longevity that have occurred during the 20th century in all of the developed and developing countries of the world. In the United States, for example, there were approximately 3 million individuals aged 65 years and older in 1900 (about 4 percent of the total population). By 1994, there were slightly more than 33.2 million individuals aged 65 or older (about 12.5 percent of the total U.S. population at the time). In the current decade (2000 to 2009), the growth of the elderly population in the United States is expected to be mild. However, between 2010 and 2030, when the baby boomer generation (those individuals born after World War II between 1946 and 1964) become the elderly generation of Americans, the number of older adults in the population will dramatically increase. By 2011, between 70 and 78 million

Clinical Management of the Elderly Patient in Pain
© 2006 by The Haworth Press, Inc. All rights reserved.
doi:10.1300/5356_17

people living in the United States will be age 65 or older—a full 20 percent of the projected population (U.S. Bureau of the Census, 1996).

Currently, about 70 percent of U.S. health care expenditures are spent on providing care for persons with chronic illnesses and the pain that frequently accompanies them. Pope and Tarlov (1991) reported that in the year 2000, 105 million people in the United States were afflicted with chronic disease, and approximately $500 billion was spent in the care of these patients. These authors estimate that by 2010, the number of Americans suffering with chronic diseases will increase to 120 million, with an annual cost to the U.S. health care system of $582 billion.

As this population shift occurs, in the United States and around the world, responding to the pain management needs of an older population will become increasingly crucial. The public will demand and researchers and clinicians alike will be expected to provide pain diagnostic and treatment services, which are responsive to the unique characteristics of pain as it presents in the elderly population. Further, pain treatment strategies of all types will need to be delivered in the most cost-efficient manner possible, as pressure will continue to mount on an already cash-strapped U.S. health care delivery system.

AGE DIFFERENCES IN PREVALENCE RATES OF CHRONIC PAIN

The prevalence of acute pain conditions (pain lasting less than six months with an essentially demonstrable physical cause explaining it) seems to be stable through the lifespan. Approximately 5 percent of the population are experiencing an acute pain condition at any one time (Kendig et al., 1996). Reports of chronic pain conditions, on the other hand, are seen to increase in prevalence up to the age of 70, and then may decline (Helme and Gibson, 2001). Several studies agree on this pattern of pain prevalence in the elderly, but differ somewhat in their estimates of prevalence rates in various groups, most likely as a result of using different sampling strategies across studies. Overall, the best studies, those incorporating samples with a wide age range, have reported a prevalence rate of 10-40 percent in early adulthood, 20-80 percent in late middle age, and 15-70 percent in the elderly (Blyth et al., 2001; Bassols et al., 1999; Kind et al., 1998; Brattberg et al., 1997). This age-related prevalence may be related to a host of psychological and expectancy variables, as well as the types of disorders suffered by patients over the lifespan.

THE NATURE OF PAIN STATES

It is especially difficult to diagnosis a specific etiology for chronic pain in elderly patients as a result of the common occurrence of multisystem disorders in this age group (Harkins, 2001). It is clear, however, that complaints of chronic musculoskeletal pain increase with age. In his review of a number of studies, Harkins (2001) concluded that the prevalence of musculoskeletal and joint pain of the neck, hip, back, and knee, as well as report of stiff joints upon awakening, is greater in older persons than younger persons, as most older people will tell you. More interesting, especially for our current purposes, was the finding that even in reviewed cases in which the prevalence of pain was not higher in the elderly group, pain intensity was reported as more severe, as were depressive symptoms and limitations in activities of daily living.

PHYSICAL DIFFERENCES IN PAIN PERCEPTION

In trying to understand the experience of pain in the elderly patient and how it may differ from the experience of younger patients, researchers have sought to examine several actual or presumed physical differences between older and younger subjects. The use of the word *subjects* is intentional here, since all of these studies have evaluated patients' responses to experimentally induced pain, so of course focus almost entirely on assessment of sensory systems. As noted by Harkins (2001) in his review of the literature and aging and pain: "For obvious reasons, laboratory and clinical studies of pain must not involve suffering, yet suffering is the hallmark of chronic pain" (p. 815).

Borrowing from the terminology used to describe changes in other sensory systems associated with age, Harkins (2001) discusses the notion of *presbyalgos,* which is defined as the effects of age systematically affecting pain sensitivity and perception. The analogy here is to the terms *presbyopia,* referring of course to the natural diminishing effects of senescence on vision, and *presbycusis,* referring to the similar phenomenon seen with the sense of audition. Given these well-known and documented effects of age on sensory systems, it might seem reasonable to assume some sort diminution of pain sensation with age. In fact, as is discussed more fully later, several studies of the report of pain states by older versus younger patients indicate that older patients often report (or complain of) less pain than younger patients, even when suffering apparently the same physical illnesses (Farrell and Gibson, 2004). However, it has been noted that changes related to vision and hearing seem to be primarily the result of accumulating damage to sensory organs involving transduction of visual and auditory stimuli, rather than changes in central nervous system mechanisms of sensation and perception of light and sound waves (Scialfa and Kline, 1996).

Overall, studies of age differences in pain perception are mixed in their findings. Some report a reduction in pain sensitivity with aging; some report an increase in pain sensitivity; and others report finding no differences at all (Harkins and Scott, 1996). In a review of the literature, Harkins (2001) discusses five components that need to be considered in the definition of presbyalgos:

1. Age-dependent loss of nociceptors
2. Changes in primary nociceptive afferents
3. Changes in centrally mediated pain mechanisms
4. Changes in descending central pain control mechanisms
5. Birth cohort differences in sociocultural history that may act to influence the meaning of pain (p. 818)

Harkins's review of studies of the first two factors, age-dependent loss of pain receptors and changes in primary nociceptive afferents, would indicate that evidence for age changes or differences in density of these nerve cells is essentially nonexistent. In studies that support differences in this regard, the effects of age tend to be very small. Further, in regard to Harkins's third and fourth components, it is noted that no studies to date have looked at possible age changes in central mechanisms of pain control in humans. Although carefully designed studies in this area would potentially be of great import, direct examination of the variables involved will be very difficult indeed. In the few studies conducted thus far that have indirectly addressed the fifth component, the possible influences of birth cohort effects on pain responses, the familiar finding that older patients often report less pain than younger people (Harkins and Scott, 1996) would seem to be more related to age differences in the meaning of chronic pain than to true differences in the physiological experience of it.

Farrell and Gibson (2004), in their review of psychosocial aspects of pain in older patients, mention their current work indicating through psychophysical studies that pain acuity may be diminished in older subjects, though the mechanisms for this remain unclear. Certainly these are interesting data to review, as are reports by Washington et al. (2000) suggesting that aging may be associated with impairment of the endogenous analgesic system. Further, the consistent reports of decreased tolerance to prolonged noxious stimulation in the elderly may be related in some way to a failing downregulation of the nociceptive system (Edwards et al., 2001; Walsh et al., 1989; Woodrow et al., 1972). Certainly, much work remains to be done in these areas, as results are often mixed and difficult to interpret, especially when they occur in the midst of other nonphysiological factors.

A review of the evidence for underlying physiological explanations for the differences of older versus younger patients' reports of the experience of their pain, Harkins (2001) concludes that geriatric pain practitioners should probably be more concerned with developing the most efficient methods to clinically evaluate and treat pain in the elderly patient than with trying to elucidate the psychophysics of it. Thus, we turn our attention to sociocultural and psychological factors that may be important in understanding the experience of pain in the older patient.

SOCIOCULTURAL FACTORS IN THE EXPERIENCE AND REPORT OF PAIN IN OLDER PATIENTS

The current population of older people (those aged 65 and above) in the United States grew up in a time that was quite different from today in many ways, including cultural mores and values. Growing up in the era between the First and Second World Wars (and in many cases serving in the Korean War), Americans, and especially American men, aspired to be the "strong silent type." It was a sign of weakness to "wear your heart on your sleeve"; rather, they were encouraged to "grin and bear it" when it came to discomforts, physical and especially emotional. This generation learned these lessons well from their own parents, who grew up during World War I, lived through the Great Depression, and came to view dogged self-sufficiency as a great virtue and dependency of any kind as a terrible weakness.

Given this backdrop, the often-reported finding that older people seem to complain less of certain types of pain may not be surprising. In their review of the literature, Harkins and Scott (1996) note several studies that have indirectly assessed the possible influence of age on pain responses. Overall, these studies suggest that the older patient tends to report less pain than younger patients, probably reflecting differences in the meaning of chronic pain to different age groups (Harkins and Scott, 1996).

Another, very different social issue related to aging and the report and experience of pain concerns the social circumstance of the individual aged chronic pain patient. Most individuals currently in this cohort are now retired from employment, following decades of working and looking forward to their golden years, a time when they would be free to pursue personal interests, enjoy greater financial flexibility, less responsibility, and so on. They expect to be able to take it easy a bit, enjoying time with their spouses, watching the grandchildren grow up, traveling, and otherwise enjoying the fruits of their labors. However, in actuality, advanced age is in many cases associated with economic hardship, decreases in mobility, impaired mental acuity, lack of purpose, death of friends or spouse, and other losses leading to social isolation, despair, and perhaps increased use of inappropriate coping devices such as alcohol. These changes in social functioning may also be expected to influence the experience and report of pain. In fact, Helme et al. (1996) have reported that increased availability of social support seemed to be related to increased reports of pain. Fordyce (1978) had earlier suggested that older persons may be more likely to complain of pain in order to receive increased social contact from friends and family, perhaps because they have limited opportunities to secure such needed supports in other ways. Further, Bradbeer et al. (2003) reported that widowhood is associated with an increased risk for pain in a sample of adult community dwellers. Although depression may well be the conduit for increased experience of pain in recently widowed people, the social isolation, lack of companionship, and decreased opportunities for social contact almost certainly enter into the mix.

Overall, the available literature on sociocultural factors affecting the experience of pain in older adults suggests that their upbringing as well as current life circumstances do significantly affect their experience and report of pain. Certainly, this is an area that is ripe for further investigation, in an effort to more fully understand the elderly patient's experience of pain.

EMOTIONAL AND PSYCHOLOGICAL FACTORS INFLUENCING PAIN EXPERIENCE

Relative to the examination of cultural factors in the experience of pain in the elderly patient, investigations of psychological and emotional factors have been more plentiful over the past several years. This work falls generally into the following categories:

1. The meaning or phenomenology of pain
2. Pain coping
3. Depression and pain
4. Anxiety states and pain

Meaning of Pain

A number of studies have provided strong evidence that the meaning ascribed to pain changes as one grows older. Older people expect that pain comes as a natural result of aging (Hofland, 1992), in a similar way that they expect a certain degree of memory loss, decreased physical stamina, sexual interest, and so on. Several studies have supported the presence of this belief among the elderly (e.g., Ruzicka, 1998; Liddell and Locker, 1997), though the finding has not been universal (e.g., Gagliese and Melzack, 1997). Further, older people differ from younger people in the importance they ascribe to the presence of mild pain (Mangione et al., 1993). Older people seem less worried about and are perhaps less likely to seek treatment for mild pain, viewing it as a concomitant of old age. However, as pain becomes more severe, older people are more likely than younger people to view their discomfort as a sign of serious or life-threatening illness and are quicker to seek appropriate medical attention (Leventhal et al., 1993; Staller, 1993). Knowing this, the pain management practitioner can more readily understand the consternation of the older patient who, upon presenting to his or her physician with a complaint of pain that has been worsening and feeling like the manifestation of some horrible disease, is told that this pain is "probably just age."

A further implication of the results of these studies is the fact that, as a result of the relatively little importance that the older patient might give to reporting mild pain, the opportunity to successfully treat a variety of diseases that begin with mild physical pain may be compromised. Thus, practitioners are well advised to remember to inquire about the presence of pain in the elderly patient, even if physical discomfort is not the primary presenting complaint.

In Western popular culture, the intimate connection between mind and body is generally not well understood. Even among physicians this is sometimes the case. For example, referrals to our behavioral medicine practice are often based on the question of whether a patient's complaints are physical or organic. This dualistic conception has been the subject of numerous writings and is certainly beyond the scope of the current discussion. What seems clear, however, is that our popular culture still expects discrete, unitary, often pharmacological solutions for whatever physical maladies they may suffer.

This, it seems, is especially true for the older patient. Gagliese and Melzack (1997) have presented data supporting the notion that although young and old alike will acknowledge that psychological factors can affect pain states, older people are less likely to appreciate a connection between pain and depression. Further, the often-discussed social stigma of acknowledging or seeking treatment for psychological problems may be especially prevalent in older patients, discouraging them further from investigating relationships between their physical pain and associated feelings of depression, anxiety, and so on.

Pain Coping Strategies

The issue of possible differences between younger and older pain patients with regard to pain coping strategies has been investigated in several studies, often yielding somewhat confusing results. The most consistent finding in this group of studies (e.g., Corran et al., 1994; McCracken, 1993) is that older persons use prayer and hope as pain coping mechanisms to a greater extent than do younger patients. It will be interesting to see as longitudinal studies become available whether this tendency toward hoping and praying as a way of coping is limited to the current cohort of older patients, or whether the differences noted reflect a developmental shift as people grow older toward a greater appreciation of and focus on religion and faith issues.

Attempts to ignore pain as a coping strategy appears to be another area in which there are differences between older and younger pain patients, at least when pain levels are mild (Watkins et al., 1999). Corran et al. (1994) have noted that attempts to ignore pain in order to cope with it seem more common in younger patients. This difference may, however, be less important to consider in the typical pain management practice, where complaints of mild pain levels are relatively rare.

Pain and Depression

The well-researched and described relationship between depression and chronic pain seems to hold regardless of patient age (Corran et al., 1997; Riley et al., 2000). A number of studies have documented consistent rates of clinical depression and individual depressive symptoms in chronic pain patients across age levels (e.g., Cossins et al., 1999; Turk et al., 1995; McCracken, 1993). According to Magni et al. (1993), chronic pain patients report a depression rate of 16.4 percent, compared with a rate of 5.7 percent for the general population, and the rate of depression among pain patients does not vary as a function of age.

These data may be somewhat unexpected, since changing rates of clinical depression and depressive symptoms are often reported as a function of age. Jorm (2000) and Henderson et al. (1998), for example, have reported that rates for depression in the general population tend to peak in late middle age and decline thereafter. The somewhat indirect observation that depression in elderly pain patients seems to mirror depression rates in younger chronic pain patients, instead of declining as it is seen to do in the wider population of older people, suggests the need to further examine the question of the effects of chronic pain states and depression in older patients. It has been suggested that such factors as increased emotional control, decreased emotional responsiveness, and a sort of psychological immunization resulting from repeated exposure over the life span to stressful life events may be responsible for decreasing depression rates in older people (Jorm, 2000). An interesting question that awaits further research is whether the existence of a chronic pain condition may counteract the effects of these factors, resulting in effectively higher rates of depression in older people suffering chronic pain conditions, when compared with their pain-free counterparts.

Finally, it has been noted that the prevalence rate for depression in elderly clinical populations ranges between 11 and 30 percent (Lyness et al., 1999; Rapp et al., 1991). In general, suicide rates for older people with serious health problems are much higher than those for relatively healthy older people. In fact, it has been estimated that 85 percent of older people committing suicide suffered an active disease, in addition to their depression, immediately preceding their death (Ouslander, 1982). Certainly, these data argue for a continued effort at understanding the relationship between pain and depression in the elderly patient. The clinician assessing the older patient's report of pain also needs to be cognizant of the need to carefully assess for depression as well, just as she or he would for all chronic pain patients—perhaps more carefully, given the older patient's possible tendency to underreport psychological symptoms, as discussed earlier.

Pain and Anxiety States

Thus far, there has not been much of an attempt in the literature to describe the relationship between chronic pain and anxiety states in the older patient. What evidence does exist would seem to indicate that older pain patients are somewhat less likely than younger ones to report concomitant anxiety symptoms with pain (Riley et al., 2000). However, this may be more related to the often-reported tendency of older people toward decreased report of negative emotional states in general, rather than a true decrease in the occurrence of anxiety symptoms in this group.

Depressive and anxiety states often occur together, and there is some evidence that generalized anxiety states may be underdiagnosed when not accompanied by depressive symptoms in older people (Lenz et al., 2001). It seems especially important to remember to assess for the presence of anxiety states, given a study by Casten et al. (1995) indicating a greater potential role for anxiety than for depression in predicting pain reports. Also, the co-occurrence of depression and anxiety may be important in predicting response to pain treatment in general, given the finding that increased psychiatric co-morbidity in general is predictive of poor response to pain treatment.

PRACTICAL ISSUES IN THE ASSESSMENT AND TREATMENT OF THE ELDERLY PAIN PATIENT

Given the foregoing discussion of the research on various physiological, sociocultural, and psychological variables affecting the response of the elderly patient to pain management treatment, I now turn to a more practical discussion of issues to consider in the assessment and treatment of these patients.

Elderly pain patients, like their younger colleagues, typically present to the pain management practitioner upon referral from a primary care physician or specialist physician after a long and exhausting search for an answer to their problem. Often, years have elapsed since the initial injury or spontaneous development of the pain problem. Many such patients have seen numerous physicians and other practitioners (e.g., physical therapists, chiropractors, psychologists) many of whom, while initially confident that they could fix the problem, became discouraged or frustrated with the patient's lack of response to their particular brand of treatment. This may well have been communicated to the patient, either directly or indirectly. Worse yet, the patient may have come to the conclusion that the pain management practitioner represents the last hope for relief. There is an old adage in psychotherapy treatment that there are only two types of patients that cannot be helped: those who believe that they cannot be helped and those who believe that the therapist is their only hope.

In addition, elderly pain patients who grew up believing in the ultimate expert power of the physician have by now often become disillusioned. They have seen one after another of their practitioners fail in their attempts to diagnose and appropriately treat their problem. They have experienced conflicting opinions regarding the nature of their problem. Sometimes they have heard one type of practitioner dismissing the efforts or authority of another. They lose faith after one "snake oil salesman" after another takes their money, fails to cure them, and then blames them for not responding to their treatment. A final insult occurs when they feel that they are being called "crazy"; that is, when they are finally referred for mental health evaluation and treatment. This, too often, is the context in which the pain management practitioner must conduct the initial evaluation of a new patient.

Over the past 20 years or so, numerous attempts have been made to develop reliable and comprehensive paper-and-pencil assessments for the chronic pain patient. Currently, such instruments as the McGill Pain

Questionnaire, the Psychosocial Pain Inventory, the Psychosomatic Symptom Checklist, the Minnesota Multiphasic Personality Inventory II, and others are receiving a lot of attention in research investigating such issues as detecting malingering, predicting treatment response, and cataloging the nature of various pain states. The reader is referred to Turner and Romano (2001) for a more in-depth discussion of these instruments in the assessment and treatment of pain syndromes.

Although some or all of these instruments may indeed be quite useful to the pain practitioner for one or more of the purposes discussed, it has been my experience that elderly pain patients in particular are often averse to doing a lot of paperwork, especially during or in advance of the initial consultation. Rather, they are is interested in telling the story of their pain experience directly to the provider. Surely, the practitioner has much to accomplish in this first session, and it would seem easier and more efficient to get the details through written instruments. However, the longer-term goal of a good doctor-patient collaborative relationship is often better served by giving patients a chance to be fully heard and an opportunity to build some initial trust in the practitioner by seeing him or her as a person who is willing (and has the time) to listen to them. In my experience, a longer initial consultation (with or without written assessment devices) pays off and saves time in the long run, produces a more willing and compliant patient, results in fewer patient complaints, and helps the patient develop realistic expectations for pain management treatment.

Psychosocial Assessment

The psychosocial assessment often begins by addressing with patients the nature of their referral to a psychologist or psychiatrist. They need to be reassured that the referral source has sent them to the mental health provider not because she or he felt that the pain was all in their head, but because she or he believed that patients can learn to use their head to deal with their pain more effectively. Sometimes, this will include a discussion between the patient and the mental health provider of the basics of the mind-body connection, using simple and direct examples of this relationship in everyday life. For example, I will sometimes ask patients if they are able to feel the physical sensation of their arm resting upon the arm of the chair on which they are sitting. When they invariably respond in the affirmative, I ask them if they had been aware of this sensation five minutes earlier in the interview. When they admit that they had not been, a discussion can ensue regarding the importance of attentional processes in pain perception.

As the initial assessment continues, patients are asked to describe the phenomenology of their pain. They are asked to describe the exact location of their pain, often by touching the areas on their bodies where the pain occurs. They are asked to describe the sensation of their pain (e.g., burning, aching, hot, tight, sharp, dull, etc.), which can be useful in indicating not only the nature of their difficulty, but also the extent to which secondary gain and other psychological factors are involved. As has become customary in pain clinics across the United States, patients are then asked to rate the intensity of their pain on the 0 to 10 scale. By the time patients are referred to a mental health professional, they are usually quite familiar with this request. Many will immediately comply, while some few others will refuse to rate their pain in this manner, noting how difficult it is to put a number on something so intricate and mercurial. When this happens, I recommend agreeing with them and asking them to instead describe the intensity of their pain in their own way. Similarly, when asked about the range of intensity of their pain, most will provide numbers, while some will begin discussing the effects of their pain on everyday functioning. Since this is one of the most important elements of the evaluation, it is useful to pursue this line of questioning as soon as it is raised. A thorough (and sometimes written) account of what activities are curtailed or prevented as a result of pain is obtained. This list is often used as treatment proceeds as a way of assessing progress in pain management treatment.

Other important information to obtain as part of the initial psychosocial pain assessment includes the patient's impressions of what treatments or activities have helped in the past and which ones have not. I try to obtain an exhaustive list of all the things that patients have tried to treat their pain in the past, along with an explanation from them regarding why they thought some treatments were useful while others were not. Patients are asked to think about and report more indirect results of their pain experience, including possible family problems, financial stressors, and legal issues. Often, these psychosocial outgrowths of the pain experience help explain a patient's less than adequate response to more traditional physically based treatments and may become foci of psychological pain management treatment in themselves.

The psychological evaluation of chronic pain patients always begins with a direct focus on their pain experience. This reassures patients that the mental health professional is indeed primarily interested in helping them to address their physical pain issues and helps build a comfortable rapport with patients. After the parameters of their pain situation are fully discussed, the assessment moves to an examination of more traditional mental health concerns. This transition in the interview can usually be easily made by explaining to patients that the practitioner knows very well that they are "more than just their pain problem" and he or she would like to get to know patients more as people. Thus the interview proceeds with an assessment of family and work history, legal history, and other psychosocial issues that are often relevant to a person's ability to learn to manage pain effectively.

The initial psychological assessment also includes a complete mental status evaluation, including assessment of attentional and memory processes, Axis I and Axis II psychiatric disorders, history of psychiatric illness and treatment in the patient and first-degree relatives, and history of alcohol and substance abuse (both illicit and prescribed drugs).

The final task in the initial psychosocial pain assessment is to develop with the patient a list of specific goals for treatment. Based on the information obtained earlier, patients may decide (with the coaching of the therapist) on such goals as achieving better family relationships, handling their emotions more effectively, and addressing reactive depressive and anxiety symptoms, in addition to learning various psychological techniques (e.g., relaxation training, biofeedback, imagery, clinical hypnosis) to reduce the intensity of their pain. As the initial session concludes, specific techniques and a time frame for meeting therapeutic goals are discussed.

Psychological Treatment Strategies

Psychological, nonpharmacological treatments for chronic pain have received considerable attention in the literature, especially over the past 30 years (Mersky and Magni, 1990). In particular, cognitive-behavioral treatment strategies have been shown in many experimental investigations to be useful to patients, both in terms of reducing or otherwise changing the patient's experience of pain, and in terms of increasing functionality—dealing with the effects that chronic pain has had on their lives. Some of these techniques are summarized in this section (for a more complete discussion, see Mersky and Magni, 1990). Thus far, research has not begun to investigate in any systematic way treatment issues and options for the elderly pain patient. Most studies merely report mean ages for study participants, though elderly patients are not typically excluded from participation in these investigations.

The first major category of psychological treatments involves those designed to help patients reduce or otherwise change their pain experience. Examples of techniques in this category include various forms of muscle relaxation training, pain imagery training, clinical hypnosis, and biofeedback.

Progressive muscle relaxation training (Wolpe, 1973) has been used extensively in the treatment of chronic pain patients. This procedure involves teaching patients to become deeply relaxed through consciously tensing and then relaxing major muscle groups throughout the body. An audiotape of the in-session exercise is typically made, and patients are instructed to practice the technique between sessions. As sessions continue, the exercise can be shortened so that patients learn to achieve a deep state of relaxation in a relatively brief period of time, so that they can successfully apply the technique throughout the day as they notice their body becoming tense. This and similar techniques can be useful in terms of reducing the secondary muscle pain that comes as a result of patients "bracing" against pain, regardless of the nature of the primary pain complaint. Further, this rather simple, very physically based strategy can be used to set the stage for more cognitively based exercises.

Various mental imagery exercises are often used in the treatment of chronic pain patients as a way of helping them to directly diminish or in some other way change their experience of pain (Mersky and Magni, 1990). Patients are taught to imagine or picture in their mind's eye various scenarios in which mastery over the pain is achieved. For example, patients may be encouraged to view themselves walking barefoot beside the ocean, seeing, hearing, feeling, and even tasting this serene and relaxing environment. They may be encouraged to give the pain a form (e.g., a hot ball) and then to imagine that ball becoming cooler and smaller. Finally, the exercise may encourage them to develop a feeling of power or control over their pain, changing its location (e.g., from stomach to fingertip), or phenomenology (e.g., from a stabbing poker to a softer feeling of moderate pressure). Generally, the patient's ability to benefit from exercises of this sort depends on a certain psychological mindedness or at least openness to attempt such techniques. Although it is not clear whether older pain patients as a group exhibit more or less ability to use these strategies, chances for success may be enhanced when they are attempted in the context of a trusting therapeutic relationship, after the patient has showed some initial positive response to more physically based techniques (e.g., progressive muscle relaxation).

Similarly, more traditional clinical hypnosis techniques have shown some usefulness in the treatment of chronic pain patients (Chaves, 1999), although they are seemingly more of an extension of imagery exercises than a distinct form of treatment. Patients can sometimes be taught to enter a lightly hypnotic state in which their perception of the pain is diminished or otherwise altered. For example, a patient, after being encouraged to relax deeply, is told to imagine the painful area of the body being placed in a bucket that contains a soothing anesthetic solution. He is encouraged through suggestion to feel the soothing effects of the imaginary solution on the affected body part, hopefully with the result that he reports feeling less pain. Further, he is taught how to achieve this state on his own, making it a quick and portable technique that he may take with him as he goes through his daily routine.

In my experience, although the more cognitively based techniques (e.g., imagery and clinical hypnosis) can be helpful with a minority of patients (perhaps 20 to 30 percent), the majority is more responsive to more physically based and grounded techniques. These treatments often seem to have more face validity to patients—they are better able to see and understand the relationship between their physical pain and the treatment technique being offered.

It is in this regard that various biofeedback techniques can often present useful treatment options for the chronic pain patient. Biofeedback basically involves the second-to-second monitoring of some specific physiological activity (e.g., muscle tension levels, temperature, heart rate, respiration rate, blood pressure, or galvanic skin response) by computerized instrumentation. This information is immediately "fed back" to the patient, who attempts to change the physical response in a desired direction. For example, when it has been determined that some component of a patient's chronic back pain involves chronic tension of the paraspinal muscles, sensors used to measure electromyographic activity are placed across the lower back in the vicinity of the pain. The patient is then taught to decrease muscle tension levels in this area by watching and reacting to the continuous information coming through the biofeedback device. It is noted that one of the strengths of these treatment techniques with chronic pain patients is the direct and apparent relationship between the presumed physical cause of the pain and the treatment technique being used. Biofeedback often has a higher face validity to the patient, and the treatment rationale is much more direct and easy for the patient to understand.

The second major category of psychological treatments for chronic pain patients involves those treatments designed to assist patients in coping with their medical condition and with the social and psychological difficulties that have grown out of their pain experience. As noted previously, anxiety and depressive states are often associated with chronic pain. Several studies over the years have been able to demonstrate that cognitive and behavioral psychotherapy for depression and anxiety management can be useful not only in reducing these psychological symptoms but in reducing the patient's suffering overall (Mersky and Magni, 1990). It is noted that tricyclic and selective serotonin reuptake inhibitor antidepressant medications can also be very useful in this regard, either alone or optimally in combination with cognitive-behavioral treatment.

Thus, one of the first exercises that I recommend with new pain patients is to have them examine a fairly exhaustive list of factors often associated with the experience of chronic pain. These factors include such things as decreases in physical activity, family problems, financial problems, legal and employment issues, difficulties with no-fault or workers' compensation insurance carriers, "getting paid for doing nothing," attention for being in pain, and feelings of anger, powerlessness, depression, and anxiety. With this list completed, a cognitive-behavioral treatment plan for addressing all of the identified factors is developed and treatment for these issues becomes an important and sometimes primary focus for the therapy.

SUMMARY

In the past several years, attention has begun to be paid to issues of particular importance in the psychosocial assessment and treatment of the elderly pain patient. This seems especially important and appropriate given the increasing numbers of elderly people (those 65 years and older) in our population.

The prevalence of chronic pain conditions increases though the life span, up until the age of 70, and then may decline. Somewhere between 15 and 70 percent of our oldest citizens suffer from chronic pain. Clearly, pain is a significant issue for a great many older people.

Efforts to examine physiological differences between older and younger people relative to their experience of pain have failed to show significant results overall. Unlike other senses such as hearing and vision, which seem to diminish over time as a result of damage or deterioration of the sense organs involved, pain perception may not change over time, at least from a physiological point of view. Psychological and sociocultural factors may play a more important role in understanding and treating pain in the elderly patient.

As with all patients, psychosocial treatment of elderly pain patients begins with a thorough assessment of their pain and psychological status. Helping patients to feel heard and understood by taking the time necessary for them to tell their story can pay off later in terms of treatment satisfaction, compliance, and outcome.

Psychological treatment of elderly pain patients is mostly concerned with being sensitive to their particular social, cultural, and psychological experience; crafting techniques known to be effective with chronic pain sufferers in general to the older patient's needs. Treatments such as relaxation training, imagery training, clinical hypnosis, biofeedback, and cognitive-behavioral psychotherapy for depressive and anxiety states can be a useful component in the overall multidisciplinary treatment of chronic pain in the older adult.

REFERENCES

Bassols A, Bosch F, Campillo M, Camellas M, Banos JE. An epidemiological comparison of pain complaints in the general population of Catalonia (Spain). *Pain* 1999; 83: 9-16.

Blyth FM, March LM, Brnabic AJ, et al. Chronic pain in Australia: A prevalence study. *Pain* 2001; 89: 127-134.

Bradbeer M, Helme RD, Yong HH, Kendig HL, Gibson SJ. Widowhood and other demographic associations of pain in independent older people. *Clin J Pain* 2003; 19(4): 247-254.

Brattberg G, Parker MG, Thorsbud M. A longitudinal study of pain: Reported pain from middle age to old age. *Clin J Pain* 1997; 13: 144-149.

Casten RG, Parmlea PA, Kleban MH, Lawton MP, Katz IR. The relationships among anxiety, depression, and pain in a geriatric institutionalized sample. *Pain* 1995; 61: 271-276.

Chaves JF. Applying hypnosis in pain management. In Krisch I, Capafons A, Cardena-Buelna E, Amigo S., eds. *Clinical Hypnosis and Self-Regulation.* Washington, DC: American Psychological Association, 1999, 227-248.

Corran TM, Farrell MJ, Helme RD, Gibson SJ. The classification of patients with chronic pain: Age as a contributing factor. *Clin J Pain* 1997; 13: 207-214.

Corran TM, Gibson SJ, Farrell MJ, Helme RD. Comparison of chronic pain experience between young and elderly patients. In Gebhart GF, Hammond DL, Jenson TS, eds. *Proceedings of the 7th World Congress on Pain, Progress in Pain Research and Management,* Vol. 2. Seattle: IASP Press, 1994, 895-906.

Cossins L, Benbow S, Wiles JR. A comparison of young and elderly patients attending a pain clinic. *Abstracts: 9th World Congress on Pain.* Seattle: IASP Press, 1999, 90.

Edwards RR, Doleys DM, Fillingim RB, Lowery D. Ethnic differences in pain tolerance: Clinical implications in a chronic pain population. *Psychosom Med* 2001; 63: 316-323.

Farrell MJ, Gibson SJ. Psychosocial aspects of pain in older people. In Dworkin RH, Breitbart WS, eds. *Psychosocial Aspects of Pain: A Handbook for Health Care Providers, Progress in Pain Research and Management,* Vol. 27. Seattle: IASP Press, 2004.

Fordyce WE. Evaluating and managing chronic pain. *Geriatrics* 1978; 33: 59-62.

Gagliese L, Melzack R. Lack of differences for age differences in pain beliefs. *Pain Res Manage* 1997; 2: 19-28.

Harkins SW. Aging and pain. In Loeser JD, ed., *Bonica's Management of Pain,* 3rd ed. Philadelphia: Lippincott, Williams, and Wilkins, 2001, 813-823.

Harkins SW, Scott RB. Pain and presbyalgos. In Birren J, ed. *Encyclopedia of Gerontology.* San Diego: Academic Press, 1996, 247-260.

Helme RD, Gibson SJ. The epidemiology of pain in older people. *Clin Geriatr Med* 2001; 17: 417-431.

Helme RD, Gibson SJ, Farrell MJ. The influence of social factors on the chronic pain experience in older people. *Abstracts: 8th World Congress on Pain.* Seattle: IASP Press, 1996, 519.

Henderson AS, Jorm AF, Rorien AE, jacomb P, christensen M, Rodgers B. Symptoms of depression and anxiety during adult life: Evidence for a decline in prevalence with age. *Psychol Med* 1998; 28: 1321-1328.

Hofland SL. Elder beliefs: Blocks to pain management. *J Gerontol Nurs* 1992; 18: 19-23.

Jorm AF. Does age reduce the risk of anxiety and depression? A review of epidemiological studies across the adult life span. *Psychol Med* 2000; 30: 11-22.

Kendig H, Helme RD, Teshuva K. *Health Status of older People Project: Data from a Survey of the Health and Lifestyles of Older Australians.* Report to the Victorian Health Promotion Foundation. Sydney: University of Sydney, 1996.

Kind P, Dolan P, Gudex C, Williams A. Variations in population health status: results from a United Kingdom national questionnaire survey. *BMJ* 1998; 316: 736-741.

Lenz EJ, Mulsant BH, Shear MK, et al. Comorbidity of depression and anxiety disorders in later life. *Depression Anx* 2001; 14: 86-93.

Leventhal EA, Leventhal H, Schaefer P, Esterling D. Conservation of energy, uncertainty reduction, and swift utilization of medical care among the elderly. *J Gerontol* 1993; 48: 78-86.

Liddell A, Locker D. Gender and age differences in attitudes to dental pain and dental control. *Com Den Oral Epidem* 1997; 25: 314-318.

Lyness JM, Caine ED, King DA, et al. Psychiatric disorders in older primary care patients. *J Gerontol Int Med* 1999; 14: 249-254.

Magni G, Marchetti M, Moreschi C, Merskey H, Luchini SR. Chronic musculoskeletal pain and depressive symptoms in the National Health and Nutrition Examination I. Epidemiologic follow-up study. *Pain* 1993; 53: 163-168.

Mangione CM, Marcantonio ER, Goldman L, et al. Influence of age on management of health status in patients undergoing elective surgery. *J Am Geriatr Soc* 1993; 41: 377-383.

McCracken LM. Age, pain, and impairment: Results from two clinical samples. *Abstracts: 7th World Congress on Pain.* Seattle: IASP Press, 1993, 99.

Mersky H, Magni G. Psychological techniques in the treatment of chronic pain. In Miller TW, ed. *Chronic Pain,* Vol. 2. Guilford, CT: International Universities Press, 1990, 367-388.

Ouslander JG. Physical illness and depression in the elderly. *J Am Geriatr Soc* 1982; 30: 593-599.

Pope A, Tarlov A. *IDM report: disability in America.* Washington, DC: National Academy Press, 1991. Available at: http://www.nap.edu/books/0309043786/html/index.html.

Rapp SR, Parisi SA, Wallace CE. Comorbid psychiatric disorders in elderly medical patients: A 1-year prospective study. *J Am Geriatr Soc* 1991; 39: 124-131.

Riley JL III, Wade JB, Robinson ME, Price DD. The stages of pain processing across the life span. *J Pain* 2000; 1: 162-170.

Ruzicka SA. Pain beliefs: what do elders believe? *J Hol Nurs* 1998; 16: 369-382.

Scialfa CT, Kline D. Vision. In Birren J, ed. *Encyclopedia of Gerontology.* San Diego: Academic Press, 1996, 605-612.

Staller EP. Interpretation of symptoms of older people. *J Aging Health* 1993; 5: 58-81.

Turner JA, Romano JM. Psychological and psychosocial evaluation. In Loesser JD, ed. *Bonica's management of pain,* 3rd ed. Philadelphia: Lippincott, Williams, and Wilkins, 2001, 329-341.

Turk DC, Okifugi A, Scharff L. Chronic pain and depression: role of perceived impact and perceived control in different age cohorts. *Pain* 1995; 61: 93-101.

Walsh NE, Schoenfeld L, Ramamurthy S, Hoffman J. Normative model for cold pressor test. *Am J Phys Med Rehab* 1989; 68: 6-11.

Washington LL, Gibson SJ, Helme RD. Age-related differences in the endogenous analgesic response to cold water inversion in human volunteers. *Pain* 2000; 89: 89-96.

Watkins KW, Shrifren K, Park DC, Morrell RW. Age, pain and coping with rheumatoid arthritis. *Pain* 1999; 82: 217-228.

Wolpe J. *The Practice of Behavior Therapy,* 2nd ed. New York: Pergamon, 1973.

Woodrow KM, Freidman GD, Siegelaub AB, Collen MF. Pain tolerance: differences according to age, sex, and race. *Psychosom Med* 1972; 34: 548-556.

Chapter 18

Use of Psychotropic Medications in Geriatric Pain Management

Guerman Ermolenko

The use of psychotropics in the augmentation and treatment of chronic pain is well documented. To date, none of the psychotropic medications discussed in this chapter have been approved by the Food and Drug Administration for use in pain management. However, numerous studies support their positive role in pain management.

ANTIDEPRESSANTS

The role of antidepressants in pain management is well established and consistent with the hypothesis of inhibitory action of serotonin and norepinephrine on descending pain pathways. In a review of 39 placebo-controlled studies, Magni (1992) reported the superiority of antidepressants in comparison to placebo in 80 percent of studies on the management of chronic pain. Although depression was the most important variable associated with persistent chronic pain (Magni, 1987, 1992) pain relief was found to be an independent action of the antidepressants (Wilson et al., 2001), which makes the use of that class of medication especially promising.

Tricyclics

The clinical role and use of tricyclic antidepressants (TCAs) is well established and documented since the early 1960s. Prior to the mid-1980s, they were the first line of treatment of depression. TCAs have been used in management of chronic pain and as an adjunct in treatment of acute types of pain including but not limited to cancer-related pain, postherpetic neuralgia, painful diabetic neuropathy, and central poststroke pain (Mattia et al., 2003).

Clinical Management of the Elderly Patient in Pain
© 2006 by The Haworth Press, Inc. All rights reserved.
doi:10.1300/5356_18

The mechanism of the analgesic effect of TCAs is most likely related to a combination of serotonin and norepinephrine reuptake inhibition in conjunction with sodium channel blockade, similar to local anesthetics and antiarrhythmic agents (Jacobson et al., 1995). They are effective (Jauhari and Bapat, 1968; Watson et al., 1998), with a response rate ranging between 40 and 70 percent, but also have a variety of contraindications and significant side effects in comparison with selective serotonin reuptake inhibitors (SSRIs) and serotonin and norepinephrine reuptake inhibitors (SNRIs). No difference was found in efficacy between tricyclics in pain management. In treatment of chronic pain, the response dose of the tricyclics is usually equal to half of the dose for depression. The response time is also shorter and pain relief may be seen within the first week (Lipman, 1996; Billings, 1994).

Due to less severe side effects, nortriptyline is considered to be the drug of choice in the geriatric population, with a starting dose of 10 mg and possible titration up to 150 mg per day. Desipramine and amitriptyline have also been used in the geriatric population with similar dosing and efficacy (Bressler and Katz, 1993; Rudorfer, Manji, and Potter, 1994; Lipman, 1996; Bryson and Wilde, 1996), but they have a higher rate of orthostatic hypotention. These agents should not be used in patients with second- or third-degree heart block, arrhythmias, or prolonged QT interval or in patients who have had a recent acute myocardial infarction (Bryson and Wilde, 1996). Since the introduction of a new group of antidepressants, SNRIs, the use of tricyclics is becoming less popular among physicians due to the safer side effect profile and comparable efficacy of SNRIs (see Table 18.1 for further information on commonly used tricyclics). Psychiatrists tend not to use TCAs as a first-line treatment due to increased side effects but also secondary to a safer outcome with other antidepressants (SSRI, SNRI) in the case of possible overdose (Phillips et al., 1997).

SNRIs

Venlafaxine was one of the first alternatives to the tricyclics as a treatment and adjunct to the treatment of different pain syndromes. This antidepressant has a dual (serotonin and norepinephrine reuptake inhibition) mechanism of action. It showed efficacy in open-label trials as well as multiple case reports in patients with fibromyalgia (response rate ~50-70 percent, $p < 0.1$), peripheral neuropathies, mixed headaches, poststroke pain, atypical facial pain, back pain, and intercostal neuralgias (Miller and Kubes, 2002; Galvez et al., 2004; Bradley et al., 2003; Adelman et al., 2000; Sayar et al., 2003; Dwight et al., 1998). The effective dosing ranged from

TABLE 18.1. Commonly used tricyclics

	Usual dose range	Anticholinergic	Sedation	Drug interactions
Nortriptyline	10-150 mg daily, titration starts at 10 mg with a slow increase as per response. Check level; do not exceed 150 μg/L due to therapeutic windows (50-150 μg/L)	Moderate	Moderate	MAOs; phenotiazines; SSRIs; Ultram; cimitidine; anticholinergics; clonidine; Type IA and IC antiarrhythmics 7-10 percent of the patients are poor metabolizers, which can lead to level increase.
Amitriptyline	25 mg up to 300 mg a day, usual maintenance dose 75-150 mg a day. Level also needs to be checked.	High	High	Same as above
Desipramine	Same dosing as amitriptyline, but low sedative effect	Moderate	Moderate	Same as above
Doxepin	10-100 mg a day, high sedation	High	High	Same as above

37.5 mg up to 300 mg per day. The effect of venlafaxine on pain was independent from its antidepressant properties. The most common side effects of venlafaxine are gastrointestinal upset (nausea and vomiting), headaches, sweating, and increased blood pressure (mostly diastolic). Venlafaxine has been widely used in the geriatric population for treatment of depressive and anxiety disorders with significant success.

The recently released duloxetine is a novel antidepressant with a similar mechanism of action as venlafaxine (SNRI) and has similar analgesic properties. In a study by Ditke et al. (2002), a 60 mg per day dose of duloxetine not only showed significant antidepressant action, but also provided substantial relief in pain measured by the VAS (visual analogue scale) (100-point scale, reduction to 28-29) when compared with a placebo. Reduction in pain was seen as early as the end of week 1 ($p < .05$) during evaluation of the back pain and continued to be significant until the end of the study at week 9 ($p < .001$). Similar results were observed on evaluation of shoulder pain ($p < .01$ at weeks 2 and 7 and $p = .083$ at week 9). Less robust but numerically superior ($p = .065-.083$) results were seen in the treatment of depressed patients with headaches and overall pain. In the treatment of depression, results were significantly better and robust ($p < .001$). In a separate trial, duloxetine was efficient in the treatment of pain associated with diabetic polyneuropathy as measured on the 24-hour Average Pain Severity scale. Starting at week 1 at doses of 60 and 120 mg per day, it was statistically superior to placebo in pain relief through the length of the study ($p < .001$ at week 12).

Mirtazapine also affects noradrenergic and serotonergic transmission. Several case series and studies (Martin-Araguz, Bustamante-Martinez, and de Pedro-Pijoan, 2003; Ansari, 2000; Brannon and Stone, 1999) showed comparable efficacy in treatment of chronic pain and headaches with tricyclics and SSRIs. Main side effects include sedation and appetite increase (lower doses, 7.5-15 mg, appeared to be more prone to cause that) which makes it a reasonable choice in geriatric depression. One should be aware of possible agranulocytosis (De Boer, 1996) when using in patients with cancer or HIV. The drug has low anticholinergic and sexual side effects, with low incidence of drug-drug interaction. Mirtazapine can be initiated at one quarter (~3.5 mg) of the 15 mg (lowest dose available) pill if used for insomnia, appetite stimulant, or as an adjunct in pain management. Dose increase can be done rather rapidly if necessary to achieve 30 mg (average therapeutic dose for depression) within 7-10 days. Combination with venlafaxine (Kelsey, 2002) appeared to be useful in management of treatment-resistant depressive disorders. No studies were found in use of antidepressant combinations for management of chronic pain.

SSRIs

SSRIs are the most commonly prescribed group of antidepressants. Since the 1980s, their role in the management of depressive disorders in the elderly has been well established in comparative studies (Bondareff et al., 2000; Flint, 1998; Robinson et al., 2000; Salzman, Wong, and Wright, 2002; Mulchahey et al., 1999; Roose et al., 2002). Due to a low side-effect profile and documented efficacy, they may merit primary consideration in treating geriatric depression. Although the comparative efficacy of SSRIs among themselves and other classes of antidepressants in the treatment of depressive disorders appears to be the same (Kroenke et al., 2001; Lawrenson et al., 2000; Bondareff et al., 2000; Robinson et al., 2000), their role in pain management is less well defined (Jung, Staiger, and Sullivan, 1997; Abdel-Salam, Baiuomy, and Arbid, 2004; Shimodozono et al., 2002; Ciaramella, Grosso, and Poli, 2000; Hickie, Scott, and Davenport, 1999).

SSRIs' use is most beneficial in mixed chronic pain with a lesser degree of efficacy in migraine, fibromyalgia, and diabetic neuropathies (Ripple et al., 2000; Jung, Staiger, and Sullivan, 1997). However, one should not hesitate to use these agents as an adjunct when depression is one of the major obstacles in proper pain control. The most common side effects are gastrointestinal upset (nausea and diarrhea, though this usually subsides with prolonged use), sexual dysfunction, insomnia, anxiety, and headaches. Less common but more problematic are hyponatremia and movement disorders.

Although SSRIs act on platelets and can extend bleeding time, no incidence of increase risk in intracranial bleeding was found (Bak et al., 2002). Dosing in treatment of pain appeared to be similar to the treatment of depressive disorders.

An average geriatric patient with chronic pain takes more than four medications, which creates a challenge in the field of pharmacodynamics and pharmacokinetics. Although the class is well tolerated as a whole, sertraline, citalopram, and escitalopram have lesser side effects and fewer drug interactions due to minimal cytochrome P450 system inhibition. They are considered to be drugs of choice for the treatment of depression in the geriatric population (see Table 18.2 for prescribing considerations and doses).

Heterocyclics

Bupropion is an antidepressant agent that, in addition to noradrenergic activities, exhibits dopamine agonist action. Seizure disorder and anorexia are major contraindications with anxiety, insomnia, and headache being the most common side effects. Practitioners should be cautious when using in patients with brain tumors or taking medications that can lower seizure threshold. The drug appears to be free from cardiotoxic side effects. Bupropion is well established in the treatment of depressive disorders and appears to be well tolerated with low side effects and minimal drug interactions. Double-blind placebo-controlled studies of bupropion SR for the treatment of neuropathic pain showed up to 73 percent response rate in comparison with placebo (Semenchuk, Sherman, and Davis, 2001). Bupropion has also been found to have a good response in treatment of patients with chronic fatigue syndrome, where pain is often a significant complaint. Case series showed efficacy in treatment of low back pain. The doses for both pain and depressive disorders range between 150 and 300 mg daily. With a new XR formulation of bupropion, medication can be used once a day without any loss in efficacy. This antidepressant should be the drug of choice in overweight patients who also want to stop smoking, as it has been used with success for smoking cessation.

Nefazodone is another antidepressant with a dual mechanism, working by inhibition of neuronal uptake of serotonin and norepinephrine. Nefazodone also antagonizes central 5-HT$_2$ receptors and alpha-1 adrenergic receptors (which may cause postural hypotension). It has a half-life of only two to four hours. Nefazodone possesses both the actions of analgesia and potentiation of opioid analgesia in the mouse hotplate assay (Semenchuk, Sherman, and Davis, 2001). The use of nefazodone has been documented in cases of diabetic neuropathies (Goodnick et al., 2000) and chronic

TABLE 18.2. Most commonly used SSRIs, SNRIs, and heterocyclics.

Antidepressant	Daily dose	Sedation/ orthostatic	Activation	Major side effects
SSRI				
Sertraline—first line for geriatrics with multiple medications	25-200 mg can be given once in a.m. or p.m.	Very low/none	Low	GI, some anxiety, sexual dysfunction, hyponatremia, serotonin syndrome, minimal inhibitor CytP450(2C19); significant interactions with MAOs, TCAs, warfarin; possible with type 1C antiarrhythmics and Ultram
Citalopram/ escitalopram—first line for geriatrics with multiple medications	10-40 mg 5-20 mg both usually given once in a.m.	None/none	Low	GI, lesser degree of anxiety, sexual dysfunction, hyponatremia, serotonin syndrome, no significant inhibition of CytP450; significant interactions with MAOs, TCAs, warfarin; possible with type 1C antiarrhythmics and Ultram
Fluoxetine—second line for geriatrics with multiple medications	10-80 mg once in a.m.	None/none	+++ Can induce anxiety and insomnia	GI, anxiety, insomnia, tremor, sexual dysfunction, hyponatremia, serotonin syndrome, potent inhibitor CytP450 2D6, moderate for 2C9, 2C19, 3A4; significant interactions with MAOs, TCAs, warfarin; possible with type 1C antiarrhythmics and Ultram. Decreases efficacy of codeine

Paroxetine—second line for geriatrics with multiple medications	10-40 mg once in p.m. 12.5-50 mg for CR formulation	Moderate/none	Very low	Same as Prozac, but also has mild to moderate anticholinergic properties; be aware of potentially severe discontinuation syndrome, less with CR formulation
Fluvoxamine—third line for geriatrics with multiple medications	25-300 mg, usually given twice or even three times a day	None/none	Low	GI, anxiety, insomnia, tremor, sexual dysfunction, hyponatremia, serotonin syndrome, potent inhibitor CytP450, 1A2, 2C19, moderate for 2C9, 3A4; significant interactions with MAOs, TCAs, antipsychotics, antihypertensive; warfarin; possible with type 1C antiarrhythmics and Ultram

SNRI

Venlafaxine, XR formulation most commonly being used—first line for geriatrics with multiple medications	37.5-300 mg at night, adequate dose is 150 mg, (doses exceeding 225 mg need to be given twice a day)	Mild/none	None	GI (nausea especially), headaches, sweating, blood pressure elevation (mostly diastolic, dose related), some anxiety, dizziness, sexual dysfunction, hyponatremia, serotonin syndrome, almost no CytP450, significant interactions with MAOs, TCAs, possible but lesser degree with type 1C antiarrhythmics and Ultram

TABLE 18.2 (continued)

Antidepressant	Daily dose	Sedation/ orthostatic	Activation	Major side effects
Duloxetine—first line for geriatrics with multiple medications	20-120mg, adequate dose is 60 mg once a day (doses exceeding 60 mg need to be given twice a day)	Mild/none	Minimal	Similar to venlafaxine GI (nausea as early as day 2), dry mouth, fatigue, insomnia, constipation, somnolence, sweating, serotonin syndrome, no CytP450, significant interactions with MAOs, possible but lesser degree with type 1C antiarrhythmics and Ultram
Mirtazapine—first line for geriatrics with multiple medications	7.5-45 mg at night (doses 45 mg and above less sedative and can be used in the morning)	High especially at lower doses/none	None, but antidepressant effect described as early as day 4	Somnolence, increase in appetite, dry mouth, agranulocytosis (rare), no CytP450 interactions, significant interactions with MAOs, serotonin syndrome, possible but lesser degree with TCAs and with Ultram
Heterocyclic				
Buproprion—first line for geriatrics with multiple medications	75-300 mg in divided doses, (150 mg and 300 mg XL formulation once a day)	None/none	+++ Can induce anxiety and insomnia	Anxiety, agitation, insomnia, headaches, tremor, anorexia (drug of choice in obese patients), nausea, seizures (less with sustained-release formulation) significant interactions with MAOs (can cause buproprion toxicity), caffeine and TCA (increase level of TCAs and risk of seizures)

Nefazodone—second to third line for geriatrics with multiple medications	25-400 mg a day in divided doses (average dose 300 mg a day)	Moderate/mild (possible asymptomatic decrease in blood pressure)	Hepatic failure, somnolence, dizziness, asthenia, insomnia, constipation, nausea, serotonin syndrome, seizures, significant interactions with MAOs, potent CytP450 3A4, dose reduction of aprazolam, zolpidem, midazolam, HIV protease inhibitors, Ca channel block; buspirone may be indicated	None (mild with high doses)
Trazodone—Use in geriatric population for sedation only	25-300 mg at night (usual dose 50-100 mg at night for insomnia)	Moderate to high/moderate especially in high doses	Somnolence, dizziness, asthenia, insomnia, constipation, nausea, serotonin syndrome, seizures, priapism, hypotension, arrhythmias, significant interactions with MAOs	None
Other			
MAO inhibitors (phenelzine, tranylcypromine, isocarboxazide) limited use in geriatrics, for depression and anxiety only	10-60 mg a day (usually at night)	Moderate/very high At least moderate anticholinergic properties	Somnolence, anxiety, dizziness, constipation, dry mouth, GI and sexual disturbances, hypotension, hypertensive crisis, serotonergic syndrome; contraindicated for use with meperidine, dextromethorphan, SSRIs, SNRIs, tyramine-containing food, bupropion, in pheochromocytoma, CHF, and severe liver diseases	Mild

headaches (ACHE, 2001) with doses ranging between 50 and 300 mg per day. The use of nefazodone has substantially decreased since 2002 due to reported severe and at times lethal cases of hepatotoxicity (Stewart, 2002; Jody, 2002). Caution needs to be exercised when used with some benzodiazepines. Doses of alprazolam, zolpidem, and midazolam need to be decreased by 50 percent due to block in metabolism (cytochrome P450 3A4) caused by nefazodone. For these reasons, the use of nefazodone in pain management is rather limited and should be utilized only when all other agents have failed.

Trazodone is an antidepressant similar in chemical structure to nefazodone. Due to the possibility of orthostatic hypotension at therapeutic doses (200-400 mg per day) the use of this drug in the elderly as an antidepressant is negligent. For this reason, trazodone is usually used as a sleeping and antianxiety aid at doses of 25-100 mg. For similar reasons, it is far less than an ideal agent for use in pain management.

Monoamine Oxidase Inhibitors

A literature search on the use of monoamine oxidase (MAO) inhibitors in pain management revealed only limited citations. Most of the data supporting their use in pain management come from basic research only (analgesic effect of MAO inhibitors; Nath et al., 1991; Bhattacharya et al., 1971; Jounela and Mattila, 1971; Jauhari and Bapat, 1968). No controlled studies or meta-analyses of case series were found. Due to multiple side effects, severe and troublesome drug interactions, and the necessity of a tyramine-free diet (tyramine is contained in foods such as aged cheeses, microbrewed beer, red wine, and chocolate) the use of MAO inhibitors has decreased substantially even for treatment of depressive disorders. On the basis of current studies and safety profile, I would not recommend using MAO inhibitors as an adjunct in the treatment of chronic or acute pain in geriatric population.

ANTIPSYCHOTICS

The use of antipsychotics in pain management has been rather limited. Most likely their analgesic properties are mediated through a serotonergic mechanism (blockade of 5-HT1A, 5-HT2A, 5-HT2C receptors) that is more prominent in atypical antipsychotics. No blinded placebo control studies have been completed to date. The use of antipsychotics in the elderly is reserved for delirium, dementia, schizophrenia, delusional disorder, and psychotic mood disorders (Alexopoulos et al., 2004). Due to higher severity and frequencies of side effects (tardive dyskinesia, extrapyramidal symptoms) of typical antipsychotics (such as haloperidol and per-phenazine) and lesser efficacy (Davis, Chen, and Glick, 2003), their use in the geriatric population is rather limited and usually reserved for the treatment of acute agitation, delirium, and schizophrenias. All atypical antipsychotics have warnings about higher risk to develop diabetes and weight gain (more case reports found with clozapine, olanzapine, and quetiapine). It is less relevant for the geriatric population as atypical antipsychotics are usually weight neutral and the risk for diabetes is equal to that of the general population. Clinicians should be aware of an increased risk of cerebrovascular accident with risperidone, olanzapine, and quetiapine in treatment of behavioral problems in patients with dementia. With the use of typical antipsychotics, the rate of tardive dyskinesia in patients 65 and older approaches 20-25 percent per year but is only 2-3 percent with atypicals (risperidone, olanzapine, quetiapine, aripiprazole, ziprasidone, and clozapine; Correll, Leucht, and Kane, 2004). Due to these constraints, almost all studies involving pain management and antipsychotics were performed on clients below the age of 65. To date, there have been several small open-label trials involving olanzapine and ziprasadone in the treatment of migraine headaches. Less study data is available regarding risperidone, quetiapine, and aripiprazole use in the field of chronic pain, though all of them have merit for use in psychosis, dementias, and delirium commonly associated with medical conditions.

Clozapine use is reserved for primary psychiatric and usually treatment-resistant conditions. Clozapine is considered to be the most side-effect-prone (sedation, seizures, siallorrhea, incontinence, anticholinergic, etc.) and toxic (cardiotoxicity with myocarditis, agranulocytosis, etc.) antipsychotic. I would not recommend using clozapine as an adjunct in chronic or acute pain management due to this high risk-benefit ratio.

Risperidone is probably the most studied atypical antipsychotic in geriatrics due to its common use in agitated dementia. In lower doses (0.25-1.5 mg per day) it is usually well tolerated with minimal sedative properties in comparison with olanzapine, quetiapine, and clozapine. Higher doses are associated with an increase of EPS (extra pyramidal symptoms) (Parkinsonism) and prolactin elevation. Several case reports (Fe-Bornstein, Watt, and Gitlin, 2002) and animal studies (Schreiber et al., 1997) suggest augmentation with risperidone in chronic pain patients with depression and anxiety who also have poor impulse control.

When dealing with patients in need of sedation, quetiapine may be a drug of choice. It has properties similar to olanzapine with a lesser degree of EPS and a short half life (T1/2) (four to six hours). Doses in geriatrics usually range between 25 and 300 mg per day, although doses above 800 mg are documented in elderly patients with schizophrenia. A small open-label trial was conducted with quetiapine in migraine headaches. Average doses were 75 mg per day. Among 24 enrolled patients, 21 reported substantial improvement (Brandes et al., 2002).

Aripiprazole is the most recently released antipsychotic, with unique pharmacological properties. It is a partial agonist/antagonist of dopamine receptors that also has potent serotonergic properties. It also has a low incidence of EPS and appears to be well tolerated in the geriatric population. Main side effects include nausea, anxiety, and headaches, which are usually transient. This antipsychotic has been widely used in the nursing home population with a dosing range of 5-30 mg per day (average 5-15 mg per day).

Most of the atypical antipsychotics were recently approved by the FDA for treatment of bipolar disorders as single agents and in combination with mood stabilizers. This will expand our knowledge and experience and hopefully will create better data for use in the management of geriatric pain.

Olanzapine

Several case reports and open-label studies involving the management of patients with acute (cancer), fibromyalgia, cluster headache, and chronic pain syndrome were identified (Khojainova, Santiago-Palma, and Gonzales, 2001; Rozen, 2001; Silberstein et al., 2002). Most of the clients had comorbid depression and/or anxiety. Olanzapine was used mostly as an adjunct. Overall, the drug was well tolerated with minimal side effects. Doses ranged between 2.5 and 10 mg daily. For pain associated with cancer treatment, eight subjects received 2.5-7.5 mg daily. All patients had a decrease in pain perception as well as opioid consumption, indicative of an independent pain reduction mechanism. Five patients with cluster headaches (Rozen, 2001) received olanzapine in the open-label trial. Four reported relief within 20 minutes postmedication intake. Doses ranged between 2.5 and 10 mg (average 5 mg) per day. Fifty patients with treatment-resistant migraine and refractory headaches were involved in another open-label trial (Silberstein et al., 2002). Doses ranged between 2.5 and 35 mg daily. As a result, 37 (74 percent) patients improved, 12 (24 percent) felt the same, and one client got worse.

Ziprasidone

A small ($N = 21$, mean age 51.7) open-label observational study evaluated efficacy of ziprasidone in the prevention of migraine headaches (Wheeler and Wheeler, 2003), none responsive to prior treatment and with or without analgesics overuse. Overall, 68.2 percent of patients improved.

A higher response rate was observed for analgesic overusers (rebounders) at 73.3 percent than for nonrebounders at 50 percent. Side effects were rather mild in intensity.

Although by itself ziprasidone does not have significant QTc interval prolongation, combination with other medications (TCAs, quinolones, antiarrhythmics, etc.) and preexisting medical problems (hypokalemia, hypomagnesemia, arrhythmias, heart block) can cause serious consequences. Because of multiple and complex medication regimens in the geriatric population, use of ziprasidone remains rather limited.

Other Psychotropics

In contemporary psychiatry, as in all medicine, the arsenal of medication is growing with each day. Anticonvulsants play an important role as mood stabilizers in a wide variety of psychiatric disorders. Chapter 11 addresses their role in pain management. At the same time I would like to mention lithium, which is one of the oldest mood stabilizers on the market. In psychiatry, we use litium for treatment and augmentation of treatment in mood disorders, schizophrenias, and disorders with poor impulse control. Use of lithium is rather limited in the geriatric population due a combination of a decrease in renal functioning, an increase of fat with decreased free water, and narrow therapeutic index lithium, which carries a great risk of becoming toxic in a short period of time. The main side effects include confusion, tremor, ataxia, GI disturbances, polyuria, polydipsia, and possible hypothyroidism (often not reversible after discontinuation of lithium). Although this medication is well studied and known in psychiatry, in the arena of pain management hard-core data are minimal (Wyant and Ashenhurst, 1979; Casacchia et al., 1981; Shimizu et al., 2000; Bussone et al., 1990; Teixeira, Pereira, and Hermini, 1995). Clinicians should always be cautious when combining lithium with indomethacin, piroxicam, other NSAIDs, angiotensin-converting enzyme inhibitors, and diuretics. Even with a single dose of NSAID, litium can reach toxic levels (above 1.2 mEq/L) and be potentially dangerous. Signs of toxicity are an increase in GI disturbances with possible nausea, vomiting and diarrhea, confusion, ataxia, and lethargy. Severe drug interactions make this drug one of the last in line for augmentation in treatment of pain in the geriatric population.

Hypnotics and anxiolytics are also one of the oldest medication classes used in psychiatry. Their action on GABA and bradykinin B1 antagonism can possibly explain their occasional pain reduction mechanism (Megarbane, Gueye, and Baud, 2003; Jones, Nisenbaum, and Reeves, 2003), although their use is rather minimal. Benzodiazepines also have a lesser role in geriatrics than in adult psychiatry due to their effect on gait and cognitive functioning. Their use (Gray et al., 2003; Stiefel and Stagno, 2004; Neutel, Walop, and Patten, 2003; Jones, Nisenbaum, and Reeves, 2003) in cases of chronic pain management is mainly limited to sedation, anxieties, and rarely for tension headaches and refractory muscle spasms. Unfortunately, they also can exacerbate depression and they are addictive. Very limited use has been described in chronic fatigue syndrome. The cross-tolerance and additive breathing center suppression make them far from ideal for augmentation in case of opioid use. If used in geriatrics, oxazepam, lorazepam, and clonazepam are considered to be the drugs of choice due to an absence of active metabolites and as a result low probability for accumulation. Still, I would recommend their use only as third or even fourth line, when at least two alternatives failed.

Buspirone is the "safe" alternative to benzodiazepines indicated for treatment of general anxiety disorder. It has been studied in chronic pain with emphasis mainly in the treatment of tension headaches and augmentation in treatment of migraines (Pakulska and Czarnecka, 2001; Mitsikostas et al., 1997). Side effects and drug interactions are mild, including mostly mild GI disturbances, headache, and dizziness. It is generally not sedative and does not negatively affect gait or cognition. Doses range from 5 mg to a total of 60 mg in divided (BID, TID) doses. Do not expect robust cessation of anxiety, especially if prior benzodiazepines were used. Due to minimal side effects and low potential for abuse, I would use buspirone as an adjunct in the treatment of chronic pain before any of the benzodiazepines.

SIGNIFICANT SIDE EFFECTS AND INTERACTIONS OF THE ANTIDEPRESSANTS

All antidepressants can increase risk for serotonin syndrome (myoclonus, rigidity, confusion, nausea, hyperthermia, autonomic instability, coma, eventual death) and decrease seizure threshold in combination with Ultram and triptans. Sedative antidepressants can potentiate somnolence in opioid-based analgesics.

Tricyclics

Tricyclics have quinidine-like effect that may worsen branch block. Be aware of preexisting heart conditions (arrhythmias, recent myocaridal infarction). Nortriptyline appeared to be safer with a minimal orthostatic hypotension which makes it among the TCAs of choice in geriatrics.

Anticholinergic side effects are present with all TCAs. This includes urinary retention, constipation, tachycardia, and possible worsening in cognition.

SSRIs

SSRIs have a more favorable side-effect profile, but have lesser utilization in pain management as single agents. Mostly they have been used as an adjunct, especially in patients with depressive and anxiety disorders. Sertraline, citalopram, and escitalopram are SSRIs of choice due to lesser drug-drug interactions. Sertraline also has a weak dopamine agonist activity, which theoretically can counteract prolactin (Sachs and Chan, 2001; Michelson, Dording, and Mischoulon, 2000; Michelson, 2000; Dording, 2000; Gordon, Whale, and Cowen, 1998) elevation, which can be important in patients with breast cancer and osteoporosis. All SSRIs have GI side effects (nausea, diarrhea), sexual dysfunction (sertraline, citalopram, and escitalopram to a lesser degree), hyponatremia, and movement disorder. Use of codeine and codeine-containing analgesics should be avoided with paroxetine and fluoxetine due to their inhibition of cytochrome P450 2D6 isoenzyme where codeine is converted to its active metabolite. Also be aware of incontinence associated with use of SSRIs (Movig et al., 2002) in the geriatric population. This problem appears to be greater with sertraline. Also be aware of serotonin syndrome between different combinations of serotonergic antidepressants.

STRATEGIES FOR COMBINED PSYCHIATRIC AND PAIN SYNDROMES

Depression and Chronic Pain

A strong correlation exists between depression and chronic pain. Each is considered to be a risk factor for the other. Use of antidepressants will bring relief not only for depression but also for pain symptoms. Simple measures such as the Geriatric Depression Scale (see Exhibit 18.1) or the Hamilton Depression scale can be of great value in judging the degree of illness. The type and class of antidepressants depend on symptoms of depression as well as concomitant pain medication. Doses need to be the same as in treatment of depressive disorders. In cases of anxious patients with poor sleep and appetite, mirtazapine (7.5-45 mg at night) can be an excellent choice. In patients requiring activation, bupropion is a drug of choice. Clients with

EXHIBIT 18.1. Geriatric depression scale.

1. Are you basically satisfied with your life?
2. Have you dropped many of your activities and interests?
3. Do you feel that your life is empty?
4. Do you often get bored?
5. Are you hopeful about the future?
6. Are you bothered by thoughts you can't get out of your head?
7. Are you in good spirits most of the time?
8. Are you afraid that something bad is going to happen to you?
9. Do you feel happy most of the time?
10. Do you often feel helpless?
11. Do you often get restless and fidgety?
12. Do you prefer to stay at home, rather than going out and doing new things?
13. Do you frequently worry about the future?
14. Do you feel you have more problems with memory than most?
15. Do you think it is wonderful to be alive now?
16. Do you often feel downhearted and blue?
17. Do you feel pretty worthless the way you are now?
18. Do you worry a lot about the past?
19. Do you find life very exciting?
20. Is it hard for you to get started on new projects?
21. Do you feel full of energy?
22. Do you feel that your situation is hopeless?
23. Do you think that most people are better off than you are?
24. Do you frequently get upset over little things?
25. Do you frequently feel like crying?
26. Do you have trouble concentrating?
27. Do you enjoy getting up in the morning?
28. Do you prefer to avoid social gatherings?
29. Is it easy for you to make decisions?
30. Is your mind as clear as it used to be?

Scoring for the Scale

Tally one point for each of these answers as below:

1. no	11. yes	21. no
2. yes	12. yes	22. yes
3. yes	13. yes	23. yes
4. yes	14. yes	24. yes
5. no	15. no	25. yes
6. yes	16. yes	26. yes
7. no	17. yes	27. no
8. yes	18. yes	28. yes
9. no	19. no	29. no
10. yes	20. yes	30. no

Cutoff: normal: 0-9; mild depressives: 10-19; severe depressives: 20-30 moderate to severe pain due to neuralgias, fibromyalgia, or back and shoulder pain can be tried on venlafaxine or duloxetine first.

For physicians who do not have wide experience in the use of antidepressants, venlafaxine, duloxetine, or SSRIs are reasonable choices to start, keeping in mind drug interactions. Follow-up consultation with a more experienced colleague or psychiatrist is highly recommended.

Chronic Fatigue Syndrome and Fibromyalgia

On the basis of current data and side-effect profile, I would recommend using the SNRI group of antidepressants. Venlafaxine and Duloxetine appear to be drugs of choice, followed by bupropion. If they fail, SSRIs should be tried with possible augmentation with atypical antipsychotics if not effective alone. In the geriatric population, sertraline, citalopram, and escitalopram should be tried first due to minimal drug interactions. Doses should be the same as used in treatment of depressive disorders.

Hypochondriasis

I cannot fail to mention the "difficult and always sick" patient. Approximately 5 percent of primary care outpatients meet the criteria for hypochondriasis. The criteria include preoccupation with an idea or fear of unfound illness despite appropriate medical workup. These beliefs are not delusional, although they cause severe distress and persist for more than six months. Often these patients have complaints of low to moderate chronic pain. No well-controlled randomized studies have been done yet. Several open-label trials as well as case reports demonstrated 40-60 percent response rate using all classes of the antidepressants. Due to significant anticholinergic side effects of the TCAs, SSRIs, and SNRIs are a more appropriate choice. Dosing is similar to that of the treatment of depressive disorder, which is also suggestive for the link in comorbidity between two conditions.

CONCLUSION

A multifaceted group approach to pain management in young patients and especially in geriatrics needs to be implemented in order to achieve proper relief and functioning. When in doubt, consultations with a psychiatrist should be scheduled. Do not rely on medication only. Psychosocial variables always need to be assessed and managed as they carry enormous value for recovery as well as for quality of life. Following the main law of medicine since Hippocrates, do not treat only the symptom but the whole human being.

BIBLIOGRAPHY

Abdel-Salam OM, Baiuomy AR, Arbid MS. Studies on the anti-inflammatory effect of fluoxetine in the rat. *Pharmacol Res* 2004; 49:119-131.

ACHE. January headache news. *Headache News* June 2001.

Adelman LC, Adelman JU, Von Seggern R, Mannix LK. Venlafaxine extended release (XR) for the prophylaxis of migraine and tension-type headache. *Headache* 2000; 40:572-580.

Alexopoulos GS, Streim J, Carpenter D, Docherty JP; Expert Consensus Panel for Using Antipsychotic Drugs in Older Patients. Using antipsychotic agents in older patients. *J Clin Psychiatry* 2004; 65(Suppl 2):5-99; discussion 100-102; quiz 103-4.

Ansari A. The efficacy of newer antidepressants in the treatment of chronic pain: A review of current literature. *Harv Rev Psychiatry* 2000; 7:257-277.

Bair MJ, Robinson RL, Eckert GJ, Stang PE, Croghan TW, Kroenke K. Impact of pain on depression treatment response in primary care. *Psychosom Med* 2004; 66:17-22.

Bak S, Trsiropoulos I, Kjaersgaard JO, et al. SSRI and risk of stroke: A population-based case control study. *Stroke* 2002; 33:1465-1473.

Bank J. A comparative study of amitriptyline and fluvoxamine in migraine prophylaxis. *Headache* 1994; 34:476-478.

Bhattacharya SK, Raina MK, Banerjee D, Neogy NC. Potentiation of morphine and pethidine analgesia by some monoamine oxidase inhibitors in albino rats. *Indian J Exp Biol* 1971; 9:257-259.

Billings JA. Neuropathic pain. *J Palliat Care* 1994; 10:40-43.

Boeker T. Ziprasidone and migraine headache. *Am J Psychiatry* 2002; 159:1435-1436.

Bondareff W, Alpert M, Friedhoff AJ, et al. Comparison of sertraline and nortriptyline in the treatment of major depressive disorder in late life. *Am J Psychiatry* 2000; 157:729-736.

Bradley RH, Barkin RL, Jerome J, DeYoung K, Dodge CW. Efficacy of venlafaxine for the long-term treatment of chronic pain with associated major depressive disorder. *Am J Ther* 2003; 10:318-323.

Brandes J, Robertson S, Starr H, Abu-Shakra S. Quetiapine for migraine prophylaxis. *Neurology* 2002; 58 (Suppl 3):A470.

Brannon GE, Stone KD. The use of mirtazapine in a patient with chronic pain. *J Pain Symptom Manage* 1999; 18:382-385.

Bressler R, Katz MD. Drug therapy for geriatric depression. *Drugs Aging* 1993; 3:195-219.

Bryson HM, Wilde MI. Amitriptyline: a review of its pharmacological properties and therapeutic use in chronic pain states. *Drugs Aging* 1996; 8:459-476.

Bussone G, Leone M, Peccarisi et al. Double blind comparison of lithium and verapamil in cluster headache prophylaxis. Headache Centre, C. Besta Neurological Institute of Milan, Italy, 1990.

Casacchia M, Cerbo R, Corona R, Boni B. Double-blind study of the effects of amitriptyline and of a combination of amitriptyline and lithium on patients with chronic primary headache. *Rev Neurol* 1981; 51:114-123.

Ciaramella A, Grosso S, Poli P. Fluoxetine versus fluvoxamine for treatment of chronic pain. *Minerva Anestesiol* 2000; 6:55-61.

Correll CU, Leucht S, Kane JM. Lower risk for tardive dyskinesia associated with second-generation antipsychotics: A systematic review of 1-year studies. *Am J Psychiatry* 2004; 161:414-425.

Davis JM, Chen N, Glick ID. A meta-analysis of the efficacy of second-generation antipsychotics. *Arch Gen Psychiatry* 2003; 60:553-564.

De Boer T. The pharmacologic profile of mirtazepine. *J Clin Psychiatry* 1996; 57: 19-25.

Dellemijn P, Fields HL. Do benzodiazepines have a role in chronic pain management? *Pain* 1994; 57:137-152.

Ditke MJ, Lu Y, Golstein D, Hayes JR, Demitrack MA. Duloxitine, 60 mg once daily, for major depressive disorder: Randomized double-blind placebo-controlled trial. *J Clin Psychiatry* 2002, 63:308-315.

Dording CM. Sexual dysfunction during SSRI continuation treatment. In: Treatment Issues with SSRIs. Program and abstracts from the 153rd Annual American Psychiatric Association Meeting, May 13-18, 2000, Chicago, Illinois. Session 1. Washington, DC: APA.

Duman EN, Kesim M, Kadioglu M, Yaris E, Kalyoncu NI, Erciyes N. Possible involvement of opioidergic and serotonergic mechanisms in antinociceptive effect of paroxetine in acute pain. *J Pharmacol Sci* 2004; 94:161-165.

Dwight MM, Arnold LM, O'Brien H, Metzger R, Morris-Park E, Keck PE Jr. An open clinical trial of venlafaxine treatment of fibromyalgia. *Psychosomatics* 1998; 39:14-17.

Fe-Bornstein M, Watt, SD, Gitlin, MC. Improvement in level of psychosocial functioning in chronic pain patients with use of risperdone. *Pain Med* 2002; 3:128-131.

Flint AJ. Choosing appropriate antidepressant therapy in the elderly: A risk-benefit assessment of available agents. *Drugs Aging* 1998; 13:269-280.

Galvez R, Caballero J, Atero M, Ruiz S, Romero J. Venlafaxine extended release for the treatment of chronic pain: A series of 50 cases. *Actas Esp Psiquiatr* 2004; 32:92-97.

Goodnick PJ. Use of antidepressants in treatment of comorbid diabetes mellitus and depression as well as diabetic neuropathy. *Ann Clin Psychiatry* 2001; 13:31-41.

Goodnick PJ, Breakstone K, Kumar A, Freund B, DeVane CL. Nefazodone in diabetic neuropathy: Response and biology. *Psychosom Med* 2000; 62:599-600.

Gordon C, Whale R, Cowen PJ. Sertraline treatment does not increase plasma prolactin levels in healthy subjects. *Psychopharmacology (Berl)* 1998; 137:201-202.

Gray SL, Eggen AE, Blough D, Buchner D, LaCroix AZ. Benzodiazepine use in older adults enrolled in a health maintenance organization. *Am J Geriatr Psychiatry* 2003; 11:568-576.

Gutierrez MA, Stimmel GL, Aiso JY. Venlafaxine: a 2003 update. *Clin Ther* 2003; 25:2138-2154.

Hamilton M. Development of rating scale for primary depressive illness. *B J Soc Clin Psychol* 1967; 6:278-296.

Hickie IB, Scott EM, Davenport TA. Are antidepressants all the same? Surveying the opinions of Australian psychiatrists. *Aust N Z J Psychiatry* 1999; 33:642-649.

Houlihan DJ. Serotonin syndrome resulting from coadministration of tramadol, venlafaxine, and mirtazapine. *Ann Pharmacother* 2004; 38:411-413. Epub 2004 Jan 23.

Jacobson LO, Bley K, Hunter JC, et al. Anti-thermal hyperalgesic properties of antidepressants in a rat model of neuropathic pain [abstr]. In: *Proceedings of the 14th annual meeting of the American Pain Society.* Glenview, IL: APS, 1995: A105.

Jauhari AC, Bapat SK. Modification by phenelzine of morphine and pethidine analgesia in mice. *Ann Med Exp Biol Fenn* 1968; 46:66-71.

Jody, JM. Important drug warning including black box information. Accessed at www.fda.gov/medwatch/SAFETY/2002/serzone_deardoc.PDF. 2002

Jones JF, Nisenbaum R, Reeves WC. Medication use by persons with chronic fatigue syndrome: Results of a randomized telephone survey in Wichita, Kansas. *Health Qual Life Outcomes* 2003; 1(1):74.

Jounela AJ, Mattila MJ. Analgesic effect of some monoamine oxidase inhibitors. *J Indian Physiol Pharmacol* 1971; 15:21-26.

Jung AC, Staiger T, Sullivan M. The efficacy of selective serotonin reuptake inhibitors for the management of chronic pain. *J Gen Intern Med* 1997; 12: 384-389.

Kelsey JE. Treatment strategies in achieving remission in major depressive disorder. *Acta Psychiatr Scand Suppl* 2002; 413:18-23.

Khojainova N, Santiago-Palma J, Gonzales GR. Pain reduction in cognitively impaired cancer patients treated with olanzapine. *Pain Med* 2001; 2:243-244.

Kroenke K, West SL, Swindle R, et al. Similar effectiveness of paroxetine, fluoxetine, and sertraline in primary care: A randomized trial. *JAMA* 2001; 286: 2947-2655.

Kwasucki J, Stepien A, Maksymiuk G, Olbrych-Karpinska B. Evaluation of analgesic action of fluvoxamine compared with efficacy of imipramine and tramadol for treatment of sciatica—open trial. *Wiad Lek* 2002; 55:42-50.

Lawrenson RA, Tyrer F, Newson RB, Farmer RD. The treatment of depression in UK general practice: Selective serotonin reuptake inhibitors and tricyclic antidepressants compared. *J Affect Disord* 2000; 59:149-157.

Lipman AG. Analgesic drugs for neuropathic and sympathetically maintained pain. *Clin Geriatr Med* 1996; 12:501-515.

Magni G. On the relationship between chronic pain and depression when there is no organic lesion. *Pain* 1987; 31:1-21.

Magni G. The use of antidepressants in the treatment of chronic pain: A review of the current evidence. *Drugs* 1992; 42:730-748.

Martin-Araguz A, Bustamante-Martinez C, de Pedro-Pijoan JM. Treatment of chronic tension-type headache with mirtazapine and amitriptyline. *Rev Neurol* 2003; 37:101-105.

Mattia C, Paoletti F, Coluzzi F, Boanelli A. New antidepressants in the treatment of neuropathic pain: A review. Rome: Institute of Anaesthesiology and Intensive Care Medicine, University of Studies La Sapienza, 2002.

Megarbane B, Gueye P, Baud F. Interactions between benzodiazepines and opioids. *Ann Med Interne* 2003; 154(Spec No 2):S64-72. French.

Michelson D. SSRI-associated sexual dysfunction: New data from prospective trials. In: *Treatment issues with SSRIs*. Program and abstracts from the 153rd Annual American Psychiatric Association Meeting, May 13-18, 2000; Chicago, IL. Session 1.

Michelson D, Dording CM, Mischoulon D. *Treatment issues with SSRIs*. Program and abstracts from the 153rd Annual American Psychiatric Association Meeting, May 13-18, 2000; Chicago, IL. Session 1.

Miller LJ, Kubes KL. Serotonergic agents in the treatment of fibromyalgia syndrome. *Ann Pharmacother* 2002; 36:707-712.

Mitsikostas DD, Gatzonis S, Thomas A, et al. Buspirone vs. amitriptyline in the treatment of chronic tension-type headache. *Acta Neurol Scand* 1997; 96: 247-251.

Movig KL, Meijer WE, Heerdink ER, Leufkens HG, Egberts AC. Selective serotonin reuptake inhibitor-induced urinary incontinence. *Pharmacoepidimiol Drug Saf* 2002; 11:271-279.

Mulchahey JJ, Malik MS, Sabai M, Kasckow JW. Serotonin selective reuptake inhibitors in the treatment of geriatric depression and related disorders. *Int J Neuropsychopharmacol* 1999; 2:121-127.

Nath C, Gurtu S, Gupta MB, Gupta GP, Srimal RC, Dhawan BN. Novel effects of MPTP: MAO-B unrelated opioidergic activity in mice. Lucknow, India: Department of Pharmacology, K.G.'s Medical College, 1991.

Nemeroff CB, Schatzberg AF, Goldstein DJ, et al. Duloxetine for the treatment of major depressive disorder. *Psychopharmacol Bull* 2002; 36:106-132.

Neutel CI, Walop W, Patten SB. Can continuing benzodiazepine use be predicted? *Can J Clin Pharmacol* 2003; 10:202-206.

O'Malley PG, Balden E, Tomkins G, Santoro J, Kroenke K, Jackson JL. Treatment of fibromyalgia with antidepressants: A meta-analysis. *J Gen Intern Med* 15: 9: 659-666.

Onghena P, Van Houdenhove B. Antidepressant-induced analgesia in chronic non-malignant pain: A meta-analysis of 39 placebo-controlled studies. *Pain* 1992; 49: 205-209.

Pakulska W, Czarnecka E. Effect of citalopram and buspirone on the antinociceptive action of analgesic drugs. *Acta Pol Pharm* 2001; 58:299-305.

Phillips S, Brent J, Kulig K, Heiligenstein J, Birkett M. Fluoxitine vs. tricyclic antidepressants: A prospective multicenter study of antidepressant drug overdoses. The Antidepressant Study Group. *J Emerg Med* 1997; 15:439-445.

Pick CG, Paul D, Eison MS, et al. Potentiation of opioid analgesia by the antidepressant nefazodone. *Eur J Pharm* 1992; 211:375-381.

Rani PU, Naidu MU, Prasad VB, Rao TR, Shobha JC. An evaluation of antidepressants in rheumatic pain conditions. *Anesth Analg* 1996; 83: 371-375.

Ripple MG, Pestaner JP, Levine BS, Smialek JE. Lethal combination of tramadol and multiple drugs affecting serotonin. *Am J Forensic Med Pathol* 2000; 21:370-374.

Robinson RG, Schultz SK, Castillo C, et al. Nortriptyline versus fluoxetine in the treatment of depression and in short-term recovery after stroke: A placebo-controlled, double-blind study. *Am J Psychiatry* 2000; 157:351-359.

Roose S, Sackeim HA, Krishnan, et al. Treatment of depression in patients over 75. Presented at: 15th Annual Meeting of the American Association for Geriatric Psychiatry; May 24-27, 2002; Orlando, FL.

Rozen TD. Olanzapine as an abortive agent for cluster headache. *Headache* 2001; 41:813-816.

Rudorfer MV, Manji HK, Potter WZ. Comparative tolerability profiles of the newer versus older antidepressants. *Drug Saf* 1994; 10:18-46.

Salzman C, Wong E, Wright BC. Drug and ECT treatment of depression in the elderly, 1996-2001: A literature review. *Biol Psychiatry* 2002; 52:265-284.

Sayar K, Aksu G, Ak I, Tosun M. Venlafaxine treatment of fibromyalgia. *Ann Pharmacother* 2003; 37:1561-1565.

Schreiber S, Backer MM, Weizman R, Pick CG. Augmentation of opioid induced antinociception by the atypical antipsychotic drug risperidone in mice. *Neurosci Lett* 1997; 228:25-28.

Schreiber S, Backer MM, Yanai J, Pick CG. The antinociceptive effect of fluvoxamine. *Eur Neuropsychopharmacol* 1996; 6:281-284.

Semenchuk MR, Sherman S, Davis B. Double-blind, randomized trial of bupropion SR for the treatment of neuropathic pain. *Neurology* 2001; 57:1583-1588.

Shiekh J, Yesavage J. Geriatric Depression Scale: Recent findings and development of a short version. In Brink T, ed. *Clinical gerontology: A guide to assessment and intervention* (pp. 427-445). New York: Haworth Press, 1996.

Shimizu T, Shibata M, Wakisaka S, Inoue T, Mashimo T, Yoshiya I. Intrathecal lithium reduces neuropathic pain responses in a rat model of peripheral neuropathy. *Pain* 2000; 85:59-64.

Shimodozono M, Kawahira K, Kamishita T, Ogata A, Tohgo S, Tanaka N. Reduction of central poststroke pain with the selective serotonin reuptake inhibitor fluvoxamine. *Int J Neurosci* 2002; 112:1173-1181.

Silberstein SD, Peres MF, Hopkins MM, Shechter AL, Young WB, Rozen TD. Olanzapine in the treatment of refractory migraine and chronic daily headache. *Headache* 2002; 42:515-518.

Stewart, DE. Hepatic adverse reactions associated with nefazodone. *Can J Clin Psychiatry* 2002; 47:375-377.

Stiefel F, Stagno D. Management of insomnia in patients with chronic pain conditions. *CNS Drugs* 2004; 18:285-296.

Teixeira NA, Pereira DG, Hermini AH. Lithium treatment prolongs shock-induced hypoalgesia. *Braz J Med Biol Res* 1995:791-799.

Watson CPN, Vernich L, Chipman M, et al. Nortriptyline versus amitriptyline in postherpetic neuralgia. *Neurology* 1998; 51:1166-1171.

Wilson KG, Mikail SF, D'Eton JL, et al. Alternative diagnostic criteria for major depressive disorder in patients with chronic pain. *Pain* 2001; 91:227-234.

Wood MR, Kim JJ, Han W, et al. Benzodiazepines as potent and selective bradykinin B1 antagonists. *J Med Chem* 2003; 46:1803-1806.

Wyant GM, Ashenhurst EM. Chronic pain syndromes and their treatment. I. Cluster headache. *Anaesth Soc J* 1979; 26:38-41.

Chapter 19

Treatment of Common Conditions

Gary McCleane

Although a wide variety of treatments are available for a range of conditions associated with pain, at some point a choice of which options provide the greatest chance of producing analgesia while having the least chance of inducing side effects must be made. This chapter includes treatment options for a variety of pain-producing disorders. The outlined options are not intended to be exhaustive and complete, but rather a basis on which treatment can be initiated and represent a personal opinion of treatment of these conditions.

Of equal importance with selecting which therapeutic agent to try first is how to decide when a treatment is unsuccessful. When that decision is made, the treatment should be withdrawn, remembering that with some agents a withdrawal reaction may be experienced.

CENTRAL POSTSTROKE PAIN

Topical

Medication and dosage	Duration	Possible side effects	Notes
Lidocaine 5 percent patch	1 day		Applied over areas of hypersensitivity

Oral

Medication and dosage	Duration	Possible side effects	Notes
Lamotrigine 300 mg/day	When full dose achieved	Skin rash Insomnia Lymphadenopathy	Dose gradually increased to reduce risk of skin rash

Clinical Management of the Elderly Patient in Pain
© 2006 by The Haworth Press, Inc. All rights reserved.
doi:10.1300/5356_19

Amitriptyline 10-150 mg/day	Dose titrated to effect	Somnolence Urinary retention Visual disturbance
Gabapentin 900-2400 mg/day	Titrated to effect	Somnolence Nausea

CERVICAL RADICULOPATHY

Topical

Medication and dosage	Duration	Possible side effects	Notes
Doxepin 5 percent cream	4 weeks	Side effects only apparent if large quantities used	
Lidocaine 5 percent patch	1 day		Over areas of hypersensitive skin

Oral

Medication and dosage	Duration	Possible side effects	Notes
Amitriptyline	Titrated to effect	Dry mouth Somnolence Urinary retention	
Oxcarbazepine 150-900 mg/day	Several days	Nausea Hyponatremia Somnolence	Side effects may be less than with carbamazepine
Lamotrigine 300 mg/day	When full dose level reached	Skin rash Insomnia Nausea Glandular swelling	Dose needs to be gradually increased to reduce risk of skin rash
Gabapentin 900-2400 mg/day	Titrated to effect	Nausea Somnolence	
Tramadol 50-200 mg/day	1 day	Nausea Somnolence	
Strong opioid	Titrated to effect	Nausea Constipation Tolerance	Controlled-release preparations preferable to immediate-release preparations

Parenteral

Medication and dosage	Duration	Possible side effects	Notes
Fosphenytoin 500 PE IM 1000 PE over 24 hours	Hours	Nausea Hyperacusis Light-headedness	
Lidocaine 500-1200 mg over 24 hours	1-3 days	Phlebitis at infusion site Light-headedness Nausea	Duration of effect can be much longer than infusion period

FIBROMYALGIA

Topical

Medication and dosage	Duration	Possible side effects	Notes
Glyceryl trinitrate patch 5 mg/24 hours	1 day	Headache Skin irritation	Can be used on several sites Suitable for localized discomfort
Lidocaine 5 percent patch	1 day		Suitable for localized discomfort

Oral

Medication and dosage	Duration	Possible side effects	Notes
Tramadol 50-200 mg/day	1 day	Constipation Nausea Tolerance	
Acetaminophen 3 g/day	1 day		
Ondansetron 4 mg TID Granisetron 2 mg QD	1 day	Constipation Headache	Can also help irritable bowel syndrome
Amitriptyline	Titrated to effect	Somnolence Dry mouth Urinary retention Visual disturbance	

Parenteral

Medication and dosage	Duration	Possible side effects	Notes
Lidocaine 500-1200 mg IV	1-3 days	Light-headedness Phlebitis at infusion site	Duration of relief can be much longer than infusion period

FRACTURE PAIN

Topical

Medication and dosage	Duration	Possible side effects	Notes
Lidocaine 5 percent patch	1 day		Applied over bone fracture
Glyceryl trinitrate patch 5 mg/24 hours	1 day	Headache	
Fentanyl patch	Titrated to effect	Constipation Nausea Tolerance	

Oral

Medication and dosage	Duration	Possible side effects	Notes
Acetaminophen 1 g QID	1 day		
NSAID	1 day	Gastric, renal, and hematological upset	
Tramadol 50-200 mg/day	1 day		
Strong opioid	Titrated to effect	Constipation Nausea Tolerance	

METASTATIC BONE PAIN

Topical

Medication and dosage	Duration	Possible side effects	Notes
Lidocaine 5 percent patch	1 day		Applied over bone deposit
Glyceryl trinitrate patch 5 mg/ 24 hours	1 day	Headache	
Fentanyl patch	Titrated to effect	Constipation Nausea Tolerance	

Oral

Medication and dosage	Duration	Possible side effects	Notes
Acetaminophen 1 g QID	1 day		
NSAID	1 day	Gastric, renal, and hematological upset	
Tramadol 50-200 mg/day	1 day		
Strong opioid	Titrated to effect	Constipation Nausea Tolerance	

MUSCLE SPASM

Oral

Medication and dosage	Duration	Possible side effects	Notes
Baclofen 10-60 mg/day	1 day		In presence of enthetic pain add NSAID
Dantrolene 25 mg/day increasing by 25 mg/week to maximum of 200 mg/day	Titrated to effect	Check liver function tests intermittently	

Others

Medication and dosage	Duration	Possible side effects	Notes
Botulinum toxin injection	1 week		Suitable when one muscle group is in spasm Can give prolonged relief of spasm

OSTEOARTHRITIS—MONOARTICULAR

Topical

Medication and dosage	Duration	Possible side effects	Notes
Capsaicin cream 0.025 percent	1 month	Burning discomfort at application site Accidental application at distant sites Sneezing	Application discomfort reduced by addition of glyceryl trinitrate
Nonsteroidal anti-inflammatory cream/ointment	1 day		
Glyceryl trinitrate patch 5 mg/ 24 hours	1 day	Headache Skin irritation	Nitrate ointment can also be used
Lidocaine 5 percent patch	1 day		
Fentanyl patch	Titrated to effect	Constipation Nausea Tolerance	May have increased effect if placed over inflamed joint

Oral

Medication and dosage	Duration	Possible side effects	Notes
NSAID	1 day	Dyspepsia, gastric ulceration Fluid retention, renal impairment Platelet dysfunction Interference with platelet effect of aspirin	

Glucosamine 1500 mg/day	3 weeks	May also increase depth of joint carti-lage with prolonged use
Acetaminophen 1 g/6 hours	1 day	Beware "hidden" acetaminophen in compound prepara-tions

Others

Medication and dosage	Duration	Possible side effects	Notes
Intra-articular steroid injection	2 days		
Intra-articular hyaluronic acid injection	3 weeks		May have chondroprotective effect
Nerve block with steroid	2 days		More appropriate when only one nerve innervates joint

OSTEOARTHRITIS—POLYARTICULAR

Topical

Medication and dosage	Duration	Possible side effects	Notes
Glyceryl trinitrate patch	1 day	Headache Skin irritation	Low-dose patches may allow applica-tion to more than one joint
Lignocaine 5 percent patch	1 day		Several patches may be used simul-taneously
Fentanyl patch	1 day	Constipation Nausea Tolerance	

Oral

Medication and dosage	Duration	Possible side effects	Notes
Nonsteroidal anti-inflammatory	1 day	Dyspepsia, gastric ulceration	
		Fluid retention, renal impairment	
		Platelet dysfunction	
		Interference with platelet effect of aspirin	
Glucosamine 1500 mg/day	3 weeks		May also increase depth of joint cartilage with prolonged use
Acetaminophen 1 g/6 hours	1 day		Beware "hidden" acetaminophen in compound preparations

Parenteral

Medication and dosage	Duration	Possible side effects	Notes
Lidocaine (IV) 500-1200 mg over 1 day	1-3 days	Phlebitis at infusion site	Duration of effect may be much longer than infusion period
		Light-headedness	

PAINFUL DIABETIC NEUROPATHY

Topical

Medication and dosage	Duration	Possible side effects	Notes
Glyceryl trinitrate patch	1 day	Headache	Useful in the presence of ischemic neuritis
		Skin irritation	
Capsaicin cream 0.025 percent	1 month	Burning discomfort at application site	Application discomfort reduced by addition of glyceryl trinitrate
		Accidental application at distant sites	
		Sneezing	

Doxepin 5 percent cream	1 month	Somnolence Dry mouth	Side effects usually apparent only when used in too large quantities
Lignocaine 5 percent patch	1 day		Several patches may be used simultaneously
Fentanyl patch	1 day	Constipation Nausea Tolerance	

Oral

Medication and dosage	Duration	Possible side effects	Notes
Amitriptyline	Titrated to effect	Dry mouth Somnolence Urinary retention	
Oxcarbazepine 150-900 mg/day	Several days	Nausea Hyponatremia Somnolence	Side effects may be less than with carbamazepine
Lamotrigine 300 mg/day	When full dose level reached	Skin rash Insomnia Nausea Glandular swelling	Dose needs to be gradually increased to reduce risk of skin rash
Gabapentin 900-2400 mg/day	Titrated to effect	Nausea Somnolence	
Tramadol 50-200 mg/day	1 day	Nausea Somnolence	
Strong opioid	Titrated to effect	Nausea Constipation Tolerance	Controlled-release preparations preferable to immediate-release preparations

Parenteral

Medication and dosage	Duration	Possible side effects	Notes
Fosphenytoin 500 PE IM, 1000 PE over 24 hours	Hours	Nausea Hyperacusis Light-headedness	

Lidocaine 500-1200 mg over 24 hours	1-3 days	Phlebitis at infusion site Light-headedness Nausea	Duration of effect can be much longer than infusion period

PERIPHERAL VASCULAR DISEASE

Topical

Medication and dosage	Duration	Possible side effects	Notes
Glyceryl trinitrate patch	1 day	Headache Skin irritation	
Capsaicin cream 0.025 percent	1 month	Burning discomfort at application site, accidental application at distant sites, sneezing	Application discomfort reduced by addition of glyceryl trinitrate
Doxepin 5 percent cream	1 month	Somnolence Dry mouth	Side effects usually apparent only when used in too large quantities
Lignocaine 5 percent patch	1 day		Several patches may be used simultaneously, useful for hypersensitivity
Fentanyl patch	1 day	Constipation Nausea Tolerance	

Oral

Medication and dosage	Duration	Possible side effects	Notes
Amitriptyline	Titrated to effect	Dry mouth Somnolence Urinary retention	Particularly where there is ischemic neuritis
Oxcarbazepine 150-900 mg/day	Several days	Nausea Hyponatremia Somnolence	Side effects may be less than with carbamazepine, useful when there is ischemic neuritis

Lamotrigine 300 mg/day	When full dose level reached	Skin rash Insomnia Nausea Glandular swelling	Dose needs to be gradually increased to reduce risk of skin rash, useful where there is ischemic neuritis
Gabapentin 900-2400 mg/day	Titrated to effect	Nausea Somnolence	Useful where there is ischemic neuritis
Tramadol 50-200 mg/day	1 day	Nausea Somnolence	
Strong opioid	Titrated to effect	Nausea Constipation	Controlled-release preparations preferable

Parenteral

Medication and dosage	Duration	Possible side effects	Notes
Lidocaine 500-1200 mg IV over 24 hours	1-3 days	Light-headedness Phlebitis at infusion site	
Phentolamine 50-100 mg over 24 hours dissolved in 1000 ml 5 percent dextrose	1-3 days	Phlebitis at infusion site Hypotension Palpitations	Can increase tissue perfusion Prolonged relief in some patients Intercurrent treatment with colloid can prevent hypotension

POSTHERPETIC NEURALGIA

Topical

Medication and dosage	Duration	Possible side effects	Notes
Capsaicin cream 0.025 percent	1 month	Burning discomfort at application site Accidental application at distant sites Sneezing	Application discomfort reduced by addition of glyceryl trinitrate
Doxepin 5 percent cream	1 month	Somnolence Dry mouth	Side effects usually apparent only when used in too large quantities

Lignocaine 5 percent patch	1 day		Several patches may be used simultaneously
Fentanyl patch	1 day	Constipation Nausea Tolerance	

Oral

Medication and dosage	Duration	Possible side effects	Notes
Amitriptyline	Titrated to effect	Dry mouth Somnolence Urinary retention	
Oxcarbazepine 150-900 mg/day	Several days	Nausea Hyponatremia Somnolence	Side effects may be less than with carbamazepine
Lamotrigine 300 mg/day	When full dose level reached	Skin rash Insomnia Nausea Glandular swelling	Dose needs to be gradually increased to reduce risk of skin rash
Gabapentin 900-2400 mg/day	Titrated to effect	Nausea Somnolence	
Tramadol 50-200 mg/day	1 day	Nausea Somnolence	
Strong opioid	Titrated to effect	Nausea Constipation Tolerance	Controlled-release preparations preferable to immediate-release preparations

Parenteral

Medication and dosage	Duration	Possible side effects	Notes
Fosphenytoin 500 PE IM, 1000 PE over 24 hours	Hours	Nausea Hyperacusis Light-headedness	
Lidocaine 500-1200 mg over 24 hours	1-3 days	Phlebitis at infusion site Light-headedness Nausea	Duration of effect can be much longer than infusion period

SCIATICA

Oral

Medication and dosage	Duration	Possible side effects	Notes
Sodium valproate 400-1000 mg/day	1 week		
Oxcarbazepine 150-900 mg/day	Several days	Nausea Hyponatremia Somnolence	Side effects may be less than with carbamazepine
Lamotrigine 300 mg/day	When full dose level reached	Skin rash Insomnia Nausea Glandular swelling	Dose needs to be gradually increased to reduce risk of skin rash
Gabapentin 900-2400 mg/day	Titrated to effect	Nausea Somnolence	

Parenteral

Medication and dosage	Duration	Possible side effects	Notes
Fosphenytoin 500 PE IM, 1000 PE over 24 hours	Hours	Nausea Hyperacusis Light-headedness	For acute use during flare-up
Lidocaine 500-1200 mg over 24 hours	1-3 days	Phlebitis at infusion site Light-headedness Nausea	Duration of effect can be much longer than infusion period

SKIN ULCERS

Topical

Medication and dosage	Duration	Possible side effects	Notes
Glyceryl trinitrate patch	1 day	Headache Skin irritation	Low-dose patches may allow application to more than one ulcer

Lignocaine 5 percent patch	1 day		Several patches may be used simultaneously
Fentanyl patch	1 day	Constipation Nausea Tolerance	Possible increased effect close to site of ulcer
Morphine solution			Analgesic effect without systemic side effects
Corticosteroid ointment			Vasculitic ulcers

TENDONITIS

Topical

Medication and dosage	Duration	Possible side effects	Notes
Glyceryl trinitrate patch	1 day	Headache Skin irritation	
Lignocaine 5 percent patch	1 day		Several patches may be used simultaneously
Capsaicin cream 0.025 percent	1 month	Burning discomfort at application site Accidental application at distant sites Sneezing	Application discomfort reduced by addition of glyceryl trinitrate
Nonsteroidal anti-inflammatory cream/ointment	1 day		

Others

Medication and dosage	Duration	Possible side effects	Notes
Corticosteroid	1-3 days	May initially exacerbate pain before reducing it	Injection into tendon sheath
Hyaluronidase 1500 IU	1-3 days		Injection into tendon sheath

TRIGEMINAL NEURALGIA

Oral

Medication and dosage	Duration	Possible side effects	Notes
Baclofen 10 mg TDS	1 day		Can be increased to 20 mg TDS
Oxcarbazepine 150-900 mg/day	Several days	Nausea Hyponatremia Somnolence	Side effects may be less than with carbamazepine
Lamotrigine 300 mg/day	When full dose level reached	Skin rash Insomnia Nausea Glandular swelling	Dose needs to be gradually increased to reduce risk of skin rash
Gabapentin 900-2400 mg/day	Titrated to effect	Nausea Somnolence	

Parenteral

Medication and dosage	Duration	Possible side effects	Notes
Fosphenytoin 500 PE IM, 1000 PE over 24 hours	Hours	Nausea Hyperacusis Light-headedness	For acute use during flare-ups
Lidocaine 500-1200 mg over 24 hours	1-3 days	Phlebitis at infusion site Light-headedness Nausea	Duration of effect can be much longer than infusion

VISCERAL PAIN

Oral

Medication and dosage	Duration	Possible side effects	Notes
Ondansetron 4 mg TID	1 day	Constipation Headache	Antiemetic and analgesic
Hyoscine 20 mg BID-QID	1 day		Where spasm features
Corticosteroids	2 days		Decreasing dose Where obstruction precipitates pain

Parenteral

Medication and dosage	Duration	Possible side effects	Notes
Lidocaine IV infusion 500-1200 mg over 24 hours	1-3 days	Light-headedness	Duration of relief can be considerably longer than infusion period

Appendix

Drug Interactions

Drug	Combined with	Interaction
Abacavir	Analgesics	Plasma concentrations of methadone possibly decreased by abacavir
ACE inhibitors and angiotensin II antagonists	Analgesics	Antagonism of hypotensive effect and increased risk of renal impairment with NSAIDs, hyperkalemia with ketorolac and possibly other NSAIDs
	Antidepressants	Possible enhanced hypotensive effect
	Muscle relaxants	Baclofen and tizanidine enhance hypotensive effect
Adrenergic neuron blockers	Analgesics	NSAIDs antagonize hypotensive effect
	Antidepressants	Tricyclics antagonize hypotensive effect
Alcohol	Analgesics	Sedative and hypotensive effect of opioid analgesics enhanced
	Antidepressants	Sedative effect of tricyclics enhanced
	Antiepileptics	CNS side effects of carbamazepine possibly enhanced.
	Muscle relaxants	Baclofen, methocarbamol, and tizanidine enhance sedative effect
Alpha-blockers	Analgesics	NSAIDs enhance hypotensive effect
Aminoglycosides	Analgesics	Indomethacin possibly increases plasma concentration of gentamycin
	Botulinum toxin	Neuromuscular block enhanced
Amiodarone	Antidepressants	Increased risk of ventricular arrhythmia with tricyclics (avoid concomitant use)
	Antidepressants	Metabolism of phenytoin inhibited
Amprenavir	Antiepileptics	Amprenavir possibly increases plasma concentration of carbamazepine

Clinical Management of the Elderly Patient in Pain
© 2006 by The Haworth Press, Inc. All rights reserved.
doi:10.1300/5356_20

Drug	Combined with	Interaction
Antacids	Analgesics	Excretion of aspirin increased in alkaline urine
	Antiepileptics	Reduced absorption of gabapentin and phenytoin
Antidepressants, tricyclic	Alcohol	Enhanced sedative effect
	Altretamine	Risk of severe postural hypotension
	Anesthetics	Risk of arrhythmias and hypotension increased
	Analgesics	Possible increased side effects with nefopam; risk of CNS toxicity increased with tramadol; possible increased sedation with opioid analgesics
	Antiarrhythmics	Increased risk of ventricular arrhythmias with drugs that prolong QTc interval, including amiodarone, disopyramide, procainamide, propafenone, and quinidine
	Antibacterials	Plasma concentrations of some tricyclics reduced by rifampicin
	Antiepileptics	Antagonism (convulsive threshold lowered); plasma concentrations of some tricyclics reduced
	Antihistamines	Increased antimuscarinic and sedative effects; increased risk of ventricular arrhythmias with terfenadine
	Antihypertensives	In general, hypotensive effect enhanced, but antagonism of effect of adrenergic neuron blockers and clonidine (and increased risk of hypertension on clonidine withdrawal)
	Antimuscarinics	Increased antimuscarinic side effects
	Antipsychotics	Increased risk of ventricular arrhythmia; increased plasma concentrations of tricyclic antidepressants and increased antimuscarinic side effects with phenothiazines and possibly clozapine
	Antivirals	Plasma concentration possibly increased by ritonavir
	Anxiolytics/ hypnotics	Enhanced sedative effects
	Beta-blockers	Risk of ventricular arrhythmias associated with sotalol increased

Drug	Combined with	Interaction
Antidepressents, trycyclic *(cont.)*	Calcium blockers	Diltiazem and verapamil increase plasma concentration of imipramine and possibly other tricyclics
	Disulfiram	Inhibition of metabolism of tricyclics
	Diuretics	Increased risk of postural hypotension
	Dopaminergics	Manufacturer advises avoid concomitant use with entacapone; CNS toxicity reported with selegiline
	Muscle relaxants	Enhanced muscle relaxant effect of baclofen
	Nitrates	Reduced effect of sublingual nitrates (owing to dry mouth)
	Sibutramine	Increased risk of CNS toxicity
	Sympathomimetics	Hypertension and arrhythmias with epinephrine; hypertension with norepinephrine; methylphenidate may inhibit metabolism of tricyclics
	Ulcer-healing drugs	Plasma concentrations of amitriptyline, doxepin, imipramine, nortriptyline, and probably other tricyclics increased by cimetidine (inhibition of metabolism)
Antidiabetics	Analgesics	Azapropazone, phenylbutazone, and possibly other NSAIDs enhance effect of sulfonylureas
	Antiepileptics	Plasma phenytoin concentration transiently increased by tolbutamide
Antifungals Imidazole Triazole	Analgesics	Metabolism of alfentanil inhibited by ketoconazole; plasma concentration of celecoxib increased by fluconazole
	Antiepileptics	Effect of phenytoin enhanced by fluconazole and miconazole; plasma concentrations of itraconazole and ketoconazole reduced by phenytoin
Antipsychotics	Analgesics	Enhanced sedative and hypotensive effect with opioid analgesics; severe drowsiness possible if indomethacin given with haloperidol
	Antidepressants	Increased risk of arrhythmias with tricyclics; increased plasma concentration and antimuscarinic side effects noted on administration of tricyclics and phenothiazines
	Antiepileptics	Antagonism (convulsive threshold reduced); carbamazepine accelerates metabolism of clozapine, haloperidol, olanzapine, and risperdal; phenytoin accelerates metabolism of clozapine and quetiapine

Drug	Combined with	Interaction
Anxiolytics	Analgesics	Opioid analgesics enhance sedative effect
Aspirin	Analgesics	Avoid concomitant use of other NSAIDs
Beta-blockers	Analgesics	NSAIDs antagonize hypotensive effect; morphine possibly increases plasma concentration of esmolol
	Antiarrhythmics	Increased risk of lidocaine toxicity with propranolol
	Muscle relaxants	Possible enhanced hypotensive effect and bradycardia with tizanidine
Bisphosphonates	Analgesics	Bioavailability of tiludronic acid increased by indomethacin
Botulinum toxin	Antibacterials	Effect enhanced by aminoglycosides
Bupropion	Antiepileptics	Carbamazepine and phenytoin reduce plasma concentration of bupropion; sodium valproate inhibits metabolism of bupropion
Calcium blockers	Antiepileptics	Effect of carbamazepine enhanced by diltiazem and verapamil; diltiazem and nifedipine increase plasma concentration of phenytoin; effect of felodipine and isradipine and probably nicardipine, nifedipine, and other dihydropyridines reduced by carbamazepine and phenytoin; effect of diltiazem and verapamil reduced by phenytoin
Carbamazepine	Alcohol	CNS side effects of carbamazepine possibly enhanced
	Analgesics	Dextropropoxyphene enhances effect of carbamazepine; effect of methadone and tramadol decreased by carbamazepine
	Antibacterials	Metabolism of doxycycline accelerated; plasma carbamazepine concentration increased by clarithromycin, erythromycin, and isoniazid (also isoniazid hepatotoxicity possibly increased); plasma carbamazepine concentration reduced by rifabutin
	Anticoagulants	Metabolism of acenocoumarol and warfarin accelerated
	Antidepressants	Antagonism of anticonvulsant effect; plasma concentration of carbamazepine increased by fluoxetine and fluvoxamine; metabolism of mianserin and tricyclics accelerated; plasma concentration increased by nefazodone

Drug	Combined with	Interaction
Carbamazepine (cont.)	Antiepileptics	Interaction includes enhanced effect, increased sedation, and reduction in plasma concentrations
	Antimalarials	Mefloquine antagonizes anticonvulsant effect
	Antipsychotics	Antagonism of anticonvulsant effect; metabolism of clozapine, haloperidol, olanzapine, and respiradone accelerated
	Antivirals	Plasma concentration of indinavir, lopinavir, nelfinavir, and saqquinavir possibly reduced; plasma concentration possibly increased by amprenavir and ritonavir
	Bupropion	Plasma concentration of bupropion reduced
	Calcium blockers	Diltiazem and verapamil enhance effect of carbamazepine; effect of felodipine, isradipine, and probably nicardapine, nifedipine, and other dihydropyridines reduced
	Cardiac glycosides	Metabolism of digoxin increased
	Cyclosporine	Metabolism accelerated
	Corticosteroids	Metabolism accelerated
	Diuretics	Increased risk of hyponatremia; acetazolamide increases plasma carbamazepine concentration
	Lithium	Neurotoxicity may occur without increased plasma concentration
	Retinoids	Plasma concentration possibly reduced by isotretinoin
	Theophylline	Metabolism of theophylline accelerated
	Thyroid hormones	Metabolism of levothyroxine and liothyronine accelerated
	Ulcer drugs	Metabolism inhibited by cimetidine
	Vitamins	Carbamazepine possibly increases vitamin D requirements
Cardiac glycosides	Analgesics	NSAIDs may exacerbate heart failure, reduce glomerular filtration rate, and increase plasma cardiac glycoside concentrations
	Antiepileptics	Metabolism of digoxin accelerated
	Muscle relaxants	Possible bradycardia with tizanidine
Chloramphenicol	Antiepileptics	Increased plasma concentration of phenytoin

Drug	Combined with	Interaction
Cholestyramine	Analgesics	Absorption of paracetamol reduced by cholestyramine
Clonidine	Antidepressants	Tricyclics antagonize hypotensive effect and also increase risk of rebound hypertension on clonidine withdrawal
Clopidogrel	Analgesics	Increased risk of bleeding with NSAIDs
Cotrimoxazole sulfonamides	Antiepileptics	Antifolate effect and plasma concentration of phenytoin increased by co-trimoxazole and possibly other sulfonamides
Cycloserine	Antiepileptics	Increased plasma concentration of phenytoin
Cyclosporine	Analgesics	Increased risk of nephrotoxicity with NSAIDs; cyclosporine increases plasma concentration of diclofenac
	Antiepileptics	Carbamazepine and phenytoin accelerate metabolism
Danazol	Antiepileptics	Inhibits metabolism of carbamazepine
Desmopressin	Analgesics	Effect of desmospressin potentiated by indomethacin
Disopyramide	Antidepressants	Increased risk of ventricular arrhythmias with tricyclics
	Antiepileptics	Plasma concentration of disopyramide reduced by phenytoin
Disulfiram	Antiepileptics	Inhibition of metabolism of phenytoin
Diuretics	Analgesics	Diuretics increase risk of nephrotoxicity of NSAIDs; NSAIDs antagonize diuretic effect; occasional reports of decreased renal function when indomethacin given with triamterene; diuretic effect of spironolactone antagonized by aspirin; aspirin reduces excretion of acetazolamide
	Antiarrhythmics	Action of lidocaine and mexiletine antagonized by hypokalemia
	Antidepressants	Increased risk of postural hypotension with tricyclics
	Antiepileptics	Increased risk of hyponatremia with carbamazepine; acetazolamide increases plasma concentration of carbamazepine; carbonic anhydrase inhibitors possibly increase risk of osteomalacia with antiepileptics such as phenytoin

Drug	Combined with	Interaction
Diuretics *(cont.)*	Muscle relaxants	Enhanced hypotensive effect with baclofen and tizanidine
Domperidone	Analgesics	Opioid analgesics antagonize effect on gastrointestinal activity; absorption of paracetamol accelerated
Erythromycin macrolides	Analgesics	Plasma concentration of alfentanil increased by erythromycin
	Antiepileptics	Clarithromycin and erythromycin inhibit metabolism of carbamazepine; erythromycin possibly inhibits metabolism of valproate; clarithromycin inhibits metabolism of phenytoin
Gabapentin	Antacids	Reduced gabapentin absorption
	Antidepressants	Antagonism of anticonvulsant effect
	Antimalarials	Mefloquine antagonizes anticonvulsant effect
Heparin	Analgesics	Aspirin enhances anticoagulant effect; increased risk of hemorrhage with intravenous diclofenac and ketorolac; possibly increased risk of bleeding with NSAIDs
H2-anaagonists	Analgesics	Cimetidine inhibits metabolism of opioid analgesics, notably meperidine
	Antiarrhythmics	Cimetidine increases plasma concentrations of flecainide and lidocaine
	Antiepileptics	Cimetidine inhibits metabolism of carbamazepine, phenytoin, and valproate
Hydralazine	Analgesics	NSAIDs antagonize hypotensive effect
	Muscle relaxants	Baclofen and tizanidine enhance hypotensive effect
Hypnotics	Antiepileptics	Metabolism of clonazepam accelerated; plasma phenytoin concentrations increased or decreased by diazepam and possibly other benzodiazepines
Imatinib	Analgesics	Caution with concomitant use of paracetamol
	Antiepileptics	Plasma concentration of imatinib reduced by phenytoin
Indinavir	Antiepileptics	Plasma indinavir concentration possibly reduced by carbamazepine and phenytoin

Drug	Combined with	Interaction
Isoniazid	Antiepileptics	Metabolism of carbamazepine and phenytoin inhibited; with carbamazepine isoniazid hepatotoxicity possibly increased
Lamotrigine	Antidepressants	Antagonism of anticonvulsant effects
	Other antiepileptics	Interactions include enhanced effect, increased sedation, and reduction in plasma concentrations
Leukotriene antagonists	Analgesics	Aspirin increases plasma concentration of zafirlukast
Levodopa	Muscle relaxants	Agitation, confusion, and hallucinations possible with baclofen
Lidocaine	Antibacterials	Increased risk of ventricular arrhythmias with quinupristin and dalfopristin
	Beta-blockers	Increased risk of myocardial depression; increased risk of lidocaine toxicity with propranolol
	Diuretics	Effect of lidocaine antagonized by hypokalemia with acetazolamide, loop diuretics, and thiazides
	Ulcer drugs	Cimetidine inhibits metabolism of lidocaine
Lithium	Analgesics	Excretion of lithium reduced by azapropazone, diclofenac, ibuprofen, indomethacin, ketorolac, mefanamic acid, naproxen, phenylbutazone, piroxicam, rofecoxib, and probably other NSAIDs
	Antiepileptics	Neurotoxicity may occur with carbamazepine and phenytoin without increased plasma lithium concentration
	Muscle relaxants	Muscle relaxant effect increased; baclofen possibly aggravates hyperkinesis
Lopinavir	Antiepileptics	Carbamazepine and phenytoin possibly reduce plasma lopinavir concentration
MAOIs	Analgesics	CNS excitation or depression with pethidine and possibly other opioid analgesics
	Antiepileptics	Antagonism of anticonvulsant effect
Mefloquine	Antiepileptics	Antagonism of anticonvulsant effect

Drug	Combined with	Interaction
Methotrexate	Analgesics	Excretion reduced by aspirin, azapropazone, diclofenac, ibuprofen, indomethacin, ketoprofen, meloxicam, naproxen, phenylbutazone, and probably other NSAIDs
	Antiepileptics	Phenytoin increases antifolate effect
Methyldopa	Analgesics	NSAIDs antagonize hypotensive effect
	Muscle relaxants	Enhanced hypotensive effect with baclofen and tizanidine
Metoclopramide	Analgesics	Increased absorption of aspirin and paracetamol; opioid analgesics antagonize effect on gastrointestinal activity
Mexiletine	Analgesics	Opioid analgesics delay absorption
	Antiarrhythmics	Increased myocardial depression with any combination of antiarrhythmics
	Antibacterials	Rifampicin accelerates metabolism
	Antiepileptics	Phenytoin accelerates metabolism
	Antihistamines	Increased risk of ventricular arrhythmias with mizolastine and terfenadine
	Antivirals	Possibly increased risk of arrhythmias with ritonavir
	Diuretics	Action of mexiletine antagonized by hypokalemia due to acetazolamide, loop diuretics, and thiazides
	Theophyllines	Plasma theophylline concentration increased
Mianserin	Antiepileptics	Antagonism; metabolism accelerated by carbamazepine and phenytoin
Moclobemide	Analgesics	CNS excitation and depression (hyper- and hypotension) with codeine, dextromethorophan, meperidine, and possibly fentanyl, morphine, and other opioid analgesics; effects of ibuprofen and possibly other NSAIDs increased
Muscle relaxants	Analgesics	Ibuprofen and possibly other NSAIDs reduce excretion of baclofen
	Antidepressants	Tricyclics enhance muscle relaxant effect of baclofen

Drug	Combined with	Interaction
Nefazodone	Antiepileptics	Plasma concentration of carbamazepine increased and plasma concentration of nefazodone reduced
Nelfinavir	Antiepileptics	Carbamazepine and phenytoin possibly reduce plasma concentration of nelfinavir
Nevirapine	Analgesics	Plasma concentration of methadone possibly reduced
NSAIDs	ACE inhibitors	Antagonism of hypotensive effect; increased risk of renal impairment and increased risk of hyperkalemia on administration with ketorolac and possibly other NSAIDs
	Anion exchange resins	Cholestyramine reduces absorption of phenylbutazone
	Antacids	Absorption of diflunisal reduced
	Antibacterials	NSAIDs possibly increase risk of convulsions with quinolones; rifampicin reduces plasma concentration of rofecoxib
	Anticoagulants	Anticoagulant effect of acenocoumarol, warfarin (and possibly phenindione) seriously enhanced by azapropazone and phenylbutazone and possibly enhanced by diclofenac, diflunisal, flurbiprofen, ibuprofen, mefanamic acid, meloxicam, piroxicam, sulindac, and other NSAIDs; increased risk of hemorrhage with IV diclofenac and ketorolac and all anticoagulants
	Antidepressants	Moclobemide enhances effect of ibuprofen and possibly other NSAIDs
	Antidiabetics	Effect of sulfonylureas enhanced by azapropazone, phenylbutazone, and possibly other NSAIDs
	Antiepileptics	Effect of phenytoin enhanced by azapropazone, phenylbutazone, and possibly other NSAIDs
	Antifungals	Plasma concentration of celecoxib increased by fluconazole
	Antihypertensives	Antagonism of hypotensive effect
	Antiplatelet drugs	Increased risk of bleeding with clopidogrel and ticlopidine
	Antipsychotics	Severe drowsiness possible if indomethacin given with haloperidol

Drug	Combined with	Interaction
NSAIDS *(cont.)*	Antivirals	Increased risk of hematological toxicity with zidovudine; plasma concentrations of piroxicam increased by ritonavir; plasma concentrations of other NSAIDs possibly increased by ritonavir
	Beta-blockers	Antagonism of hypotensive effect
	Bisphosphonates	Bioavailability of tiludronic acid increased by indomethacin
	Cardiac glycosides	NSAIDs may exacerbate heart failure, reduce GFR, and increase cardiac glycoside concentration
	Corticosteroids	Increased risk of gastrointestinal bleeding and ulceration
	Cyclosporine	Increased risk of nephrotoxicity; cyclosporine increases plasma concentration of diclofenac
	Cytotoxics	Excretion of methotrexate reduced by aspirin, azapropazone, diclofenac, ibuprofen, indomethacin, ketoprofen, meloxicam, naproxen, phenylbutazone, and probably other NSAIDs
	Desmopressin	Effect potentiated by indomethacin
	Diuretics	Risk of nephrotoxicity of NSAIDs increased; NSAIDs antagonize diuretic effect; indomethacin and possibly other NSAIDs increase risk of hyperkalemia with potassium-sparing diuretics
	Lithium	Excretion of lithium reduced by azapropazone, diclofenac, ibuprofen, indomethacin, and possibly other NSAIDs
	Muscle relaxants	Ibuprofen and possibly other NSAIDs reduce excretion of baclofen
	Theophylline	Rofecoxib possibly increases plasma concentration of theophylline
	Thyroid hormones	False low total plasma thyroxine concentration with phenylbutazone
	Ulcer drugs	Plasma concentration of azapropazone possibly increased by cimetidine; plasma concentration of lornoxicam increased by cimetidine; risk of CNS toxicity with phenylbutazone increased by misprostol

Drug	Combined with	Interaction
NSAIDS *(cont.)*	Uricosurics	Probenecid delays excretion of indomethacin, ketoprofen, ketorolac, and naproxen
	Vasodilators	Risk of bleeding associated with ketorolac increased by pentoxifylline; possible increased risk of bleeding with pentoxifylline and other NSAIDs
Opioid analgesics	Alcohol	Enhanced sedative and hypotensive effect
	Antiarrhythmics	Delayed absorption of mexiletine
	Antibacterials	Rifampicin accelerates metabolism of methadone; erythromycin increases plasma concentration of alfentanil
	Anticoagulants	Dextropropoxyphene may enhance effect of acenocoumarol and warfarin
	Antidepressants	CNS excitation or depression if meperidine and possibly other opioid analgesics given to patients receiving MAOIs; tramadol increases risk of CNS toxicity with SSRIs and tricyclics; possibly increased sedation with tricyclics; plasma concentration of methadone increased by fluvoxamine
	Antiepileptics	Dextropropoxyphene enhances effect of carbamazepine; effect of methadone and tramadol decreased by carbamazepine; phenytoin accelerates methadone metabolism
	Antipsychotics	Enhanced sedative and hypotensive effect
	Antivirals	Methadone possibly increases plasma concentration of zidovudine; plasma concentration of dextropropoxyphene and pethidine increased by ritonavir; plasma concentration of other opioid analgesics possibly increased by ritonavir
	Anxiolytics	Enhanced sedative effect
	Beta-blockers	Morphine possibly increases plasma concentration of esmolol
	Dopaminergics	Hyperpyrexia and CNS toxicity reported if meperidine given to patients receiving selegiline
	Metoclopramide	Antagonism of gastrointestinal effects
	Ulcer drugs	Cimetidine inhibits metabolism of opioid analgesics, notably meperidine

Drug	Combined with	Interaction
Oxcarbazepine	Antidepressants	Antagonism of anticonvulsant effect
	Antimalarials	Mefloquine antagonizes anticonvulsant effect; chloroquine and hydroxychlorquine occasionally reduce seizure threshold
Paracetamol	Anion exchange resins	Cholestyramine reduces absorption of paracetamol
	Anticoagulants	Prolonged regular use of paracetamol possibly enhances warfarin
	Metoclopramide	Accelerates absorption of paracetamol
Pentoxifylline	Analgesics	Increased risk of bleeding with ketorolac; possible increase in risk of bleeding with other NSAIDs
Phenindione	Analgesics	Anticoagulant effect enhanced by aspirin and possibly other NSAIDs; increased risk of hemorrhage with IV diclofenac and ketorolac
Phenytoin	Analgesics	Plasma phenytoin concentration increased by aspirin, azapropazone, and possibly other NSAIDs
	Antacids	Reduced phenytoin absorption
	Antiarrhythmics	Amiodarone increases plasma phenytoin concentration; phenytoin reduces plasma concentrations of disopyramide, mexiletine, and quinidine
	Antibacterials	Plasma phenytoin concentration increased by chloramphenicol, clarithromycin, cycloserine, isoniazid, and metronidazole; plasma phenytoin concentration and antifolate effect increased by co-trimoxazole and trimethoprim and possibly by other sulfonamides; plasma phenytoin concentration reduced by rifampicin; plasma concentration of doxycycline reduced by phenytoin; plasma phenytoin concentration possibly altered by ciprofloxacin
	Anticoagulants	Metabolism of acenocoumarol and warfarin accelerated
	Antidepressants	Antagonism of anticonvulsant effect; fluoxetine and fluvoxamine increase plasma phenytoin concentration; phenytoin reduces plasma concentration of mianserin, paroxetine, and tricyclics

Drug	Combined with	Interaction
Phenytoin *(cont.)*	Antidiabetics	Plasma phenytoin concentration transiently increased by tolbutamide
	Antifungals	Plasma phenytoin concentration increased by fluconazole and miconazole; plasma concentration of itraconazole and ketoconazole reduced
	Antimalarials	Mefloquine antagonizes anticonvulsant effect; chloroquine and hydroxychloroquine occasionally reduce convulsive threshold; increased risk of antifolate effect with pyrimethamine
	Antiplatelet drugs	Plasma phenytoin concentration increased by aspirin
	Antipsychotics	Antagonism of anticonvulsant effect; phenytoin accelerates metabolism of clozapine and quetiapine
	Antivirals	Plasma concentration of indinavir, lopinavir, nelfinavir, and saqquinavir possibly reduced; plasma phenytoin concentrations increased or decreased by zidovudine
	Anxiolytics	Diazepam and possibly other benzodiazepines increase or decrease plasma phenytoin concentrations
	Bupropion	Plasma concentration of bupropion decreased
	Calcium blockers	Diltiazem and nifedipine increase plasma concentration of phenytoin; effect of felodipine, isradipine, nisoldipine, and probably nicardapine, nifedipine, and other dihydropyridines, diltiazem, and verapamil reduced
	Cardiac glycosides	Metabolism of digoxin accelerated
	Corticosteroids	Metabolism of corticosteroids accelerated
	Cyclosporine	Metabolism of cyclosporine accelerated
	Cytotoxics	Reduced absorption of phenytoin; increased antifolate effect with methotrexate; plasma concentration of imatinib reduced by phenytoin
	Disulfiram	Plasma phenytoin concentration increased
	Diuretics	Increased risk of osteomalacia with carbonic anhydrase inhibitors

Drug	Combined with	Interaction
Phenytoin *(cont.)*	Folic acid	Plasma phenytoin concentration possibly reduced by folic acid
	Lithium	Neurotoxicity may occur without increased plasma lithium concentration
	Sympathomimetics	Plasma phenytoin concentration increased by methylphenidate
	Theophylline	Metabolism of theophylline accelerated
	Thyroid hormones	Metabolism of levothyroxine and liothyronine accelerated; plasma phenytoin concentration possibly increased by levothyroxine and liothyronine
	Ulcer drugs	Cimetidine inhibits metabolism; sulcralfate reduces absorption; esomeprazole and possibly omeprazole enhance effect of phenytoin
	Uricosurics	Plasma phenytoin concentration increased by sulfinpyrazone
Probenecid	Analgesics	Aspirin antagonizes effect; excretion of indomethacin, ketoprofen, ketorolac, and naproxen delayed and increased plasma NSAID concentrations
Procainamide	Antidepressants	Increased risk of ventricular arrhythmias with tricyclics
Proton pump inhibitors	Antiepileptics	Effects of phenytoin enhanced by esomeprazole and possibly omeprazole
Quinidine	Antidepressants	Increased risk of ventricular arrhythmias with tricyclics
	Antiepileptics	Phenytoin accelerates metabolism
Quinine	Antiarrhythmics	Plasma concentration of flecainide increased
Quinolones	Analgesics	Possible increased risk of convulsions with NSAIDs
	Antiepileptics	Ciprofloxacin possibly alters plasma concentrations of phenytoin
Retinoids	Antiepileptics	Plasma concentration of carbamazepine possibly reduced by isotretinoin
Rifamycins	Analgesics	Metabolism of methadone accelerated; rifampicin reduces plasma concentration of rofecoxib
	Antidepressants	Metabolism of some tricyclics accelerated by rifampicin

Drug	Combined with	Interaction
Rifamycins *(cont.)*	Antiepileptics	Metabolism of phenytoin accelerated; plasma concentration of carbamazepine reduced by rifabutin
Ritonavir	Analgesics	Plasma concentration of dextropropoxyphene, pethidine, and piroxicam increased; plasma concentrations of other opioid analgesics and NSAIDs possibly increased; plasma concentration of methadone decreased
	Antidepressants	Plasma concentration of tricyclics possibly increased
Selegiline	Analgesics	Hyperpyrexia and CNS excitation with meperidine
	Antidepressants	CNS toxicity reported with tricyclics
Sulcralfate	Antiepileptics	Reduced absorption of phenytoin
Sulfinpyrazone	Analgesics	Aspirin antagonizes uricosuric effect
	Antiepileptics	Plasma concentration of phenytoin increased
Sympathomimetics	Antidepressants	With tricyclics, administration of epinephrine and norepinephrine may cause hypertension and arrhythmias; methylphenidate may inhibit metabolism of tricyclics
	Antiepileptics	Methylphenidate increases plasma concentrations of phenytoin
Temozolomide	Antiepileptics	Valproate increases plasma concentration of temozolomide
Tetracyclines	Antiepileptics	Carbamazepine and phenytoin increase metabolism of doxycycline
Theophylline	Analgesics	Rofecoxib possibly increases plasma concentration of theophylline
	Antiepileptics	Plasma theophylline levels reduced by carbamazepine and phenytoin
Thyroid hormones	Analgesics	False low plasma thyroxine concentration with phenylbutazone
	Antiepileptics	Carbamazepine and phenytoin accelerate metabolism of levothyroxine and liothyronine; plasma concentration of phenytoin possibly increased by levothyroxine and liothyronine
Tibolone	Antiepileptics	Carbamazepine and phenytoin accelerate metabolism
Ticlopidine	Analgesics	Increased risk of bleeding with NSAIDs
Trimethoprim	Antiepileptics	Plasma concentration and antifolate effect of phenytoin increased

Drug	Combined with	Interaction
Valproate	Analgesics	Aspirin enhances effect
	Anion exchange resins	Cholestyramine possibly reduces absorption
	Antibacterials	Erythromycin possibly inhibits metabolism; plasma concentration reduced by meropenem
	Anticoagulants	Anticoagulant effect of acenocoumarol and warfarin possibly increased
	Antidepressants	Antagonism of anticonvulsant effects
	Antimalarials	Mefloquine antagonizes anticonvulsant effect; chloroquine and hydroxychloroquine occasionally reduce convulsive threshold
	Antipsychotics	Antagonism of anticonvulsant effect
	Antivirals	Plasma concentration of zidovudine possibly increased
	Bupropion	Metabolism of bupropion inhibited
	Cytotoxics	Plasma concentration of temozolomide increased
	Ulcer drugs	Cimetidine inhibits metabolism
Warfarin	Analgesics	Aspirin increases risk of bleeding; anticoagulant effect seriously enhanced by azapropazone and phenylbutazone and possibly other NSAIDs; anticoagulant effect possibly enhanced by dextropropoxyphene and by prolonged use of paracetamol
	Antiepileptics	Reduced anticoagulant effect with carbamazepine; anticoagulant effect possibly increased by valproate; both reduced and enhanced effects reported with phenytoin

Glossary

allodynia: Pain due to a stimulus that does not normally provoke pain.

analgesia: Absence of pain in response to stimulation that would normally be painful.

anesthesia dolorosa: Pain in an area or region that is anesthetic.

causalgia: A syndrome of sustained burning pain, allodynia, and hyperpathia after a traumatic nerve lesion, often combined with vasomotor and sudomotor dysfunction and later trophic changes.

central pain: Pain initiated or caused by a primary lesion or dysfunction in the central nervous system.

cluster headache: Unilateral, excruciatingly severe attacks of pain, principally in the ocular, frontal, and temporal areas, recurring in separate bouts with daily, or almost daily, attacks for weeks to months, usually with ipsilateral lacrimation, conjuctival injection, photophobia, and nasal stuffiness and/or rhinorrhea.

complex regional pain syndrome (CRPS) type I: CRPS type I is a syndrome that usually develops after an initiating noxious event, is not limited to the distribution of a single peripheral nerve, and is apparently disproportionate to the inciting event. It is associated at some point with evidence of edema, changes in skin blood flow, abnormal sudomotor activity in the region of the pain, or allodynia or hyperalgesia.

complex regional pain syndrome (CRPS) type II: Burning pain, allodynia, and hyperpathia usually in the hand or foot after partial injury of a nerve or one of its major branches.

dysesthesia: An unpleasant abnormal sensation, whether spontaneous or evoked.

hyperalgesia: An increased response to a stimulus that is normally painful.

Clinical Management of the Elderly Patient in Pain
© 2006 by The Haworth Press, Inc. All rights reserved.
doi:10.1300/5356_21

hyperesthesia: Increased sensitivity to stimulation, excluding the special senses.

hyperpathia: A painful syndrome characterized by an abnormally painful reaction to a stimulus, especially a repetitive stimulus, as well as an increased threshold.

hypoalgesia: Diminished pain in response to a normally painful stimulus.

hypoesthesia: Decreased sensitivity to stimulation, excluding the special senses.

meralgia paresthetica: Hypoesthesia and painful dysesthesia in the distribution of the lateral femoral cutaneous nerve.

neuralgia: Pain in the distribution of a nerve or nerves.

neuritis: Inflammation of a nerve or nerves.

neurogenic pain: Pain initiated or caused by a primary lesion, dysfunction, or transitory perturbation in the peripheral or central nervous system.

neuropathic pain: Pain initiated or caused by a primary lesion or dysfunction in the nervous system.

neuropathy: A disturbance of function or pathological change in a nerve: in one nerve, mononeuropathy; in several nerves, mononeuropathy multiplex; if diffuse and bilateral, polyneuropathy.

nociceptor: A receptor preferentially sensitive to a noxious stimulus or to a stimulus that would become noxious if prolonged.

noxious stimulus: A stimulus that is damaging to normal tissue.

pain: An unpleasant sensory and emotional experience associated with actual or potential tissue damage, or described in terms of such damage.

pain threshold: The minimum amount of noxious stimulation required to first elicit the report of pain.

pain tolerance: The intensity at which a person seeks to withdraw from any further noxious stimulation.

paresthesia: An abnormal sensation, whether spontaneous or evoked.

peripheral neuropathic pain: Pain initiated by a primary lesion or dysfunction in the peripheral nervous system.

radicular pain: Pain perceived as arising in a limb or the trunk wall caused by ectopic activation of nociceptive afferent fibers in a spinal nerve or its roots or other neuropathic mechanisms.

radiculopathy: Objective loss of sensory and/or motor function as a result of conduction block in axons of a spinal nerve or its roots.

referred pain: Pain perceived as occurring in a region of the body topographically distinct from the region in which the actual source of pain is located.

trigeminal neuralgia: Sudden, usually unilateral, severe brief stabbing recurrent pains in the distribution of one or more branches of the fifth cranial nerve.

Index

Clinical Management of the Elderly Patient in Pain
© 2006 by The Haworth Press, Inc. All rights reserved.
doi:10.1300/5356_22

Order a copy of this book with this form or online at:
http://www.haworthpress.com/store/product.asp?sku=5356

CLINICAL MANAGEMENT OF ELDERLY PATIENTS IN PAIN

_____in hardbound at $59.95 (ISBN-13: 978-0-7890-2619-4; ISBN-10: 0-7890-2619-8)

_____in softbound at $34.95 (ISBN-13: 978-0-7890-2620-0; ISBN-10: 0-7890-2620-1)

Or order online and use special offer code HEC25 in the shopping cart.

COST OF BOOKS_____

☐ **BILL ME LATER:** (Bill-me option is good on US/Canada/Mexico orders only; not good to jobbers, wholesalers, or subscription agencies.)

POSTAGE & HANDLING_____
(US: $4.00 for first book & $1.50 for each additional book)
(Outside US: $5.00 for first book & $2.00 for each additional book)

☐ Check here if billing address is different from shipping address and attach purchase order and billing address information.

Signature_____

SUBTOTAL_____

☐ **PAYMENT ENCLOSED: $**_____

IN CANADA: ADD 7% GST_____

☐ **PLEASE CHARGE TO MY CREDIT CARD.**

STATE TAX_____
(NJ, NY, OH, MN, CA, IL, IN, PA, & SD residents, add appropriate local sales tax)

☐ Visa ☐ MasterCard ☐ AmEx ☐ Discover
☐ Diner's Club ☐ Eurocard ☐ JCB

Account # _____

FINAL TOTAL_____
(If paying in Canadian funds, convert using the current exchange rate, UNESCO coupons welcome)

Exp. Date_____

Signature_____

Prices in US dollars and subject to change without notice.

NAME_____

INSTITUTION_____

ADDRESS_____

CITY_____

STATE/ZIP_____

COUNTRY_____ COUNTY (NY residents only)_____

TEL_____ FAX_____

E-MAIL_____

May we use your e-mail address for confirmations and other types of information? ☐ Yes ☐ No We appreciate receiving your e-mail address and fax number. Haworth would like to e-mail or fax special discount offers to you, as a preferred customer. **We will never share, rent, or exchange your e-mail address or fax number.** We regard such actions as an invasion of your privacy.

Order From Your Local Bookstore or Directly From
The Haworth Press, Inc.
10 Alice Street, Binghamton, New York 13904-1580 • USA
TELEPHONE: 1-800-HAWORTH (1-800-429-6784) / Outside US/Canada: (607) 722-5857
FAX: 1-800-895-0582 / Outside US/Canada: (607) 771-0012
E-mail to: orders@haworthpress.com

For orders outside US and Canada, you may wish to order through your local sales representative, distributor, or bookseller.
For information, see http://haworthpress.com/distributors

(Discounts are available for individual orders in US and Canada only, not booksellers/distributors.)

PLEASE PHOTOCOPY THIS FORM FOR YOUR PERSONAL USE.
http://www.HaworthPress.com   BOF06